PHARMACOLOGY – RESEARCH, SAFETY TESTING AND REGULATION

CIPROFLOXACIN

BIOSYNTHESIS, APPLICATIONS, AND ADVERSE EFFECTS

PHARMACOLOGY – RESEARCH, SAFETY TESTING AND REGULATION

Additional books and e-books in this series can be found
on Nova's website under the Series tab.

PHARMACOLOGY – RESEARCH, SAFETY TESTING AND REGULATION

CIPROFLOXACIN

BIOSYNTHESIS, APPLICATIONS, AND ADVERSE EFFECTS

MOHAMED SAID ATTIA
EDITOR

nova science publishers
New York

NOTICE TO THE READER

Library of Congress Cataloging-in-Publication Data

ISBN: 978-1-53614-534-2
Library of Congress Control Number: 2018958576

Published by Nova Science Publishers, Inc. † New York

CONTENTS

Preface		**vii**
Chapter 1	The Challenge of Improving the Bioavailability of Ciprofloxacin by Supramolecular Engineering *Graciela Pinto Vitorino and María Rosa Mazzieri*	**1**
Chapter 2	Ciprofloxacin-Silica/Hydroxyapatite Nanoparticles: Release Profile, *In Vitro* Biocompatibility, Bactericidal Efficiency and Cytocompatibility Studies *Gracielle Ferreira Andrade and Edésia Martins Barros de Sousa*	**37**
Chapter 3	Distribution of Ciprofloxacin in the Peripheries *Janis Vella, Kevin Cassar, Lilian M. Azzopardi, Anthony Serracino-Inglott and Godfrey LaFerla*	**77**
Chapter 4	Ciprofloxacin and Bacterial Pathogens: Correlation to Microbial Resistance *Neveen M. Saleh, Mohamed M. Abd-Almouty and Mona I. Mabrouk*	**111**

Chapter 5 Methods of Analysis, New Applications and Common Adverse Effects of Some Fluoroquinolones **155**
Vania Maslarska, Stanislav Bozhanov and Magdalena Kondeva

Chapter 6 Ciprofloxacin: Analytical Methods of Analysis for Monitoring It in the Environment **203**
Lucas Moreira Silva, Marcos Vinicius Foguel and Maria Del Pilar Taboada Sotomayor

Chapter 7 Fluorescence Detection of Ciprofloxacin **265**
Subhankar Singha

About the Editor **295**

Index **297**

PREFACE

It's my pleasure to present this book, which is authored by a distinct group of scientists working in the field of Pharmacology, drug delivery, nanotechnology and analytical chemistry. This book is the first book that focused on the properties, bioavailability and assessment of the antibiotic ciprofloxacin either in body fluids or in the environmental samples and its multiple applications in treatment of diseases and it is also one of the most important books in this area because of the importance of this antibiotic. These characteristics are summarized in preparation of solid forms of ciprofloxacin, including multi-component systems to overcome their biopharmaceutical restrictions such as ciprofloxacin with amino acids and polymers to improve solubility and/or permeabilty, and ciprofloxacin-silica/hydroxyapatite nanoparticles to carry ciprofloxacin, besides their bactericidal efficacy, these systems are promising candidates for bone infection treatment. The bacterial resistance of ciprofloxacin, usually mediated by mutations in bacterial enzymes (gyrA, gyrB), topoisomerase IV (parC and parE) and how to overcome them. The evaluation of the ciprofloxacin in real samples by a regression model that can help predict and calculate the individual dose of ciprofloxacin for patients with foot infections, as well as its assessment in the wastewater. Many technological aspects are also presented. This book will benefit researchers whose are related to these topics of research. The material is presented in clear and organized form and contains many published and unpublished work. This book took 9 months for completing the publishing process and contains a summary of distinct research work related to Pharmacology, drug delivery, nanotechnology and analytical chemistry. Finally I would like to thank all those who contributed to the completion of this work and also extends my thanks to the publishing house that oversaw this great work.

Editor
Prof. Dr. Mohamed Said Attia (M. S. Attia), Ph.D
Professor of Analytical Chemistry
Chemistry Department, Faculty of Science, Ain Shams University, Egypt

In: Ciprofloxacin
Editor: Mohamed Said Attia
ISBN: 978-1-53614-534-2

Chapter 1

THE CHALLENGE OF IMPROVING THE BIOAVAILABILITY OF CIPROFLOXACIN BY SUPRAMOLECULAR ENGINEERING

Graciela Pinto Vitorino[1,*] and María Rosa Mazzieri[2]
[1]Química Medicinal, Departamento de Farmacia, Facultad de Ciencias Naturales y Ciencias de la Salud, Universidad Nacional de la Patagonia San Juan Bosco, Comodoro Rivadavia, Chubut, Argentina
[2]Departamento de Ciencias Farmacéuticas, Facultad de Ciencias Químicas, Universidad Nacional de Córdoba, Pabellón Ciencias 2, Ciudad Universitaria, Córdoba, Argentina

ABSTRACT

As ciprofloxacin (CIP) is a poorly soluble drug, it displays unfavorable bioavailability. To date, attempts to improve its solubility have mainly been focused on the manipulation of its features in the solid state. CIP can exist as a zwitterion or a unionized form, with both crystal structures having been described independently. It has been shown to be able to convert a zwitterion into the other form after being heated to its

* Corresponding Author Email: gpinto@unpata.edu.ar.

melting point whereas the reverse transformation occurred when a unionized species was exposed to high humidity. Furthermore, CIP exists as both anhydrous and hydrous forms, with the former being the most soluble.

Since amorphous types are usually more soluble than crystalline solids, there have been several attempts to transform one into the other. CIP has been amorphized by spray drying in pure water. In addition, using an amorphous solid dispersion methodology, multicomponent amorphous solids were obtained when CIP was formulated with amino acids and polymers.

Some of these formulations have been shown to improve solubility and/or permeabilty. Moreover, different cocrystals and salts have been prepared with drugs, and generally recognized as safe compounds. These are hippuric, maleic, barbituric, 4-hydroxybenzoic, aspartic, glutamic, succinic, maleic, adipic, salicylic, lactic and phosphoric acids, and other compounds such as norfloxacin, diflunisal, indoprofen and saccharin. Metal complexes have also been prepared using aluminum, magnesium, zinc, iron (III), bismuth, copper, cadmium and cobalt.

This review presents a brief description of the results obtained from methodologies frequently employed to prepare solid forms of CIP, including multicomponent systems. Their reported characterization and physicochemical properties are also summarized. Although not all the investigations on the solid state of CIP have been performed with the aim of overcoming its biopharmaceutical limitations, we have incorporated most of these in this revision as we consider they may be of interest.

Keywords: ciprofloxacin, supramolecular engineering, solid state

LIST OF ACRONYMS

ALA: alanine

APIs: Active Pharmaceutical Ingredients

ARG: arginine

ASD: Amorphous Solid Dispersions

ASP: aspartic acid

BCS: Biopharmaceutic Classification Systems

CA: citric acid

CIP: Ciprofloxacin

CIP-CA: ciprofloxacin with citric acid

CIP-DIF: ciprofloxacin with diflunisal
CIP-FA: ciprofloxacin with fumaric acid
CIP-HA: ciprofloxacin and hippuric acid
CIP-INDP: ciprofloxacin with indoprofen
CIP-LA: ciprofloxacin with Lactate
CIP-MA: ciprofloxacin with maleic acid
CIP-SA: ciprofloxacin with salicylic acid
CYS: cysteine
DIF: diflunisal
FA: fumaric acid
FQ: fluoroquinolone
FTIR: Fourier transform infrared spectroscopy
GLU: glutamic acid
GLY: glycine
GRAS: generally regarded as safe
HA: hippuric acid
H_2ba: barbituric acid
4HBA: 4-hydroxybenzoic acid
HPMCAS: hydroxypropyl methylcellulose acetate succinate
HSM: Hot Stage Microscopy
H_2tba: 2-thiobarbituric
INDP: indoprofen
LA: lactic acid
MA: maleic acid
NOR: norfloxacin
P*XRD:* powder X ray diffraction
SA: salicilic acid
SAC: saccharin
SCXRD: single crystal X ray diffraction
SER: serine
ssNMR: solid state nuclear magnetic resonance
TG-DSC: thermogravimetry and differential scanning calorimetry
VT-P*XRD:* variable temperature powder X ray diffraction

1. Introduction

Ciprofloxacin (CIP), 1-cyclopropyl-6-fluoro-1,4-dihydro-4-oxo-7-(1-piperazinyl)-3-quinoline carboxylic acid is a second generation fluoroquinolone (FQ) which was first marketed in 1986 (Figure 1).

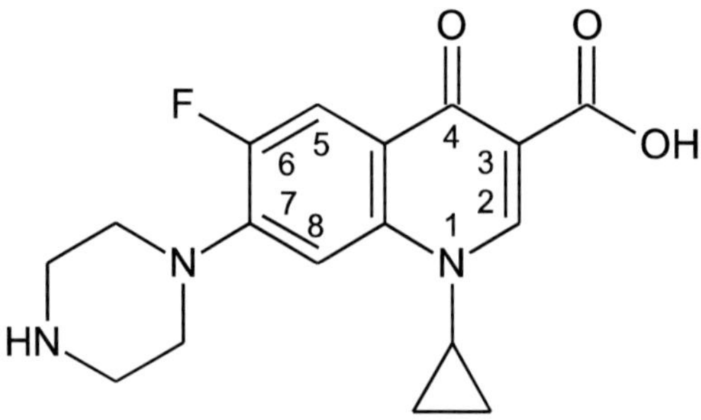

Figure 1. Molecular structure of CIP.

CIP is a wide spectrum antibiotic that is active against Gram-positive and Gram-negative bacteria, and also effective against atypical organisms such as *Legionella pneumophila*, *Chlamydia trachomatis*, *Mycobacterium tuberculosis*, and *Mycoplasma hominis*. It is used in the treatment of various infectious diseases, both in human and veterinary medicine, including those that affect the urinary and respiratory tract, bones, joints and abdomen [1, 2]. CIP is the most widely used FQ, which is marketed either as free base (oral suspensions) or as hydrochloride salt (in tablets). The mechanism of action of FQs, involves the inhibition of the intracellular enzymes DNA-gyrase and Topoisomerase IV [3, 4].

2. Physicochemical Properties

Although CIP has several potentially ionizable functional groups, only two of these, the carboxylic acid at position 3 and the NH on piperazine at position 7, are pharmaceutically relevant. The ionization of CIP can be described by the scheme displayed in Figure 2, showing that four different microspecies can be found in solution (unionized, zwitterion, and positively and negatively charged) depending on the pH [5, 6].

As can be seen in Figure 2, while the uncharged and zwitterionic microspecies predominate at neutral pH, the positive microspecies predominates at acidic pH whereas the negative microspecies prevails at basic pH. In the solid state, CIP can exist as a zwitterion and/or as a unionized molecule.

There is an extensive literature showing that the values for pK_1 and pK_2 of CIP are approximately 5.90-6.15 and 7.41-8.89, respectively (Table 1).

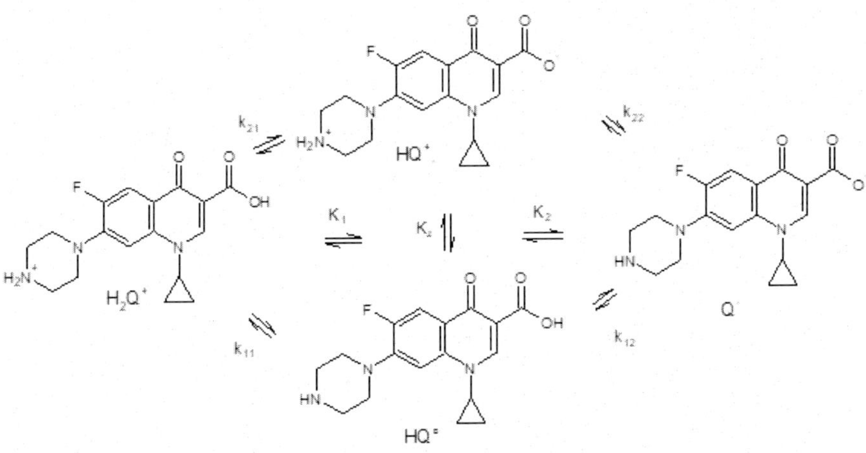

Figure 2. Microspeciation equilibrium of CIP (HQ°: unionized, HQ^{+}-: zwitterion, H_2Q^+: cation, Q^-: anion).

Table 1. pK_1 and pK_2 values reported for CIP

pK_1	pK_2	Reference
6.00	8.80	[7]
6.09	8.74	[3]
6.14	7.41	[8]
6.15	8.66	[9]
5.90	8.89	[10]

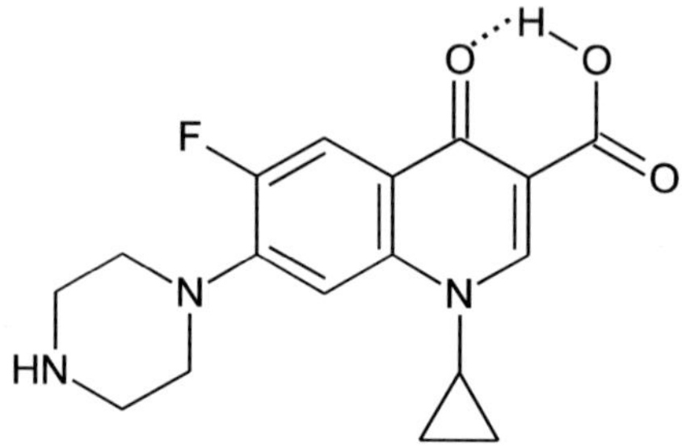

Figure 3. Intramolecular hydrogen bonding between the carboxylic acid and the keto function.

The value of pK_1 for CIP, and for the FQs in general, is higher than that usually observed for carboxylic acid, with this decrease in acidity having been attributed to the formation of an intramolecular hydrogen-bond between the carboxylic acid and the keto function at position 4, resulting in the stabilization of protonated species (Figure 3).

The zwitterionic nature of CIP molecule results in a U-shaped pH solubility profile with a high solubility at pH < 5 and pH > 10. The lower solubility range is between pH 5 and 10, particularly at physiological pH (7.4), and has a value of 0.06 and 0.08 mg/mL at 25 and 37°C, respectively [11-13]. CIP is also poorly soluble in other common solvents such as ethanol, methanol, propanol, dichloromethane, acetone, and chloroform [14].

There is a broad agreement that a poor pH-solubility behavior may lead to a suboptimal bioavailability, especially when high doses are administered to the patient. This drug is predominantly absorbed in the proximal part of the gastrointestinal tract, mainly by passive diffusion [15, 16]. In addition, precipitation of the dissolved drug might occur after being transferred from the stomach to the upper intestine. Also, as oral absorption of CIP is influenced by the poor dissolution rate, high doses (250-1000 mg) are required with the reported absolute bioavailability of orally administered CIP varying widely (between 56% and 77%) [17-19].

Due to its low solubility and low permeability, which are both properties that conspire against a good bioavailability [6, 20], CIP is classified as class IV according to the Biopharmaceutic Classification Systems (BCS).

3. Solid Forms of CIP

The low aqueous solubility and dissolution rates of certain drugs are major pharmaceutical concerns, due to their unfavorable impact on bioavailability and therapeutic effectiveness. A solution to this problem is one of the greatest challenges faced by scientist today, who must develop new methods in order to improve pharmaceutical performance. It is in this context that crystal engineering arises as an emerging and promising approach, which is focused on making crystals with "a purpose," and which may be useful for supramolecular synthesis. In particular, one of the most explored strategies in recent years is the search for new solid-state forms of old active pharmaceutical ingredients (APIs), without altering their pharmacological activities [21, 22]. Some examples of these are polymorphs, salts, hydrates, solvates and cocrystals. Each one of these solid modifications may print different pharmaceutical properties on a specific API. Consequently, to find the optimal pharmaceutical solid-state form requires a broad screening during the initial phase of drug development [21].

Currently, there are numerous useful methods for solid state characterization, particularly those that impact on pharmaceutical properties, such as single crystal X ray diffraction (SCXRD), powder X ray diffraction (P*XRD)*, variable temperature powder X ray diffraction (VT-P*XRD),* Fourier transform infrared spectroscopy (FTIR), thermogravimetry and differential scanning calorimetry (TG-DSC), solid state nuclear magnetic resonance (ssNMR) and hot stage microscopy (HSM).

The different solid forms of CIP that have been reported to date are described below. It should be noted that not all of these were studied with the aim of overcoming biopharmaceutical limitations of the APIs. Nevertheless, they are also included in this review when we consider it to be of interest to researchers working in this area.

3.1. CIP Ionized and Noionized in Solid State

Anhydrous CIP usually exists in its more stable zwitterionic form in the solid state ($HQ^{\pm}$, Figure 2). However, the crystalline unionized form (HQ°, Figure 2) has also been prepared, with both structures and the interchange between them having been investigated by several researchers [23, 24, 28, 29].

Mahapatra et al. (2010) reported on the SCXRD of $HQ^{\pm}$, in which intermolecular ionic bonds are formed between the positively charged nitrogen of 7-piperazine and the negatively charged 3-carboxylate oxygen of two neighboring molecules. This head-to-tail interaction produces a one-dimensional supramolecular chain of molecules. In addition, adjacent chains are connected by strong intermolecular $NH_2^{+}\cdots O^{-}$ hydrogen bonds, thereby forming two-dimensional layers. In this way, each CIP is linked to both neighboring and adjacent molecules, resulting in a tetramer-like structure. Other intermolecular interactions involve C−H π−π between the aromatic rings and between these rings and cyclopropyl. All of these interactions render a dense packing of the zwitterionic molecules in the crystal structure, which is the cause of poor CIP solubility [23].

Fabbiani et al. described the crystal structure of HQ°, where a distinctive O−H···O intramolecular H-bond is formed between the hydrogen of the 3-carboxylic acid and the neighboring 4-ketone oxygen (Figure 3). The intermolecular prominent interactions of the unionized crystaline form of CIP involve an N−H···N bond between the secondary amine groups of neighboring molecules, generating a dimer. In addition, intermolecular interactions between the carbonyl oxygen of the 3-carboxylic acid and various C−H groups are present [24]. A unique weak halogen C−H···F intermolecular bond was also reported in the crystal structures of both HQ° and $HQ^{\pm}$ [11, 25].

In order to try to corroborate the ionization state of the solid state of CIP, FTIR was used. The spectrum of the ionizated drug contained two peaks, at 1650-1510 cm^{-1} and at 1400-1280 cm^{-1}, corresponding to the asymmetric and symmetric vibrations of the carboxylate ion (COO^{-}), respectively. In contrast, a definite absorption maximum was found between 1680 and 1760 cm^{-1} at the FTIR spectrum of HQ°, which corresponded to the unionized COOH group. The peak at approximately 1618 cm^{-1} in the spectrum of CIP has been assigned to the C=O stretch of the 4-ketone carbonyl. NH_2^+ stretching vibrations presented absorptions at 2400–2600 cm^{-1}, with similar bands being found in the FTIR spectra of CIP salts, in which the piperazine secondary amine is ionized [28]. These characteristic signals are used to distinguish between no-ionic or zwitterionic species in the solid state of CIP [26, 27].

CIP has the ability to interchange between unionized and zwitterionic forms in the solid state. Several studies have described this behavior, with Messallati et al. (2016) demonstrating by P*XRD* and FTIR that upon being heated to a temperature near its melting point the zwitterionic form of CIP transfered a proton from the protonated piperazine amino group to the carboxylate anion [28]. Likewise, Turel et al. (1996) found that the FTIR carboxylate absorbance bands of the drug disappeared and were replaced by the characteristic peaks of 3-carboxylic acid and 4-carbonyl when the solid was heated to 270°C (before the drug melts or begins to decompose) [29]. This can be explained by the conversion of a zwitterion to the unionized form, which was found to be the case for CIP hexahydrate upon heating to 280°C [27]. Similarly, Mahapatra et al. (2010) claimed that heating CIP up to 250°C resulted in the reversible formation of unionized CIP, as shown by P*XRD* [23]. In contrast, Mesallati et al. (2016) demostrated the converse interchange, with unionized CIP being converted to the crystalline zwitterionic form on being exposed to a high humidity atmosphere in the solid state [28].

Finally, as the experimental results described above have demonstrated, the crystal structures of unionized and zwitterionic CIP differ quite substantially. Aditionally, their interchange in the solid state can involve a reorientation of the molecules as well as a proton transfer. All of these findings were also confirmed by Mesallati et al. (2016) by using computational methods [28].

3.2. Hydrates and Anhydrates

Hydrates and solvates are multicomponent crystalline molecular adducts that contain API and water (hydrate) or other solvents (solvate). They are incorporated in the crystal lattice structure and often establish H bonds and coordinate covalent bonds with the APIs. Hydrates are the most frequent type of solvated organic compounds, and can be formed by different stoichiometric relationships. The presence of water molecules affects the intermolecular interactions and the degree of crystalline disorder, thereby impacting on the free energy, thermodynamic parameters, solubility, dissolution rate, solid state stability and the bioavailability of hydrated APIs [30].

The first CIP-hydrate reported was the hexahydrate CIP.6H_2O in 1997. Its crystal structure revealed a clearly zwitterionic form of the molecule [27]. Later, Mafra et al. (2012) isolated and determined the structure of two new CIP channel hydrates (forms II and III) that had the same framework but different stoichiometries, which were 3.7 and 4.8 hydrates for II and III, respectively. Moreover, those authors demonstrated that the anhydrate transforms into II after a simple exposure to water vapor (RH > 90%) or upon suspension in water. In addition, the *PXRD* data showed that II converts back to the anhydrate at ~60 [31].

The anhydrous CIP was described by Li et al. (2006) and compared with its hydrates by TG-DSC and P*XRD*. The powder dissolution profiles of the two crystal forms of CIP indicated that the anhydrous form had a significantly higher dissolution rate than its hydrate and achieved its maximum concentration within 1 min. However, immediately after a peak concentration was reached, the dissolution rate started to decrease to almost 50% by the end of the 60 min experiment [36]. This behavior may have been caused by the crystallization of the CIP hydrate, which has a significantly lower solubility [13].

Mahapatra et al. (2010) obtained the SCXRD of the anhydrous form of CIP, which crystallizes in the triclinic P-1 space group. Its hygroscopic characteristics on heating were analyzed by VT-*PXRD*, and an irreversible conversion between the anhydrous and the hydrated form of CIP was corroborated [28].

3.3. Solvates

Only two solvates of CIP could be found in the literature. Li et al. (2006) reported the SCXRD analysis of CIP methanol hemisolvate. In the crystal lattice, this drug exists as a zwitterion and the methanol molecule is disordered across a twofold rotation axis [32]. Fabianni et al. (2011) also reported on a solvate constituted by zwitterionic CIP and 2,2-difluoro-ethanol in a 2:3 stoichiometric relationship [33].

3.4. CIP Amorphization

Amorphous solids are more soluble than their crystalline counterparts, as the lack of strong intermolecular interactions produces the most energetic solid state, with less energy therefore being required by the molecules to enter the solution. However, for the same reason, this type of solid is intrinsically unstable and prone to crystallization. In the same way, amorphous drugs are more hygroscopic than crystals, due to their irregular arrangement and large free volume.

Thus, water can be absorbed into the internal structure of the material rather than just being adsorbed to the surface. Consequently, this absorption of water can negatively affect the drug solid stability by increasing the rate of crystallization, which results in a reduction in its disolution [34].

Pure amorphous CIP is difficult to obtain, due to its low solubility, strong crystal lattice and thermal degradation of the drug. However, despite these difficulties, Mesallati et al. (2016) were the first to report the successful preparation of pure amorphous CIP. Although they attempted several techniques, only spray drying in pure water resulted in a completely amorphous product. Moreover, while many processing methods generated the zwitterionic form of CIP, spray drying in an ethanol/water mixture produced the unionized form. The characterization of these solid materials was examined by P*XRD*, FTIR, and TG-DSC [28].

Due to the necessity of improving the stability, dissolution rate and bioavailability of amorphous drugs, interest in the formation of amorphous solid dispersions (ASD) has increased in the pharmaceutical field. An ASD is defined as a dispersion of a drug in a solid matrix, where the matrix is constituted by a polymer or a small molecule, with the latter being named a coamorphous system [35, 36].

Mesallati et al. obtained and characterized ASD of CIP with aminoacids and with polymeric substances [11, 37]. They studied the possibility of forming amorphous formulations with CIP and amino acids, which were able to improve the physical stability of the amorphous drug form. The aminoacids selected were aspartic acid (ASP), glutamic acid (GLU), cysteine (CYS), arginine (ARG), glycine (GLY), alanine (ALA) and serine (SER) (Figure 4), and they were able to prepare ASD of CIP with ASP, GLU, CYS and ARG. The characterization by FTIR and ssNMR confirmed the formation of an amorphous salt linked by ionic unions between the positively charged piperazine amino group of CIP and the negatively charged α-carboxylate groups of the amino acids. These salts were then stored in dry conditions and remained amorphous for at least 10 months, except for CIP-CYS, which showed some evidence of crystallization after 12 months. Significant improvements in the solubility of CIP were observed for all the ASDs, particularly among those and the corresponding physical mixtures. However, an increase in the solubility was not always matched by a rise in the permeability of the samples. While CIP-ASP and CIP-GLU showed the greatest solubility enhancement, they were also significantly less permeable than pure crystalline CIP. In contrast, CIP-CYS and CIP-ARG significantly improved the permeability of CIP, but they had a lower effect on its solubility. In addition, by using another method, semicrystalline solid dispersions were obtained with CIP and GLY, ALA and SER [37].

Mesallati et al. (2017) obtained Amorphous Solid Dispersions (ASDs) of CIP with the acidic polymers Eudragit L100, Eudragit L100-55, Carbopol and hydroxypropyl methylcellulose acetate succinate (HPMCAS) by ball milling. All of these were polymeric drug salts, formed by the interaction between the positively charged secondary amine of CIP with carboxylate groups of the polymers. They demonstrated that ASDs constitued with HPMCAS increased the proportion of CIP available for diffusion through bacterial cell membranes, thereby provoking a decrease in the minimal inhibitory concentration and minimal bactericidal concentration. These authors proposed that ASDs could be promising to use in order to obtain CIP formulations with an improved solubility, bioavailability, and antibacterial activity [11].

The formation of ASDs is a subject of recent development and is of much interest to the pharmaceutical sciences However, further studies of the interactions at a molecular level are still necessary.

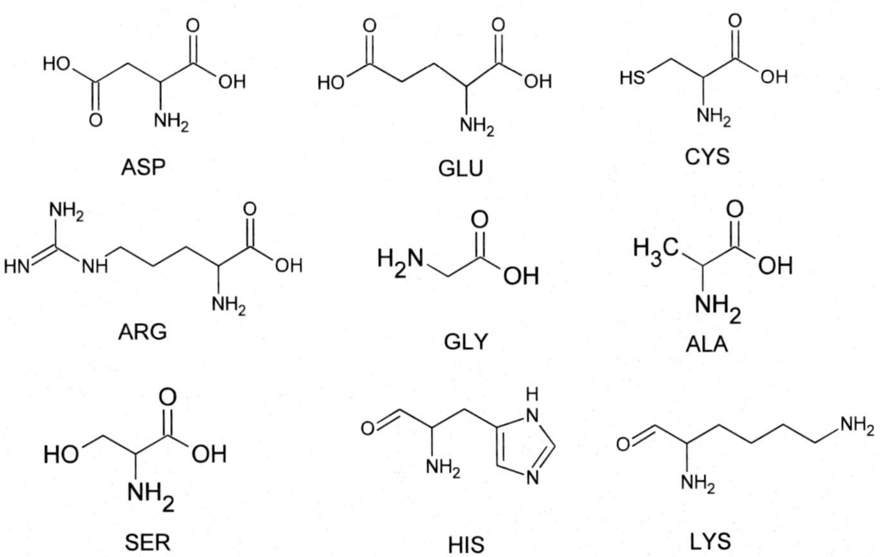

ASP: aspartic acid, GLU: glutamic acid, CYS: cysteine, ARG: arginine, GLY: glycine, ALA: alanine, SER: serine.

Figure 4. Chemical structures of the aminoacids used to study the formation of ASD.

4. Cocrystals and Salts of CIP

The definition of the cocrystal is a topic still being debated, both in the chemical and legal sense. Izutsu et al. (2016) defined cocrystals as "crystalline solids composed of stoichiometric ratios of multiple ingredients that form the crystal lattice by non-ionic interactions" [38]. Pharmaceutical cocrystals are composed of an API and other components called former or conformers crystals. Cocrystals offer new possibilities for exploring solid forms, since they are not limited to ionizable drugs. However, coformer selection is one of the major challenges in cocrystal developments. Coformers must be safe for human consumption and should be able to interact with the API through non-covalent bonds [39]. Preferably, the coformers are chosen from the list of generally regarded as safe (GRAS) substances, which was elaborated by USA Food and Drug Administration and has over 3000 substances, including food additives, preservatives, excipients, vitamins, minerals, amino acids, bio-molecules, and their APIs [40].

A pharmaceutical salt is integrated by an ionizable API (cationic, anionic or zwitterionic) and a molecular or atomic counterion, with salification being the most common method employed to improve their aqueous solubility and bioavailability. Nowadays, about 50% of these drugs are sold as salts [41]. However, in recent times, the difference between a salt and cocrystal is being reviewed by researchers, since there might exist a continuum linking cocrystals and salts, based on the extent of proton transfer between acidic and basic components. Frequently, when the proton is on the base, the crystalline acid–base complex is a salt whereas when the proton remains on the acid it is usually a cocrystal. It has also been observed that when the ΔpKa between the acid and the base is more than 3.75, a salt is formed. However, a neutral cocrystal results when the pKa difference is less than zero. Finally, the proton will have an intermediate hydrogen bonding character when the transition range falls between 0 and 3.75, with this intermediate situation leading to either a salt or a cocrystal [37, 42].

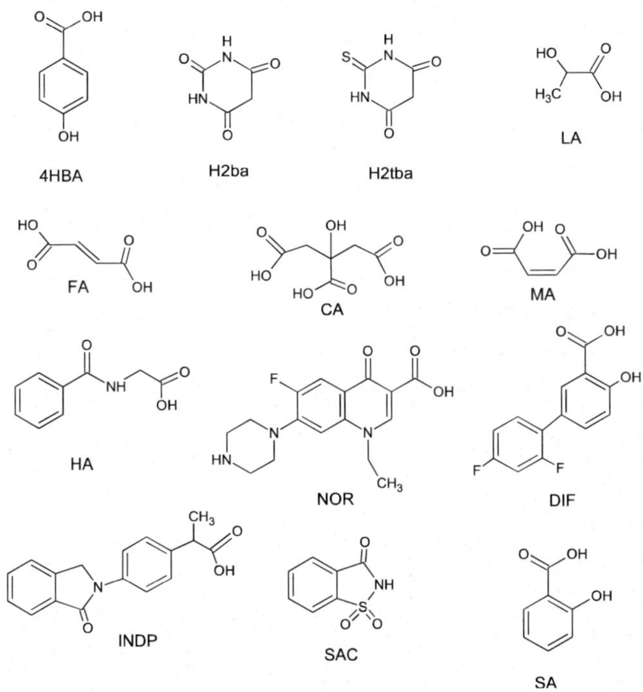

Figure 5. Chemical structure of the coformers employed for obtaining the cocrystals and salts of CIP described in this chapter. 4HBA: 4-hydroxybenzoic acid, H_2tba: 2-thiobarbituric, H_2ba: barbituric acid, LA: lactic acid, FA: fumaric acid, CA: citric acid, MA: maleic acid, HA: hippuric acid, NOR: norfloxacin, DIF: diflunisal, INDP: indoprofen, SAC: saccharin and SA: salicilic acid.

Although CIP has two ionizable groups that are able to react with acid or base, the only useful pharmaceutical salts are obtained from the neutralization of its 7-piperazinic amino group (pKa 8.74) with an acid compound. In fact, as mentioned above, most of drug products containing CIP are compounded by CIP hydrochloride (CIPHCl).

Products such as salts or cocrystals may exist in variable stoichiometric proportions with respect to the API and the counterion or conformer, with the resulting arrangement of molecules determining the physicochemical properties of the solids. Hence, the molar ratio of APIs and the coformer, as well as the type of coformer, should all be taken into account when synthesizing complexes of APIs. However, although a large number of polybasic organic acids react with CIP to generate salts in variable proportions, few reports of CIP salts in different proportions have been published.

Solvent evaporation is a typical method for salt screening, but the use of large quantities of solvents may imply a high cost and also lead to environmental pollution. However, solvent drop grinding (SDG; Trask et al., 2006), which requires little solvent, has been reported to be an effective technique for preparing salts. Indeed, due to the the low cost and environmental protection of SDG, this method has attracted increasing attention among researchers [43].

Some examples of the CIP salts and cocrystals reported in the literature are described below, with the chemical structure of the coformers being summarized in Figure 5.

4.1. CIP and 4-Hydroxybenzoic Acid

Cocrystallization of hydrochloride salt of CIP was successfully achieved by using 4-hydroxybenzoic acid (4HBA) as the coformer (Figure 5). The cocrystal, CIPHCl−4HBA has been obtained by different methodologies, including slurry conversion, SDG, crystallization by solvent evaporation, and reaction crystallization. Bulk solids of these cocrystals are stable in acidic solutions and can be stored for a month under thermal/relative humidity stress conditions without undergoing phase conversion.

The CIPHCl salts feature secondary ammonium groups that commonly interact with chloride ions in the crystal. Analysis of the structure of CIPHCl−4HBA has revealed significant variations in the supramolecular interactions between the ionic components compared to crystals of CIPHCl. A dense packing was observed in CIPHCl-4HBA, with the ions being closely bound, resulting in a solid with lower thermodynamic solubility and dissolution rate compared to the starting CIPHCl$\cdot$1.34H_2O salt. These findings have highlighted the utility of chloride ion as a hydrogen bonding acceptor, and revealed that cocrystals of salts can exhibit important and useful alterations to the physicochemical properties which are of interest. However, the prediction of the final structure-property result is not straightforward [23].

4.2. CIP with 2-Thiobarbituric Acid and Barbituric Acid

CIP crystallizes with 2-thiobarbituric (H_2tba) and barbituric acid (H_2ba) from an aqueous solution to yield two salts, $CIPH_2(Htba)\cdot 3H_2O$ (I) and $CIPH_2(Hba)\cdot H_2O$ (II), and also a salt cocrystal $CIPH_2(Hba)$ $(H_2ba)\cdot 3H_2O$ (III). The compounds have been structurally characterized by SCXRD. The numerous intermolecular hydrogen bonds N–H···O and O–H···O formed by the water molecules, Htba−/Hba− and $CIPH_2^+$ ions, and H_2ba molecules stabilize the crystal structures of I to III. These hydrogen bonds form a 2D plane network in the salts of I and II and a 3D network in the salt cocrystal of III, with different π-π interactions in I, II or III. The compounds were characterized by P*XRD*, TG-DSC and FTIR, which revealed that their dehydration process stopped at temperatures of 130°C-150°C and with their oxidative decomposition being in the range 250°C to 275°C [44].

4.3. Salt of CIP Hydrochloride 1.34-Hydrate

Turel et al. (2003) determined the crystal structure of $CIPHCl\cdot 1.34.H_2O$, which crystallizes in the $P2_1/C$ spatial group [45]. Later, Liu et al. (2005) obtained different crystal behavoirs of this salt by cooling, dilution and salting out crystallization [46].

4.4. Salt of CIP Lactate

Prasanna et al. (2001), with the aim of analyzing the role of weak interactions in the crystal structure of the salt of CIP with lactate (CIP-LA) (Figure 5), crystallized the product from methanol by slow evaporation of the solvent. The characterization of the material was performed by SCXRD, with the crystal structure of CIP-LA·1.5 H_2O found to have channels running along the crystallographic *b*-axis and π-stacks of CIP moieties linked through water molecules. A ten-membered hydrogen bonded pattern was formed by centrosymmetrically related lactate and water molecules filled the center of the channel. The structure also had a C-H···F intramolecular interaction and an intramolecular hydrogen bonding [47].

4.5. Salts with Fumaric, Citric and Maleic Acid

Zhang et al. (2016) selected pharmaceutical organic acids to react with CIP in different proportions and reported the synthesis of four new salts. Two of these were salts of CIP with fumaric acid in proportions of 2:1 and 1:1 (2:1CIP-FA, and 1:1CIP-FA, respectively). Another salt was obtained from CIP with citric acid, resulting in a 2:1CIP-CA, and finally the reaction of CIP with maleic acid yielded a 1:1CIP-MA [48]. The chemical structures of the coformers used are shown in Figure 5. These salts were characterized by P*XRD* and DSC, with the 3D molecular structures showing that the water molecules involved in hydrogen bondings and π–π stacking between the quinoline rings played important roles in stabilizing the crystal structures of these salts.

Curious findings involving the solubility behavoir of the above described salts were reported by Zhang et al. (2016) [48]. Usually, as the molar ratio of a basic insoluble drug and the soluble acid in the salt decreases, the solubility of the salt improves. However, the 2:1CIP-FA was observed to be four times more soluble than 1:1CIP-FA; and the 2:1CIP-CA salt also had a higher solubility, which turned out to be similar to 2:1CIP-FA. With the objective of investigating this uncommon phenomenon, a comparison between the crystal structures of compounds was made, with two similar characteristics being observed in the 2:1CIP-FA and 2:1CIP-CA salts. The acid molecules were linked together to form a hydrophilic layer and the CIP molecules formed a hydrophobic layer, which were arranged alternately to form a sandwich-like structure. However, a different array in 1:1CIP-FA salt and 1:1CIP-MA salt was found, with the acid molecules located in voids enclosed by CIP molecules. As the water molecules permeated more easily into the sandwich-like structure, this caused it to disintegrate in pure water. Consequently, both 2:1 salts showed a better solubility in pure water than those with a proportion of 1:1. On the other hand, the 1:1CIP-MA salt was loosely arranged and had a lower density than the 1:1CIP-FA salt, so the 1:1CIP-MA salt was more soluble. In fact, all the synthesized salts revealed a greater solubility than CIP. Furthermore, the largest enhancement of solubility in pure water was displayed by the 2:1CIP-FA salt, which was approximately 50-fold more soluble than CIP [48]. In addition, three polymorfic salts of CIP with MA were published by Sutov et al. (2016) and will be described in section 4.10 [49].

4.6. Salt with Hippuric Acid

Chadha et al. (2016) prepared a salt of CIP and hippuric acid (CIP-HA) with a stoichiometry 1:1 using the SDG procedure (Figure 5). A single crystal was obtained by the vapor diffusion technique and the new phase was analyzed using FTIR, DSC and P*XRD*, with structural parameters being determined using SCXRD. The solubility and the intrinsic dissolution rate of the salt were measured in buffer solution at pH 1.2 and also in water (pH 6.3). A 22-fold solubility improvement was demonstrated along with a faster dissolution rate than CIP. Pharmacokinetic studies on rats have revealed higher plasma concentration of CIP-HA than that CIP. Also, synergistic activity has been reported [50].

4.7. Salt with Norfloxacin

In our laboratory, we have obtained and characterized a new multicomponent molecular complex, CIP-NOR, which originated from the heteroassociation of CIP and norfloxacin (NOR) in the solid state. NOR is another FQ of the second generation (Figure 5). Both APIs are in a 1:1 molecular relation, producing a mutually hydrated salt with an interesting supramolecular structure (Figure 6). This arrangement is isostructural with a hydrated phase of CIP, as described by Fabianni et al. (2011) [37].

Experimental data related to melting temperatures, DSC profiles, and P*XRD* patterns have shown that the physical properties of CIP-NOR are different from those of pure components. In the crystal, the molecules of CIP and NOR are ionized, and interact by stacking with adjacent molecules. In addition to N−H····O hydrogen bonding linking the molecules in linear chains, there is π-stacking between each fluorophenyl residue. Also, there is a complex and very extensive hydrogen bonding scheme in the resulting crystal structure, with water molecules being highly disordered. The propensity for heteroassociation between CIP and NOR under the conditions described above gave rise to a salt, which was reported for the first time between FQs [51]. Interestingly, when antibacterial activity was evaluated, some combinations of CIP and NOR showed not only additivity but even more synergistic activity [52].

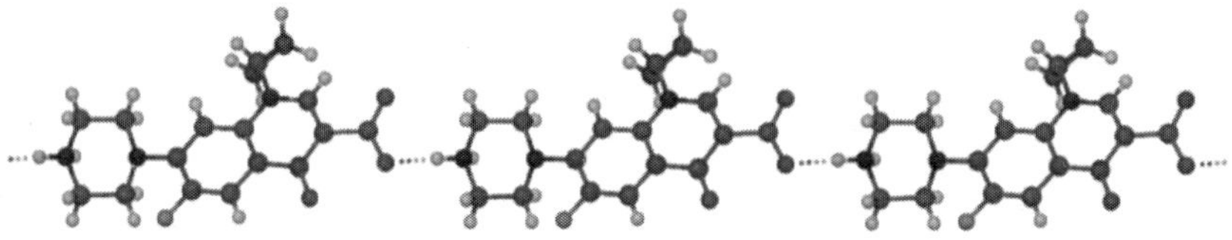

Figure 6. Linear hydrogen bonded chains of CIP and NOR.

4.8. Salts with Diflunisal and Indoprofen

Bag et al. (2014) described the synthesis and characterization of two salts of CIP with the non-steroidal anti-inflammatory drugs diflunisal (CIP-DIF) and indoprofen (CIP-INDP-H_2O), whose chemical structures are shown in Figure 5. Single crystals were obtained by SDG and by fast evaporation of the solvent, with the characterization of the materials being performed by SCXRD, TG-DSC and HSM. In the salts, ionic interactions between the protonated piperazine of CIP and the carboxylate ion of the coformers were reported [53].

4.9. Salts with Amino Acids

Elshaer et al. evaluated the formation of salts between CIP and amino acids. The ones selected for this study were cationic (ARG, LYS and HIS) and anionic (ASP and GLU) (Figure 4). The authors found that CIP formed salts with ASP and GLU when freeze dried in a 1:1 molar ratio. For both of these amino acids, the positively charged piperazine amino group of CIP was found to form an ionic interaction with a carboxylate group of ASP or GLU. These results were confirmed by FTIR, NMR and DSC studies. Molecular dynamic simulations have shown that the hydrophobic interaction between CIP molecules decreases in the presence of the acidic amino acids and generates stable salts, resulting in increasing CIP solubility. However, these authors were not able to form salts with the basic amino acids ARG, LYS and HIS [54].

4.10. Polymorphic Salts of CIP

Polymorphism is the ability of a compound to crystallize in more than one crystal structure, and this is of great importance for overcoming solubility shortcomings in pharmaceutical solids [55]. Because of the different polymorphs of a given crystalline API, there may be differences in the physicochemical properties such as melting temperature, solubility, stability, dissolution rate and bioavailability. Although polymorphism is of constant interest for researchers worldwide, the phenomenon remains largely unpredictable, especially for multicomponent crystals. Therefore, a crucial step at all stages of pharmaceutical development and manufacture must be the identification and characterization of any possible polymorphic forms, as well as the study of their thermodynamic stability.

To date, there have not been described polymorphic forms of CIP. This behavior makes a difference with NOR (the structural analog of CIP), for which at least four polymorphic forms have been identified [56, 57]. However, some polymorphic salts of CIP have been reported and are described briefly below:

4.10.1. CIP and Maleic Acid

Surov et al. (2016) reported that the pharmaceutical salt of CIP with maleic acid (CIP-MA) exists in three polymorphic forms (I, II and III) and one hydrate, and their crystal structures were determined by SCXRD. In fact, CIP-MA is still the only example of a polymorphic system among the FQ salts, for which structural information for three polymorphs is available. The mechanochemical reaction for the salt formation consists of the rapid growth of the kinetic form III and its conversion into stable polymorphic II. However, the mechanochemical synthesis of I requires seeding, which indicates a high activation barrier of nucleation of form I. The stability relationships between the polymorphs were studied by using a number of experimental and theoretical methods, with the results establishing the following order of stabilities of the polymorphs: form I (thermodynamically the most stable), followed by II and then III [46].

4.10.2. CIP and Saccharinate

Saccharin (SAC), the well known artificial sweetener, is a crystalline solid that is very soluble in water. It has acid properties (pka=1.6) and has been classified by FDA as an indirect additive used in food contact substances (Figure 5) [58]. Therefore, most of its features make it a coformer that is worthy of consideration as a possible way of improving CIP biopharmaceutic shortcomings.

Two polymorphic forms of CIP saccharinates (CIP-SAC) have been reported by Garro Link et al. (2011). These are aducts with stoichiometry 1:1 and can be synthesized by straightforward methods [59].

Recently, Singh et al. (2017) reported and characterized a new polymorph of CIP saccharinate (CIP-SAC III) by TG-DSC, FTIR and P*XRD*, which was obtained by SDG with ethanol. Validation of the crystal structure of CIP-SAC III was carried out using P*XRD* data, with the experimental ssNMR chemical shifts being correlated with those obtained from computational calculations. The resulting improved aqueous solubility and dissolution profile, along with an increased oral bioavailability and synergistic antibacterial activity of CIP-SAC III, makes it a potential candidate for the pharmaceutical industry. The authors attributed these improved biopharmaceutical properties to the higher absorption and distribution in comparison with CIP [60].

4.10.3. CIP and Salicilic Acid

Nagalapalli et al. (2014) carried out the synthesis, SCXRD structure analysis, and the Hirshfeld surface analyses of a molecular salt of CIP with salicylic acid (CIP-SA), with the chemical structure of SA being shown in Figure 5. The formation of CIP-SA was further characterized and confirmed by FTIR analysis. It was demonstrated that the crystal structure of this salt was mainly stabilized by the following hydrogen bonding, N^{+}–H···O–, O–H···O, C–H···F, and also by π-π interactions. A 3D Hirshfeld surface analysis and 2D fingerprint maps analysis revealed that N–H···O and O–H···O hydrogen bonding intermolecular interactions were more prominent in the salt [61].

Our final comment on pharmaceutical polymorphism is related to statistics performed by Cruz-Cabeza et al. (2015), which revealed that one out of three compounds in the Cambridge Structural Database are polymorphic. Thus these statistics explain the importance of polymorphism as a central theme of materials science [50]. However, despite this, the polymorphism of the FQ multicomponent crystals has not yet been thoroughly studied, and further investigations are now needed to explore the potential of these systems.

5. METAL COMPLEX WITH CIP

Three of the chemical features present in the CIP structure (3-carboxylic acid, the basic NH at 7-piperazinyl ring, and the carbonyl oxygen at the 4-position) make CIP a good ligand to bind metal ions. Indeed, a wide variety of metal complexes in which it can act as bidentate, unidentate or as a bridging ligand have been synthesized and reported. In the polymeric complexes in solid state, multiple modes of coordination are simultaneously possible, with CIP acting as a ligand in the form Q^- in basic conditions, and in the $HQ^{\pm}$ form in neutral, slightly acidic or slightly basic media. In contrast, in a strongly acidic medium, CIP form ionic complexes of the H_2Q^+ form.

Table 2. Selected chelates of CIP

Metal	Compound	Reference
VO^{2+}	$[VO(CIP)_2]SO_4.10H_2O$	[63]
Fe^{3+}	$[Fe(CIP)(nta)]\ 3.5H_2O$	[64]
Al^{3+}	$(CIP.HCl)_3\ Al$	[14]
Cu^{2+}	$[Cu(CIP)_2Cl_2].6H_2O$	[65]
	$[Cu(CIP)(H_2O)_3]SO_4.2H_2O$	[66]
	$[Cu_2(cip)_2(bpy)_2(pip)]\cdot 6H_2O$ (bpy=2,2'-bipyridyl, pip= piperazinyl anion)	[67]
	$[Cu(HCIP)_2(ClO_4)_2].6H_2O$	[68]
	$[Cu^{II}(CIP)_2(Cu^{I}Cl_2)_2]$	[69]
	$[Cu(HCIP)_2](NO_3)_2.6H_2O$; $[Cu(phen)(CIP)](NO_3).4H_2O$; $Cu(phen)(HCIP)(NO_3)_2.H_2O$	[70]
Cd^{2+}	$[Cd(HCIP)_2(Cl)_2].4H_2O$	[62]
Co^{2+}	$[Co(CIP)_2(H_2O)_2].9H_2O$	[71]
Ce^{3+}	$[Ce(CIP)_2(H_2O)_4]Cl(H_2O)_{3.25}(C_2H_5OH)_{0.25}$	[72]
Mg^{2+}	$(CIPH_2)_2\text{-}[Mg(H_2O)_6](SO_4)_2.\ 6H_2O$	[73]
	$[Mg(CIP)_2]\cdot 2.5H_2O$	[74]
	$[Mg(CIP)_2(H_2O)_2]\cdot 2H_2O$	[75]
	$[Mg(H_2O)_2(CIPH)_2](NO_3)_2\cdot 2H_2O$	[76]
	$[Mg\text{-}(CIPH)_3](SO_4)\cdot 5H_2O$	[64]
Bi^{3+}	$(CIPH_3)(CIPH_2)[BiCl_6].2H_2O$	[77]
	$[Bi(CIP)_3(H_2O)_2]$	[78]
	$(CIPH_3)_2[Bi_2Cl_{10}].4H_2O$	[79]
Zn^{2+}	$[Zn(CIP)_2(H_2O)_2].8H_2O$	[62]
	$[Zn(CIPH)(Hbtc)].\ H_2O$ (btc:1,3,5-benzenetricarboxylate)	[80]
	$[Zn_2(CIPH)_2(odpa)]$ (odpa: 4,4´-oxydiphthalate)	[69]
	$[Zn2(CIPH)_2(bptc)].\ 4H_2O$ (bptc: 3,3´,4,4´-benzophenonetetracarboxylate)	[69]
	$(CIP)_2\cdot ZnCl_4\cdot 2H_2O$;$([Zn(CIP)_2]\cdot 3H_2O)$	[81]

Many of the complexes reported above were created with the aim of studying the experimental and theoretical charge density of various metal-quinolone crystals, and this has contributed to the elucidation of the intricate mechanisms of action of the quinolone drugs and the role of metal ions in these processes. The antibacterial activity of several of these complexes has been analyzed, and some examples of the published complexes of CIP are displayed in Table 2.

CONCLUSION

CIP is a wide spectrum antibiotic that can be used in the treatment of multiple infectious diseases in both human and veterinary medicine. The main disadvantage of this drug, however, is its poor solubility, which is one of the principal causes of its unfavorable biopharmaceutical properties. Attempts to improve its solubility have largely been focused on manipulation of its solid state features, in particular those that impact on its pharmaceutical properties, using state-of-the-art chemical engineering along with the aid of numerous useful methods for obtaining solid state characterization.

The simple and versatile chemical structure of CIP, its chemical and physical stability, and its clinical importance make this drug an interesting candidate to focus scientific efforts on due to its pharmaceutical potential as a solid.

We predict that the study of the solid state of this drug will continue to grow rapidly, with more CIP solid forms being reported. Hopefully, most of these will be useful for new therapeutic options, implying a broader commercialization of drug products containing CIP.

REFERENCES

[1] Appelbaum, Peter C. and Pamela A. Hunter. 2000. "The fluoroquinolone antibacterials: past, present and future perspectives." *Int. J. Antimicrob. Agents*. 16:5−15.

[2] Gutiérrez-Castrellón, Pedro, Luisa Díaz-García, Agustín de Colsa-Ranero, Juan Cuevas-Alpuche and Irma Jiménez-Escobar. 2015. "Efficacy and safety of ciprofloxacin treatment in urinary tract infections (UTIs) in adults: a systematic review with meta-analysis." *Gac. Med. Mex.* 151:225-44.

[3] Shen, Linus L., William Kohlbrenner, Debra Weigl, and John Baranowski. 1989. "Mechanism of quinolone inhibition of DNA gyrase. Appearance of unique norfloxacin binding sites in enzyme-DNA complexes." *J. Biol. Chem.* 264:2973–2978.

[4] Khodursky, Arkady B., and Nicholas R. Cozzarelli. 1998. "The mechanism of inhibition of topoisomerase IV by quinolone antibacterials." *J. Biol. Chem.* 273:27668–27677.

[5] Ross, Diana L., and Chistopher M. Riley. 1992. "Physicochemical Properties of the Fluoroquinolone Antimicrobials. II. Acid Ionization Constants and Their Relationship to Structure." *Int. J. Pharm.* 83:267-272.

[6] Ross, Diana L., and Chistopher M. Riley. 1994. "Dissociation and complexation of the fluoroquinolone antimicrobials -an update." *J. Pharm. Biomed. Anal.* 12:1325-1331.

[7] Belal, Fathalla, Abdulrahman A. Al-Majed, and Abdulrahman M. Al-Obaid. 1999. "Methods of Analysis of 4-quinolone Antibacterials." *Talanta* 50:765-86.

[8] Lee, Dong-Sun, Hee-Jung Han, Kun Kim, Won-Bong Park, Jung-Kil Cho, and Jae-Hyun Kim. 1994. "Dissociation and Complexation of Fluoroquinolone Analogues." *J. Pharm. Biomed. Anal.* 12:157-164.

[9] Yu, Xuanqiang, Gail Zipp, and G. W. Ray Davidson III. 1994. "The Effect of Temperature and pH on the Solubility of Quinolone Compounds: Estimation of Heat of Fusion." *Pharm. Res.* 11:522-527.

[10] Drakopoulos, Anargiros I. and Pinelopi C. Ioannou. 1997. "Spectrofluorimetric Study of the Acid-Base Equilibria and Complexation Behavior of the Fluoroquinolone Antibiotics Ofloxacin, Norfloxacin, Ciprofloxacin and Pefloxacin in Aqueous Solution." *Anal. Chim. Acta.* 354:197-204.

[11] Mesallati, Hanah, Anita Umerska, Krzysztof J. Paluch, and Lidia Tajber. 2017. "Amorphous polymeric drug salts as ionic solid dispersion forms of ciprofloxacin." *Mol. Pharm.* 14:2209–2223.

[12] Tehler, Ulrika, Jonas H. Fagerberg, Richard Svensson, Mats Larhed, Per Artursson, and Christel A. S. Bergström. 2013. "Optimizing solubility and permeability of a biopharmaceutics classification system (BCS) class 4 antibiotic drug using lipophilic fragments disturbing the crystal lattice." *J. Med. Chem.* 56:2690−2694.

[13] Fallati, Claudia S., Amelia A. Ahumada, and Rubén H. Manzo. 1994. "El Perfil de Solubilidad de la Ciprofloxacina en Función del pH." *Acta Farm. Bon.* 13:73-77.

[14] Zhang, Cong-Liang, Fang Zhao, and Yan Wang. 2010. "Thermodynamics of the solubility of ciprofloxacin in methanol, ethanol, 1-propanol, acetone, and chloroform from 293.15 to 333.15K." *J. Mol. Liq.* 156:191−193.

[15] Harder, Sebastian, Uwe Fuhr, Dieter Beermann, and Horst Staib. 1990. "Ciprofloxacin absorption in different regions of the human gastrointestinal tract. Investigations with the hf-capsule." *Br. J. Clin. Pharmacol.* 30:35-39.

[16] Zakelj, Simon, Katja Sturm, and Albin Kristl. 2006. "Ciprofloxacin permeability and its active secretion through rat small intestine in vitro." *Int. J. Pharm.* 313:175-180.

[17] Li, Xianwen, Feng Zhi, and Yiqiao Hu. 2006. "Investigation of excipient and processing on solid phase transformation and dissolution of ciprofloxacin." *Int. J. Pharm.* 328:177-82.

[18] Hoffken, Gert, Hartmut Lode, Claus Prinzing, Klaus Borner, and Peter Koeppe. 1985. "Pharmacokinetics of Ciprofloxacin after Oral and Parenteral Administration." *Antimicrob. Agents Ch.* 27:375-379.

[19] Brunner, Martin, Heino Stass, Jan-Georg Moller, Claudia Schrolnberger, Boban Erovic, Ursula Hollenstein, Markus Zeitlinger, Hans Georg Eichler, and Markus Muller. 2002. "Target site concentrations of ciprofloxacin after single intravenous and oral doses." *Antimicrob. Agents Ch.* 46:3724-3730.

[20] Breda, Susana A. Alvaro F. Jimenez-Kairuz, Rubén H. Manzo, and María E. Olivera. 2009. "Solubility behavior and biopharmaceutical classification of novel high-solubility ciprofloxacin and norfloxacin pharmaceutical derivatives." *Int. J. Pharm.* 371:106–113.

[21] Cerreia Vioglio, Paolo, Michele R. Chierotti, and Roberto Gobetto. 2017. "Pharmaceutical aspects of salt and cocrystal forms of APIs and characterization challenges." *Adv. Drug Deliv. Rev.* 117:86–110.

[22] Wouters, Johan, and Luc Quéré. 2012. *Pharmaceutical Salts and Co-crystals.* UK:RSCPublishing.

[23] Mahapatra, Sudarshan, Katharigatta N. Venugopala, and Tayur N. Guru Row. 2010. "A Device to Crystallize Organic Solids: Structure of Ciprofloxacin, Midazolam, and Ofloxacin as Targets." *Cryst. Growth Des.* 10:1866−1870.

[24] Fabbiani, Francesca P. A., Birger Dittrich, Alastair J. Florence, Thomas Gelbrich, Michael B. Hursthouse, Werner F. Kuhs, Norman Shankland, and Heidrun Sowa. 2009. "Crystal structures with a challenge: high-pressure crystallization of ciprofloxacin sodium salts and their recovery to ambient pressure." *Cryst Eng Comm.* 11:1396−1406.

[25] Wassvik, Carola M., Anders G. Holmén, Rieke Draheim, Per Artursson, and Christel A. S. 2008. "Bergström, C. A. Molecular Characteristics for Solid-State Limited Solubility." *J. Med. Chem.* 51:3035−3039.

[26] Dorofeev, V. L. 2004. "The betainelike structure and infrared spectra of drugs of the fluoroquinolone group." *Pharm. Chem. J.* 38:698−702.

[27] Turel, Iztok, Peter Bukovec, and Miguel Quirós. 1997. "Crystal structure of ciprofloxacin hexahydrate and its characterization." *Int. J. Pharm.* 152: 59−65

[28] Mesallati, Hanah, Naila A. Mugheirbi, and Lidia Tajber. 2016. "Two Faces of Ciprofloxacin: Investigation of Proton Transfer in Solid State Transformations." *Cryst. Growth Des.* 16:6574–6585.

[29] Turel, Iztok and Peter Bukovec. 1996. "Comparison of the thermal stability of ciprofloxacin and its compounds." *Thermochim. Acta* 287:311−318.

[30] Healy, Anne Marie, Zelalem A. Worku, Dinesh Kumar, and Atif M. Madi. 2017. "Pharmaceutical solvates, hyd rates and amorphous forms: A special emphasis on cocrystals." *Adv. Drug Deliv. Rev.* 117:25-46.

[31] Mafra, Luis, Sergio M. Santos, Renée Siegel, Inês Alves, Felipe A. Almeida Paz, Dmytro Dudenko, Hans W. Spiess. 2012. "Packing Interactions in Hydrated and Anhydrous Forms of the Antibiotic Ciprofloxacin: a Solid-State NMR, X-ray Diffraction, and Computer Simulation Study." *J. Am. Chem. Soc.* 134:71−74.

[32] Li, Xian W., Yong Ch. Hu, Y. Gao, Geoffrey G. Z. Zhang, and Roger F. Henry. 2006. "A methanol hemisolvate of ciprofloxacin." *Acta Cryst.* E62:o5803-o5805.

[33] Fabbiani, Francesca P. A. Jean-Baptiste Arlin, Gernot Buth, Birger Dittrich, Alastair J. Florence, Regine Herbst-Irmer, and Heidrun Sowa. 2011. "Inter-molecular inter-actions, disorder and twinning in ciprofloxacin-2,2-difluoro-ethanol (2/3) and ciprofloxacin-water (3/14.5)." *Acta Cryst.* C67: o120−o124.

[34] Aso, Yukio, Sumie Yoshioka, Jiang Zhang, J., and George Zografi. 2002. "Effect of Water on the Molecular Mobility of Sucrose and Poly(vinylpyrrolidone) in a Colyophilized Formulation as Measured by ^{13}C-NMR Relaxation Time." *Chem. Pharm. Bull.* 50:822−826.

[35] Dengale, Swapnil J., Holger Grohganz, Thomas Rades, and Korbinian Löbmann. 2016. "Recent advances in co-amorphous drug formulations." *Adv. Drug Deliv. Rev.* 100:116-125.

[36] Dhirendra, K., S. Lewis, N. Udupa, and K. Atin. 2009. "Solid dispersions: a review." *Pak. J. Pharm. Sci.* 22:234-246.

[37] Mesallati, Hanah, Daryl Conroy, Sarah Hudson, and Lidia Tajber. 2017. "Preparation and characterization of amorphous ciprofloxacin-amino acid salts." *Eur. J. Pharm. Biopharm.* 121:73–89.

[38] Izutsu, Ken-ichi, Tatsuo Koide, Noriyuki Takata, Yukihiro Ikeda, Makoto Ono, Motoki Inoue, Toshiro Fukami, and Etsuo Yonemochif.

2016. "Characterization and Quality Control of Pharmaceutical Cocrystals." *Chem. Pharm. Bull.* 64:1421–1430.

[39] Qiao, Ning, Mingzhong Li, Walkiria Schlindwein, Nazneen Malek, Angela Davies, Gary Trappitt. 2011. "Pharmaceutical cocrystals: An overview." *Int. J. Pharm.* 419:1–11.

[40] Thakuria, Ranjit, and Bipul Sarma. 2018. "Drug-Drug and Drug-Nutraceutical Cocrystal/Salt as Alternative Medicine for Combination Therapy: A Crystal Engineering Approach." *Crystals* 8:101-140.

[41] Serajuddin, Abu T. M. 2007. "Salt formation to improve drug solubility." *Adv. Drug Deliv. Rev.* 59:603-616.

[42] Aitipamula, Srinivasulu, Rahul Banerjee, Arvind K. Bansal, Kumar Biradha, Miranda L. Cheney, Angshuman Roy Choudhury, Gautam R. Desiraju, Amol G. Dikundwar, Ritesh Dubey, Nagakiran Duggirala, et al. 2012. "Polymorphs, Salts, and Cocrystals: What's in a Name?" *Cryst. Growth Des.* 12:2147–2152.

[43] Trask, Andrew V., and William Jones. 2005. "Crystal Engineering of Organic Cocrystals by the Solid-State Grinding Approach." *Top. Curr. Chem.* 254: 41–70.

[44] Golovnev, Nikolay N., Maxim S. Molokeev, Maxim K. Lesnikov, and Victor V. Atuchin. 2017. "Two salts and the salt cocrystal of ciprofloxacin with thiobarbituric and barbituric acids: The structure and properties." *J. Phys. Org. Chem.* Accessed February 2, 2018. doi.org/10.1002/poc.3773.

[45] Turel, Iztok, and Amalija Golobic. 2003. "Crystal Structure of Ciprofloxacin Hydrochloride 1.34-Hydrate." *Anal. Sci.* 19:329-330.

[46] Liu, Yong, Jingkang Wang, and Qiuxiang Yin. 2005. "The crystal habit of ciprofloxacin hydrochloride monohydrate crystal." *J. Cryst. Growth* 276: 237-242.

[47] Prasanna, M. D., and Tayur N. Guru Row. 2001. "Hydrogen bonded networks in hydrophilic channels: crystal structure of hydrated Ciprofloxacin Lactate and comparison with structurally similar compounds." *J. Mol. Struct.* 559:255-261.

[48] Zhang, Guoshun, Li Zhang, Dezhi Yang, Na Zhang, Lan He, Guanhua Duc, and Yang Lu. 2016. "Salt screening and characterization of ciprofloxacin." *Acta Cryst.* B72:20–28.

[49] Surov, Artem O., Andrei V. Churakov, and German L. Perlovich. 2016. "Three Polymorphic Forms of Ciprofloxacin Maleate: Formation Pathways, Crystal Structures, Calculations, and Thermodynamic Stability Aspects." *Cryst. Growth Des.* 16:6556-6567.

[50] Chadha, Renu, Pawanpreet Singh, Sadhika Khullar, and Sanjay K. Mandal. 2016. "Ciprofloxacin Hippurate Salt: Crystallization Tactics, Structural Aspects, and Biopharmaceutical Performance." *Cryst. Growth Des.* 16:4960-4967.

[51] Pinto Vitorino, Graciela, Norma R. Sperandeo, Mino R. Caira, and María R. Mazzieri. 2013. "A Supramolecular Assembly Formed by Heteroassociation of Ciprofloxacin and Norfloxacin in the Solid State: Co-Crystal Synthesis and Characterization." *Cryst. Growth Des.* 13:1050-1058.

[52] Pinto Vitorino, Graciela, María C. Becerra, Gustavo D. Barrera, Mino R. Caira, and María R. Mazzieri. 2017. "Cooperative behaviour of fluorquinolone combinations against *Escherichia coli* and *Staphylococcus aureus*." *Biol. Pharm. Bull.* 40: 758–764.

[53] Bag, Partha P., Soumyajit Ghosh, Hamza Khan, Ramesh Devarapalli, and C. Malla Reddy. 2014. "Drug–drug salt forms of ciprofloxacin with diflunisal and indoprofen." *Cryst. Eng. Comm*, 16:7393-7396.

[54] ElShaer, Amr, Defang Ouyang, Peter Hanson, and Afzal R. Mohammed. 2013. "Preparation and evaluation of aminoacid based salt forms of model zwitterionic drug ciprofloxacin." *Pharm. Drug Deliv. Res.* 2:1–10.

[55] Cruz-Cabeza, Aurora J., Susan M. Reutzel-Edens, and Joel Bernstein. 2015. "Facts and fictions about polymorphism." *Chem. Soc. Rev.* 44:8619-8635.

[56] Barbas, Rafael, Rafael Prohens, and Cristina Puigjaner. 2007. "A new polymorph of norfloxacin. Complete characterization and

relative stability of its trimorphic system." *J. Therm. Anal. Calorim.* 89:687–692.

[57] Bratu, I., G. Borodi, I. Kacsó, Z. Moldovana, C. Filip, F. Dragan, M. Vasilescu, and S. Simon. 2011. "New solid form of Norfloxacin: Structural studies." *Spectroscopy* 25:53–62.

[58] FDA. U.S. Food and Drug Administration. https://www.accessdata.fda.gov/scripts/fdcc/?set=IndirectAdditives (accessed March 2018).

[59] Garro Linck, Yamila, Ana K. Chattah, R. Graf, Carolina B. Romañuk, María E. Olivera, Rubén H. Manzo, Gustavo A. Monti, and H. W. Spiess. 2011. "Multinuclear solid state NMR investigation of two polymorphic forms of Ciprofloxacin-saccharinate." *Phys. Chem. Chem. Phys.* 13:6590–6596.

[60] Singh, Pawanpreet, and Renu Chadha. 2017. "A new polymorph of ciprofloxacin saccharinate: Structural characterization and pharmaceutical profile." *J. Pharm. Biomed. Anal.* 146:7–14.

[61] Nagalapalli, Ravikumar, and Shankar Yaga Bheem. 2014. "Synthesis, Crystal Structure, and Hirshfeld Surface Analysis of Ciprofloxacin-Salicylic Acid Molecular Salt." *J. Cryst.* Article ID 936174, 5 pages. doi:10.1155/2014/936174.

[62] Uivarosi, Valentina. 2013. "Metal Complexes of Quinolone Antibiotics and Their Applications: An Update." *Molecules* 18:11153-11197.

[63] Rehder, Dieter, Joao Costa Pessoa, Carlos F. G. C. Geraldes, M. Margarida C. A. Castro, Themistoklis Kabanos, Tama´s Kiss, Beate Meier, Giovanni Micera, Lage Pettersson, Maria Rangel, et al. 2002. "In vitro study of the insulin-mimetic behaviour of vanadium (IV, V) coordination compounds." *J. Biol. Inorg. Chem.* 7:384–396.

[64] Wallis, Steven C., Lawrence R. Gahan, Bruce G. Charles, and Trevor W. Hambley. 1995. "Synthesis and X-ray structural characterization of an iron(III) complex of the fluoroquinolone antimicrobial ciprofloxacin, $[Fe(CIP)(NTA)]_3 \cdot 5H_2O$ (NTA-Nitrilotriacetato)." *Polyhedron* 14:2835-2840.

[65] Turel, Iztok, Ivan Leban, and Natasa Bukovec. 1994. "Synthesis, characterization, and crystal structure of a copper(II) complex with

quinolone family member (ciprofloxacin): bis(1)-cyclopropyl-6-fluoro-1,4-dihydro-4-oxo-7-piperazin-1ylquinoline-3-carboxylate) copper(II) chloride hexahydrate." *J. Inorg. Biochem.* 56:273-282.

[66] Turel, Iztok, Ljubo Golic, and Osar L. Ruiz Ramirez. 1999. "Crystal structure and characterization of a new copper(II)-ciprofloxacin (cf) complex $[Cu(cf)(H_2O)_3]SO_4.2H_2O$." *Acta Chim. Slov.* 46:203-211.

[67] Wu, Guangguo, Guoping Wang, Xuchun Fu, and Longguan Zhu. 2003. "Synthesis, Crystal Structure, Stacking Effect and Antibacterial Studies of a Novel Quaternary Copper (II) Complex with Quinolone." *Molecules* 8:287-296.

[68] Jiménez-Garrido, N., Lourdes Perelló, Rubén M. Ortiz, Gloria Alzuet, Marta González-Alvarez, E. Cantoón, Malvaliu Liu-González, M. García-Granda, and M. Pérez-Priede. "Antibacterial studies, DNA oxidative cleavage, and cristal structures of Cu(II) and Co(II) complexes with two quinolone family members, ciprofloxacin and enoxacin." *J. Inorg. Biochem.* 99:677–689.

[69] Drevenšek, Petra, Tatjana Zupančič, Boris Pihlar, Roman Jerala, Uwe Kolitsch, Andreja Plaper, and Iztok Turel. 2005. "Mixed-valence Cu(II)/Cu(I) complex of quinolone ciprofloxacin isolated by a hydrothermal reaction in the presence of L-histidine: Comparison of biological activities of various copper–ciprofloxacin compounds." *J. Inorg. Biochem.* 99:432–442.

[70] Hernández-Gil, J., L. Perelló, Rubén M. Ortiz, Gloria Alzuet, Mirta González-Álvarez, and Malvaliu Liu-González. 2009. "Synthesis, structure and biological properties of several binary and ternary complexes of copper(II) with ciprofloxacin and 1,10 phenanthroline." *Polyhedron* 28:138–144.

[71] López-Gresa, M. P., Rubén M. Ortiz, L. Perelló, J. Latorre, Malvaliu Liu-González, S. García-Granda, M. Pérez-Priede, and E. Cantón. 2002. "Interactions of metal ions with two quinolone antimicrobial agents (cinoxacin and ciprofloxacin). Spectroscopic and X-ray structural characterization. Antibacterial studies." *J. Inorg. Biochem.* 92:65–74.

[72] Li, Jia-Bin, Pin Yang, Fei Gao, Gao-Yi Han, and Kai-Bei Yu. 2001. "Novel Lanthanide Complexes of Ciprofloxacin: Synthesis, Characterization, Crystal Structure and in vitro Antibacterial Activity Studies." *Chin. J. Chem.* 19:598-605.

[73] Turel, Iztok, Ivan Leban, Marija Zupancic, Peter Bukovec, and Karl Gruber. 1996. "An Adduct of Magnesium Sulfate with a Member of the Quinolone Family (Ciprofloxacin)." *Acta Cryst.* C52:2443-2445.

[74] Drevenšek, Petra, Natasa Poklar Ulrih, Andreja Majerle, and Iztok Turel. 2006. "Synthesis, characterization and DNA binding of magnesium–ciprofloxacin (cfH) complex $[Mg(cf)_2]\cdot_2.5H_2O$." *J. Inorg. Biochem.* 100:1705–1713.

[75] Turel, Iztok, A. Šonc, Marija Zupančič, K. Sepčić, and T. Turk. 2000. "Biological activity of some magnesium(II) complexes of quinolones." *Met. Based Drugs* 7: 101–104.

[76] Turel, Iztok, Petra Zivec, Andrej Pevec, Sarah Tempelaar, and George Psomas. 2008. "Compounds of Antibacterial Agent Ciprofloxacin and Magnesium – Crystal Structures and Molecular Modeling Calculations." *Eur. J. Inorg. Chem.* 23:3718–3727.

[77] Turel, Iztok, Ivan Leban, and Natasa Bukovec. 1997 "Crystal structure and characterization of the bismuth(III) compound with quinolone family member (ciprofloxacin). Antibacterial study." *J. Inorg. Biochem.* 66:241-245.

[78] Shaikh, Anwar R., R. Giridhar, Francis Megraud, and M. R. Yadav. "Metalloantibiotics: Synthesis, characterization and antimicrobial evaluation of bismuth-fluoroquinolone complexes against *Helicobacter Pylori*." *Acta Pharm.* 59:259–271.

[79] Turel, Iztok, Ljubo Golic, Peter Bukovec, and Marija Gubina. 1998. "Antibacterial tests of Bismuth(III)–Quinolone (Ciprofloxacin, cf) compounds against Helicobacter pylori and some other bacteria. Crystal structure of $(cfH_2)_2[Bi_2Cl_{10}]\cdot 4H_2O$." *J. Inorg. Biochem.* 71:53-60.

[80] Xiao, Dong-Rong, En-Bo Wang, Hai-Yan An, Yang-Guang Li, and Lin Xu. 2007. "Syntheses and Structures of Three Unprecedented

Metal-Ciprofloxacin Complexes with Helical Character." *Cryst. Growth Des.* 7:506-512.

[81] Zupancic, Marija, Iztok Turel, Peter Bukovec, Andrew J. P. White, and David J. Williams. 2001. "Synthesis and Characterization of Two Novel Zinc(II) Complexes with Ciprofloxacin. Crystal Structure of $[C_{17}H_{19}N_3O_3F]_2 \cdot [ZnCl_4] \cdot 2H_2O$." *Croat. Chem. Acta* 74:61-74.

In: Ciprofloxacin
Editor: Mohamed Said Attia
ISBN: 978-1-53614-534-2

Chapter 2

CIPROFLOXACIN-SILICA/HYDROXYAPATITE NANOPARTICLES: RELEASE PROFILE, *IN VITRO* BIOCOMPATIBILITY, BACTERICIDAL EFFICIENCY AND CYTOCOMPATIBILITY STUDIES

Gracielle Ferreira Andrade*, PhD
and Edésia Martins Barros de Sousa, PhD
Centro de Desenvolvimento da Tecnologia Nuclear,
CDTN, Belo Horizonte, MG, Brazil

ABSTRACT

The difficulty in treating diseases affecting bone tissue, such as osteomyelitis, motivates the development of devices that enable targeted delivery of drugs. Thus, the development of systems that can operate more efficiently against infections and also ensure bone integration as well as regeneration have been be of great interest for pharmaceutical

---

* Corresponding Author Email: graciellefandrade@yahoo.com.br.

technology. Among all the inorganic support materials, ordered mesoporous materials based on silica have been intensively studied as candidate systems for controlled drug release due to their high surface area, high ordering of the mesopores and pore size in the nanometer scale. Several synthesis routes for mesoporous silica-based materials have been carried out in order to develop devices for biological application due to their bioactive properties and their biocompatibility. Ordered mesoporous materials have a network of channels and well-defined pore size ranging from 2 to 30 nm, with structural diversity of pores, high surface area (400 – 1,000 $m^2.g^{-1}$). Pore structure is important to make these materials suitable for the incorporation and of a variety of molecules into the matrix, and for their subsequent release. Among their applications are the use of these materials as antibiotic delivery systems, and as osteogenic systems to be used in bone treatment. The synthesis of silica with calcium phosphate *in situ*, which is a mineral present in large amounts in bone tissue, can offer interesting aspects for an improved biological activity of these materials. Furthermore, the incorporation of ciprofloxacin enables the development of a promising and efficient system for the treatment of infected tissues. Ciprofloxacin is a drug with broad spectrum of action and can be used in the treatment of bone infection. Acting against gram-positive and gram-negative bacteria, it has shown high action against *Staphylococcus aureaus*, the main causative bacteria of osteomyelitis. In addition, bactericidal efficacy of these particles was tested against microorganisms present in bone infections, and our composites had bactericidal efficiency comparable to free-ciprofloxacin. In summary, taking into account the great potential of these nanoparticle structures to carry ciprofloxacin, besides their bactericidal efficacy, these systems are promising candidates for bone infection treatment.

Keywords: ciprofloxacin, drug delivery, silica/hydroxyapatite nanoparticles, nanocomposites, biocompatibility, bactericidal efficacy

1. Introduction

The impact of bone diseases has increased significantly in the last decades around the world (Gong et al. 2015). The treatment of bone infections is difficult to perform due to the intrinsic characteristics of the bone tissue as bones are poorly perfused organs and lack permeability to drugs. Thus, it is necessary to investigate new forms of local molecule delivery for a decrease or eradication of possible toxicity generated by a systemic therapy with antimicrobial agents (Arcos and Vallet-Regí 2010; Huh and Kwon 2011b; Patzakis 2003).

The combination of nanotechnology and biology can elucidate several biomedical problems, and can revolutionize the field of health and medicine (Curtis and Wilkinson 2001). Developments in medicine based on nanotechnology promise important advances in diagnosis, therapeutics, molecular biology and bioengineering. Nanotechnology implies the manufacture of materials at the atomic level to attain unique properties, which can be suitably manipulated for the desired applications (Shrivastava et al. 2007). Today, the use of nanosystems is very plausible for the delivery of biomolecules and for numerous disease treatments, such as those based on liposomes and nanoparticles (Hartmann 2005). The multidisciplinary character of this theme contributes in a very significant way to reveal this new horizon of science.

In this context, many nanomaterials have been studied as potential candidates for various types of applications. One of them, ordered mesoporous silica, consists of silicate based compounds that, although amorphous, have highly organized pore structures with nanometric dimensions, which give these materials very interesting textural characteristics such as high thermal stability, tuneable pore size with narrow distribution in the nanometre range and high surface area (Ulrike Ciesla 1999).

These materials may have different applications such as adsorption, catalysis (Ren et al. 2017), electronics (Florek and Kleitz, n.d.), and as molecule reservoirs and carriers (Andreza De Sousa et al. 2010; Vallet-Regí et al. 2006). Each application depends on the qualities provided by their nanometric structure, as well as their organization in the macrostructure. In this way, the synthesis, modification and control of these materials in this scale represent the access to new properties and diversified behaviour. All these characteristics make nanostructured mesoporous materials promising candidates for applications in the areas related to bionanotechnology. In addition, the possibility of selectively modifying these materials to be used for specific applications provides a large area to be explored, taking into account their intrinsic characteristics (Gracielle Ferreira Andrade et al. 2013; Vallet-Regí et al. 2007).

The nanocomposite based mesoporous silica materials, when submitted to the *in situ* synthesis, carried out with sources of calcium and phosphorus, form a composite of silica with apatite which presents a multiplicity of applications in the medical area by adding properties of both materials (A Sousa, Souza, and Sousa 2008; Gracielle F. Andrade et al. 2015). The biocompatibility of the two materials, the adsorption capacity of molecules in the silica pores and the established bioavailability of hydroxyapatite represent excellent properties which justify the formation of this nanocomposite and its possible application in bone repair (Vallet-Regí et al. 2007).

In addition, by promoting changes on their surfaces, these materials can acquire targeted functionality as well as allow the storage of molecules, and may promote, for example, the protection of these molecules during absorption in the human body (I. Kim et al. 2011). Mesoporous silica materials may serve as barriers to unwanted degradation or metabolization of the drugs, thus keeping the dose within the range of therapeutic efficacy and leading to a decrease in undesired effects (Rámila et al. 2003).

Applications for silica-based materials in medicine and biotechnology as devices for bone repair and as a drug delivery system have been shown. Both the structure and the chemical composition promote final characteristics and interesting properties for this type of application. Therefore, adequate combination of synthetic techniques, the various possibilities of superficial modification, as well as their bioactive behaviour with the ability to carry molecules, make these materials excellent candidates for the development of devices for tissue engineering (Vallet-Regí and Balas 2008).

Ciprofloxacin can be successfully loaded onto the nanocomposite, due to its high surface area and pore volume. Moreover, it can be delivered to the bone region due to the presence of apatites, since the composition of these materials is similar to the vertebrate bone structure, and thus can be released in a specific region (Gracielle Ferreira Andrade et al. 2017).

In this context, many efforts have been made using these mesoporous materials in order to develop devices with biomedical applications that aggregate the two main uses, that is, as drug delivery systems and to promote regeneration of bone tissue (Vallet-Regí et al. 2006).

In this work, the recent developments in nanocomposites based on mesoporous materials and hydroxypaptite will be overviewed. Two categories of nanoparticles are described: (1) mesoporous silica nanoparticles and (2) mesoporous silica with hydroxyapatite nanocomposite included. The recent progress and applications of each one of these materials in the biomedical field and ciprofloxacin delivery system are reported.

2. CIPROFLOXACIN

Ciprofloxacin is the most widely used antibiotic for bacterial bone infections caused by *Staphylococcus aureus, Staphylococcus epidermidis, Pseudomonas aeruginosa* and *Proteus mirabilis.* It is an antibiotic of the 2nd generation of the quinolone drug group (Figure 1). The first compounds of 2nd generation appeared in the decade of the 1980s, with the combination of a fluorine atom (C-6 position) and a piperazinyl group (C-7 position) (norfloxacin, ciprofloxacin, ofloxacin). This combination led to a greater spectrum of action and an outstanding enhancement of antibacterial activity, resulting in better activity against Gram (-) bacteria, and also allowing them to cover some Gram (+) species with the addition of functional groups (Sharma et al. 2010; Overbeck et al. 1995).

Ciprofloxacin shows a wide spectrum of antimicrobial activity and a good penetration in many tissues, including bone tissue. The minimum inhibitory concentration of ciprofloxacin is low (0.25 – 2 $\mu g.mL^{-1}$) for the *Staphylococcus aureus*, which is a quite common pathogen in osteomyelitis, a bone infection. Ciprofloxacin is also very efficient against many gram-negative microorganisms, such as the *Enterobacteriaceae*, which are frequently responsible for bone infections, which demand prolonged treatment using antibiotics (Desevaux 2002).

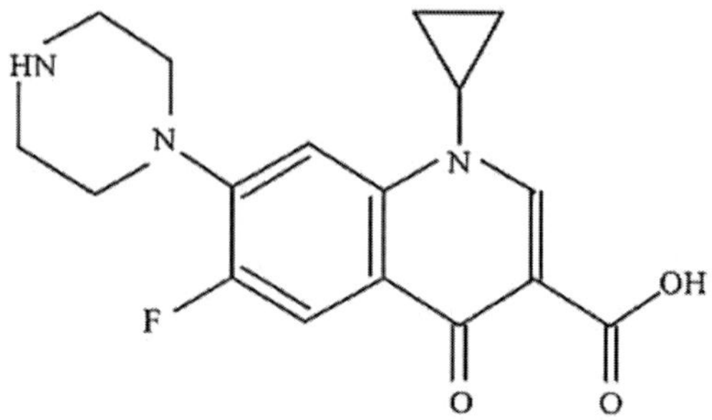

Figure 1. Structure of ciprofloxacin.

Fluoroquinolone antibiotics act by directly inhibiting DNA synthesis through their activity against DNA gyrase and Topoisomerase IV. These are essential enzymes that maintain negative supercoiling of DNA (DNA gyrase) or separated interlocked daughter DNA strands formed during replication, facilitating segregation into the daughter cells (Topo IV) (RANG, H. P. e DALE 2001). These molecules are selective for the bacterial enzymes, since they differ structurally from the mammalian enzyme. Zhang *et al.* (Zhang et al. 2010) specify that the inhibition occurs in subunits A of the DNA gyrase, responsible for the division of the double strand of chromosomes.

The *in vivo* behavior of fluoroquinolones is significantly affected by their physicochemical properties, in particular by their ability to be ionized as a function of pH, and to form complexes with metal ions (Drakopoulos and Ioannou 1997). Fluoroquinolones may form complexes with certain cations such as Al^{3+}, Mg^{2+}, Fe^{3+}, Ca^{2+}, Cu^{2+}e Au^{3+}.

The presence of charged centers in many drugs may be essential for their biological activity and their passage through cell membranes. Many drugs have ionizable groups and exhibit zwitterionic characteristics, which consist of electrically neutral chemical compounds, but have opposite charges on different non-adjacent atoms, which can interact intra- and intermolecularly, directly influencing their physicochemical properties (Pistos, Koutsopoulou, and Panderi 2004).

According to Barbosa et al. (Barbosa J, Barrón D 1999), it is possible find the fluoroquinolones in the forms: (a) protonated (in acidic media); (b) zwitterionic (in neutral or weakly acid media); (c) and as an anion (in alkaline media), where the ionization constants refer to the protons 3-carboxyl and 7-piperazine.

Ciprofloxacin is a zwitterionic fluorquinolone at physiological pH with bactericidal action. Ciprofloxacin has two proton receptor functional groups, corresponding to two chemical ionization equilibria, in a physiologically normal pH range. The carboxyl group, which is in the 3-position, protonates in a slightly acidic medium, pKa 6. The group associated with the nitrogen (N) at the 4-position of the piperazine ring (attached to the 7-position of the quinolonic ring) deprotonates in an alkaline medium, pKa 8.8. There are four sites for potential protonation / dissociation processes in the molecule: in addition to the carboxyl group, and the N4 ', mentioned above, the other nitrogen atom of the piperazine ring, N1' and the nitrogen atom in the aromatic nucleus N1.

3. Silica/Hydroxyapatite Nanocomposite - Biomaterial

Biomaterials are synthetic or natural materials, which are used as a whole or as part of a system for treating, enlarging or replacing tissues, organs or bodily functions. When in contact with the biological system, they interact with it in a way that causes the least toxic reaction possible. This definition originated in the 1982 Consensus Conference on Biomaterials for Clinical Applications. Thus, it is a non-toxic material used as a medical device characterized by interaction with the biological system (Williams 1987).

Among all the characteristics that a biomaterial must have, the biocompatibility is the most important, because the biofunctionality of the material can only be manifested if it is compatible with biological systems. Biocompatibility is not only the absence of rejection but also involves the interaction between the implant and the adjacent tissue. Therefore, it is possible to distinguish biocompatible biomaterials as bioactive, bioinert and bioreabsorbed (Khademhosseini and Langer 2016).

The field of bioceramics appeared in the late 1960s, as an effort to overcome some biocompatibility problems associated with the metallic implants used in orthopedic surgeries at that time (Arcos and Vallet-Regí 2013). The first generation of bioceramics, called inert ceramics, were represented by alumina (Al_2O_3) and zirconia (ZrO_2), which had an important role as a material to replace bone tissue due to their low reactivity (V. J. SHIRTLIFF 2003). Until then, the replacement was regarded as having low tissue response, perhaps because the only expected responses were inflammatory responses and rejection of the material.

However, the discovery of bioglass (Bioglass) by Prof. Hench in 1969 led to new insights regarding the reactivity of tissue implant surfaces (Hench 2006). Great scientific efforts have resulted in a deep understanding of bioactive materials based on silica, especially those synthesized with chemical routes such as the sol-gel process (Pereira and Hench 1996) in ternary (SiO_2-CaO-P_2O_5) and binary systems (SiO_2-CaO). Bioglass, vitro-ceramic and some calcium phosphates are examples of these materials (Vallet-Regi et al. 2003).

Due to the diversity offered by mesoporous silica and hydroxyapatite, it is possible to join two materials that have interesting characteristics and that together complement each other, enabling the application in the medical area. These materials have the capacity of drug loading and promoting bone repair, due to their pore structure, surface area and bioactivity. As important characteristics, these materials have a high surface area due to the presence of nanostructured pores resulting from the mesoporous silica, and bioactivity and biocompatibility owing to both the silica and the hydroxyapatite (Shi et al. 2008).

Therefore, these materials are considered as bioactive because they provide a chemical bond between the implanted material and the bone tissue (osseointegration). Bioactive ceramics bind to and integrate with living bone in the body without the formation of fibrous tissue around them and, in some cases, may induce a specific biological response at the interface with living tissue (LeGeros 2002; Díaz et al. 2006). Due to the chemical similarity between these materials and the bone mineral part, the bone tissues bind to them. The inorganic bone matrix is composed of carbonated hydroxyapatite. Accordingly, the vast majority of bioactive materials are based on ceramics and glasses containing silicate ions and calcium phosphates (Cassidy 2015; Juhasz and Best 2012). This allows the osteoconduction by means bone cells covering. When the bioactive material is deployed in the body, a series of biochemical and biophysical reactions occurs at the implant and tissue interface. These reactions eventually result in an interfacial bond of chemical and physical nature (L. L. Hench 1993).

In a previously paper, a study with two bioceramic materials, namely SBA-16 (*Santa Barbara Amouphous-16*) and HA/SBA-16, mesopouros silica and hydroxyapatite composite were presented. Figure 2 shows scanning electronic microscopy (SEM) images demonstrating the morphology of these matrices. The materials present spherical shaped particles and the HA/SBA-16 sample also reveals the presence of smaller crystals around the particles (Gracielle Ferreira Andrade et al. 2014).

The other report proposed to assess the potential of matrices as biomaterials for tissue engineering applications described by Andrade *et al.* (Gracielle F. Andrade et al. 2015). The data generated indicated two compositions with very interesting properties, such as porosity and stability. In addition, the cytocompatibility and biological effects of those compositions have been evaluated using stem cells. The source of stem cells used was adipose-derived stem cells (ASCs). The adipose tissue, derived from the embryonic mesoderm, besides its functions of energy reserve, involvement in the metabolism of fats and some steroid hormones, is currently a source of stem cells as proposed by Zuk *et al.*(Zuk et al. 2001). This source of stem cells has advantages in relation to, for example, bone marrow-derived cells: ease of stromal isolation, accessibility and abundance of production, and the fact that it is possible to isolate a large number of cells (Mizuno et al. 2009).

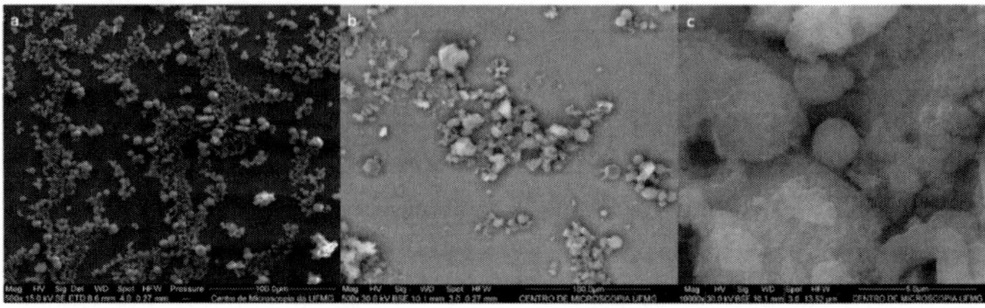

Figure 2. SEM of SBA-16 (a), HA/SBA-16 (b) and HA/SBA-16 in higher magnification (c).

The osteogenic differentiation in the presence of the particles was evidenced by the extracellular matrix mineralization (ECM) staining protocol of von Kossa. The proposed method involved cells cultured for 21 days in basal medium (BM - DMEM) or osteogenic medium (OM), in comparison to tissue culture polystyrene (TCPS) or in the presence of SBA-16 or HA/SBA-16. Secretion of calcified extracellular matrix was confirmed as black nodules with von Kossa staining. Cells cultured in BM-DMEM did not mineralize ECM. However, ASCs cultured in OM or DMEM in the presence of HA/SBA-16 showed mineral accumulation in the ECM, compatible with osteogenic differentiation into functional osteoblasts (Figure 3). These results indicated that the cells cultured with SBA-16 and HA/SBA-16 were successfully differentiated into the osteogenic phenotype and that HA/SBA-16 functioned as an osteogenic differentiation induction component in the system (Gracielle F. Andrade et al. 2015).

According to KOKUBO et al. (Kokubo,T; Kim, HM 2000), one of the requirements a biomaterial must possess in order to bind to bone is the formation of a biologically active apatite layer between the material and bone interface, known as bone-like apatite. This layer of apatite is similar to the mineralized phase of bone tissue in composition and structure. It promotes the signalling of proteins and cells to initiate the cascade of events that results in the formation of bone structure. That is, osteoblasts, bone cells responsible for the production of bone tissue, preferentially proliferate and differentiate producing apatite and collagen on the apatite layer previously formed. This process favours the union of the implant with the bone. When this occurs, a chemical bond is formed between the bone and the apatite layer, and this reduces the interfacial energy between them (Kokubo, Kim, and Kawashita 2003).

Vallet-Regì et al. evaluated the bioactive performance of mesoporous silica materials observing the growth of a layer of apatite on the mesoporous silica surface immersed in simulated fluid solution (SBF). The effective presence of silanol groups in the mesoporous silica wall provides these characteristics of bioactivity. The material presented a potential for bone regeneration, besides allowing the adsorption of bioactive molecules in its pores that may have contributed to this bioactivity process (Vallet-Regí and Balas 2008).

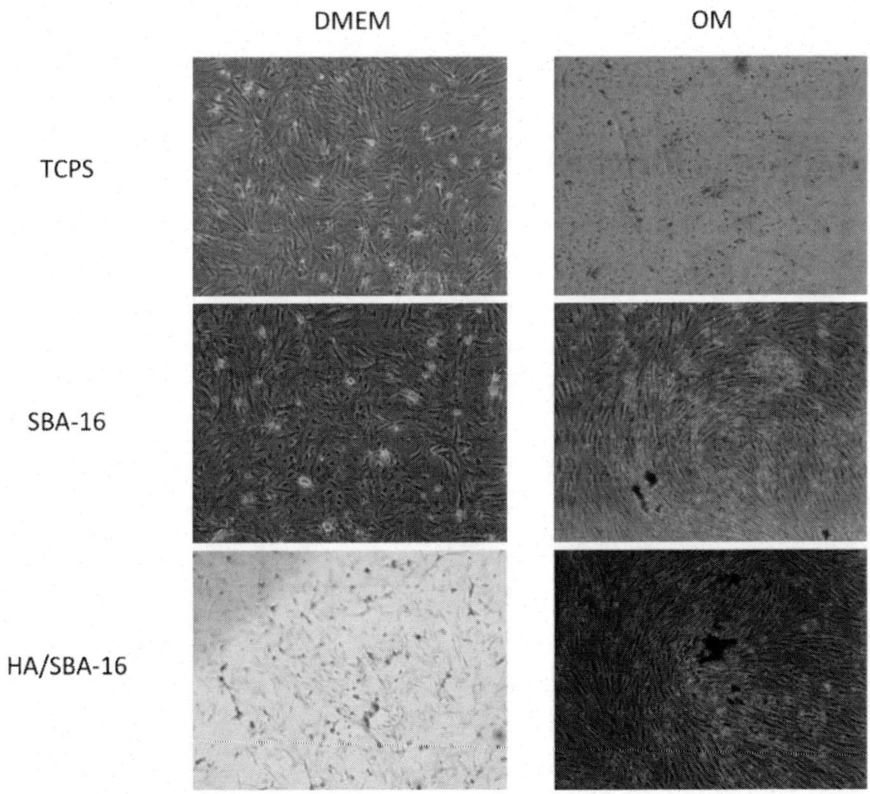

Figure 3. Analysis of the osteogenic differentiation of ASC cultured in TCPS, SBA-16 and HA/SBA-16 as assessed by von Kossa staining during osteogenic differentiation.

Thus, the synthesis of mesopouros silica integrating other chemical compounds like hydroxyapatite provides an extremely attractive matrix to form nanocomposites, which have been widely used as bone-tissue regeneration systems (Tang, Li, and Chen 2012; H. W. Kim, Knowles, and Kim 2004). Additionally, drug delivery system based on this nanocomposites can also be developed to enhance bone ingrowth and regeneration during the treatment of bone defects, besides presenting characteristics such as excellent biocompatibility, bioactivity, low susceptibility to immune response, and resistance to lipases (Wu and Chang 2012; Valente et al. 2016). Moreover, these nanocomposites can not only improve the resistance of therapeutic agents against enzymatic degradation, but also provide the possibility of transporting biomolecules to specific regions in a controlled manner (Dasgupta et al. 2010).

4. *In Vitro* Biocompatibility and Cytocompatibility Studies

Calcium phosphate ceramics (hydroxyapatite) and silica-based bioactive glasses are the most representative components of the bioceramics class. Bioactive materials have high reactivity due to their outstanding values of surface area, porosity and presence of silanol groups. In physiological fluids, these materials lead to the crystallization of an apatite-phase, similar to the inorganic component of bones (Hench 1991). Additionally, the calcium phosphate nanoparticles that growth within an organized silica structure is chemically and structurally similar to the bone mineral phase (S. M. Best et al. 2008).

Bioactive ceramics bind to and integrate with living bone in the body without forming fibrous tissue around them, thus providing a direct bonding by bridging host tissue with implants (Larry L. Hench 2004). Futhermore, some bioglass compositions can promote the activation of genes that stimulate the regeneration of bone tissue (Arcos and Vallet-Regí 2013).

The nanocomposite silica/hydroxyapatite obtained by sol-gel process has demonstrated excellent bioactivity. The release of calcium and silicon ions may contribute to the modulation of cellular attachment by promoting the control the cell cycle of the osteoprogenitor cells (Patricia Valerio et al. 2004). In addition, ionic products of degradation of silica species have shown osteoinductive properties.

In order to be used in their full potential and to consolidate their application as engineered tissues, bioceramic materials can be associated with stem cells and their differentiation-derived cell types, such as osteoblasts (Langer and Vacanti 1993).

SBA-16 and HA/SBA-16 were evaluated by their cytotoxicity with the tetrazolium salt MTT (3-(4,5-dimethiol-2-thioazolyl)-2,5-diphenyl tetrazolium bromide) assay (Figure 4), which is based on the reduction of tetrazolium salt to formazan crystals by the dehydrogenases present in living cells mitochondria and other cell components (Berridge, Herst, and Tan 2005). The results showed that adipose-derived stem cells (ASCs) cultured in the presence of both biomaterials were capable of metabolizing MTT into formazan crystals, which demonstrated their viability and proliferation. In addition, MTT metabolization was higher in cells cultured in the presence of HA/SBA-16 compared to SBA-16, indicating that hydroxyapatite presence increased cytocompatibility of material (Gracielle F. Andrade et al. 2015).

In the same article, the production of bone alkaline phosphatase (AP), a biochemical marker of bone metabolism, which we can define as a substance that shows bone formation or resorption, was also used to verify the biocompatibility and osteogenic differention (Gracielle F. Andrade et al. 2015). Since formation is dependent of the action of osteoblasts, formation markers (bone alkaline phosphatase) actually measure products from the action of these cells. The formation markers are all products of osteoblastic synthesis. Bone alkaline phosphatase is a specific glycoprotein found on the surface of osteoblasts. Its function has not yet been fully elucidated, but its role in skeletal mineralization is confirmed. The activity of bone alkaline phosphatase as bone marker, provides useful information on bone remodelling in osteoporosis, Paget's disease and the follow-up of preventive therapies and hormone replacement or other anti-absorption therapies (P Valerio et al. 2005).

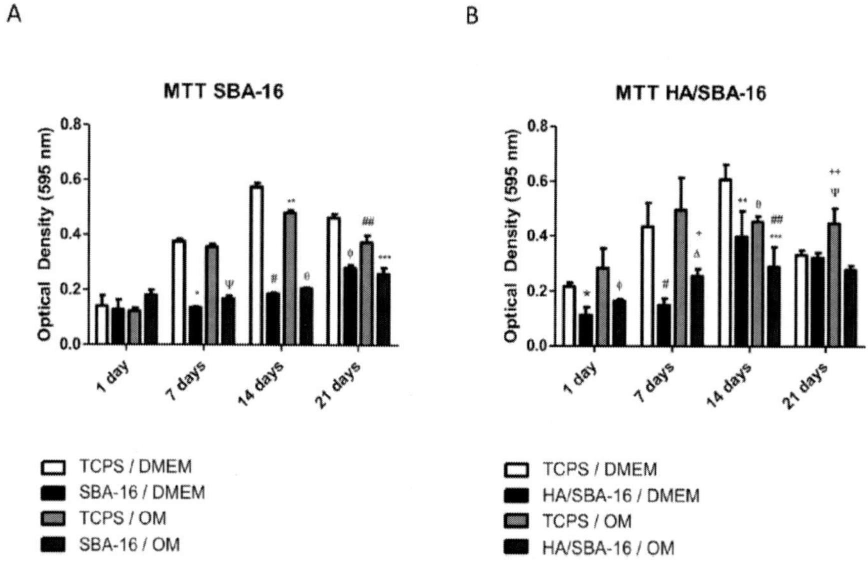

Figure 4. Cytotoxicity of ASCs seeded on SBA-16 (A) and HA/SBA-16 (B) composites as assessed by 3-(4,5-dimethylthiazol- 2-yl)-2,5-diphenyltetrazolium bromide assay during osteogenic differentiation. The results demonstrate the viability and possible proliferation of ASC seeded on the different scaffolds as a function of time in basal medium (DMEM) or in Osteogenic Medium (OM), in comparison to tissue culture polystyrene (TCPS). Data is represented as mean – standard deviation. In A: $^{*}p < 0.05$ compared to TCPS/DMEM at day 7. $^{\#}p < 0.05$ compared to TCPS/DMEM at day 14. $^{\Phi}p < 0.05$ compared to TCPS/DMEM at day 21. $^{**}p < 0.05$ compared to TCPS/DMEM at day 14. $^{\#\#}p<0.05$ compared to TCPS/DMEM at day 21. $^{\Psi}p < 0.05$ compared to TCPS/OM at day 7. $^{\theta}p < 0.05$ compared to TCPS/OM at day 14. $^{***}p < 0.05$ compared to TCPS/OM at day 21. In B:$^{*}p < 0.05$ compared to TCPS/DMEM at day 1. $^{\#}p < 0.05$ compared to TCPS/DMEM at day 7. $^{**}p < 0.05$ compared to TCPS/DMEM at day 14. $^{\Psi}p <0.05$ compared to TCPS/DMEMat day 21. $^{\Phi}p < 0.05$ compared to TCPS/OM at day 1. $^{\Delta}p < 0.05$ compared to HA/SBA-16/DMEM at day 7. $^{+}p < 0.05$ compared to TCPS/OM at day 7. $^{***}p < 0.05$ compared to HA/SBA-16/DMEM at day 14. $^{\#\#}p < 0.05$ compared to TCPS/OM at day 14. $^{++}p < 0.05$ compared to HA/SBA-16/DMEM at day 21. $^{\theta}p < 0.05$ compared to TCPS/DMEM at day 14 (Gracielle F. Andrade et al. 2015).

Studies have already shown that the production of alkaline phosphatase by osteoblasts in contact with different biomaterials has an altered behaviour, depending on the composition of these biomaterials (S. Best et al. 1997). Moreover, the qualitative and quantitative verification of the secretion of this enzyme is an important parameter for analysis of the effects caused on bone tissue, since it reflects the osteoblastic activity (Ohgushi et al. 1993). An increase in the production of alkaline phosphatase has been demonstrated when the osteoblasts are in the presence of apatites (Nishio et al. 2000) and of bioactive glass with 45% silica (Xynos et al. 2000).

The cell alkaline phosphatase detection assay used to verify AP activity of ASCs cultured in the presence SBA-16 and HA/SBA-16 composites was the NBT / BCIP (Invitrogen, São Paulo, SP, Brazil). This assay is based on the alkaline phosphatase created by the cells, which cleaves the phosphate group of the BCIP substrate (Bromo-chloro-indole phosphate). The reaction produces a proton, which associated with NBT (nitro blue tetrazole), generates an insoluble purple precipitate.

The results presented in Figure 5 demonstrated that ASCs cultured in the presence of SBA-16 presented smaller amounts of AP activity than control groups (Figure 5A). On the other hand, ASCs cultured in the presence of HA/SBA-16 showed similar or higher levels of AP activity as cells in TCPS groups (Figure 5B). Those results suggest that, in contrast to SBA-16, the HA/SBA-16 biomaterial induced an increase in AP production/activity of ASCs (Gracielle F. Andrade et al. 2015).

It was possible to conclude, based on the results presented, that cells cultured with nanocomposites were viable and successfully differentiated into the osteogenic phenotype. The nanocomposite consisting of a silica/hydroxyapatite composite functioned as an osteogenic differentiation inductor when in contact with adipose-derived stem cells (ASCs). Therefore, nanocomposites obtained by nucleation and growth of inorganic phase calcium phosphate within mesoporous silica are an excellent alternative as biomaterial for tissue engineering applications, since they maintained adipose-derived stem cells viability while allowing/promoting osteogenic differentiation.

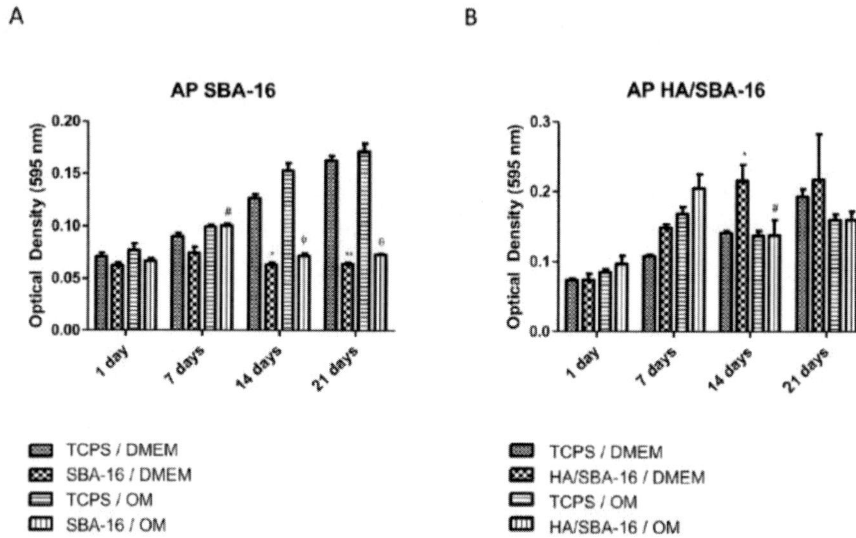

Figure 5. Alkaline Phosphatase (AP) assay of the ASC seeded on SBA-16 (A) and HA/SBA-16 (B) particles as assessed by NBT-BCIP assay during osteogenic differentiation. The results are indicative of osteogenic differentiation of ASC seeded on the different scaffolds as a function of time in basal medium (DMEM) or in Osteogenic medium (OM), in comparison to tissue culture polystyrene (TCPS). In A: $^{*}p < 0.05$ compared to TCPS/DMEM at day 14. $^{**}p < 0.05$ compared to TCPS/DMEM at day 14. $^{\#}p < 0.05$ compared to SBA-16/DMEM at day 7. $^{\phi}p < 0.05$ compared to TCPS/OM at day 14. $^{\theta}p < 0.05$ compared to TCPS/OM at day 21. In B: $^{*}p < 0.05$ compared to TCPS/DMEMat day 14. $^{\#}p < 0.05$ compared to HA/SBA-16/DMEM at day 14.

5. Ciprofloxacin Loaded in Silica/HA and Its Release Profile

Prolonged administration of systemic antibiotics is usually required to treat bacterial bone infection, since the systemic administration of antibiotics does not always allow for an efficient concentration of the drug at the infected site. This leads to the administration of high and repeated antibiotic doses in the attempt to produce acceptable concentrations in the affected region. Thus, local antibiotic release using nanoparticles is a promising procedure for drug delivery (Nayak, Bhattacharyya, and Sen 2011; Mäkinen et al. 2005).

In order to have the best control in the release of the ciprofloxacin and to obtain a greater adsorption thereof, a combination of bioactivity and different materials is necessary to create the nanocomposite. Therefore, in a previous study, a mesoporous silica particles/hydroxyapatite (HA/SBA-16) hybrid drug carrier was produced by homogeneously incorporating calcium and phosphate salt into silica particles. SBA-16 and HA/SBA-16 were investigated for their structural and physicochemical characteristics. Furthermore, *in vitro* assays indicated that the as-synthesized HA/SBA-16 nanocomposite and SBA-16 can be used as an attractive and promising drug delivery system (Gracielle Ferreira Andrade et al. 2014; Gracielle F. Andrade et al. 2015).

Interesting results were observed when the amount of ciprofloxacin incorporated into the SBA-16 and HA/SBA-16 silica network samples was studied by UV-VIS spectroscopy. The results revealed that the HA/SBA-16 composite presented the higher ciprofloxacin incorporation rate (15.1% w/w), as compared to the SBA-16 sample (5.5% w/w).

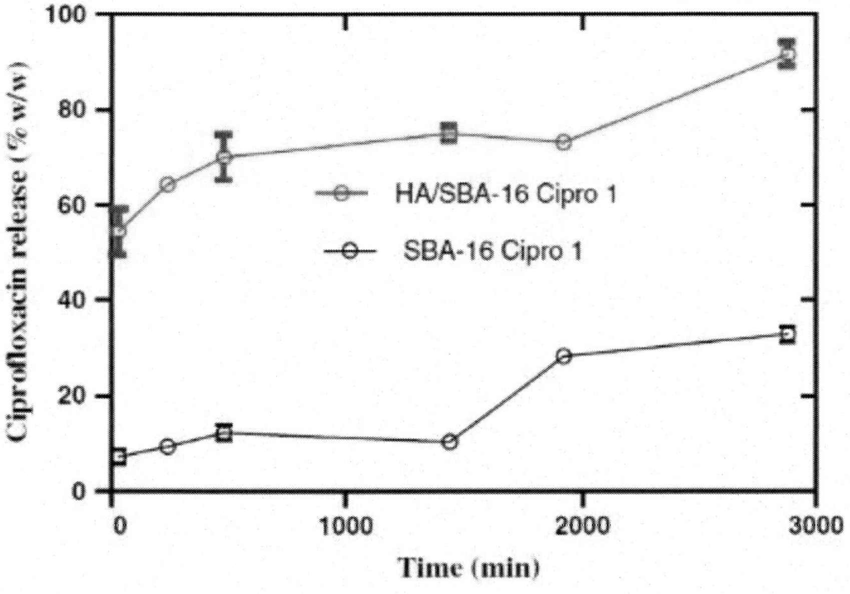

Figure 6. Ciprofloxacin release profiles from SBA-16 and HA/SBA-16 samples.

Furthermost, the release of ciprofloxacin was studied as a function of time for SBA-16 and HA/SBA-16 samples (Figure 6). The maximum release achieved in 24 h for the SBA-16 sample was approximately 32%, as compared to the HA/SBA-16 samples, which reached 93%, a level even greater than the pure sample. Based on these results it was possible to prove the matrices capacity for loading and releasing ciprofloxacin (Gracielle Ferreira Andrade et al. 2014). Therefore, ciprofloxacin was successfully loaded onto particles and gradually released in 24 h, which represented a relatively high and constant amount of drug release.

Based on the results presented in the paper (Gracielle Ferreira Andrade et al. 2014), it was found that both the pore volume and the surface interaction do in fact affect the rate and amount of drug released from the particles. The highest loading and release from the HA/SBA-16 is attributed to the increase in pore volume and the decrease in interactions between the composite surface and the entrapped ciprofloxacin molecules, since the crystals developed in the process can promote the *in situ* formation of larger pores. Moreover, in a solution of simulated body fluid (SBF) at pH 7.3, the carboxylic acid of the ciprofloxacin molecules was found to be dissociated, while the nitrogen of the piperazinyl ring is protonated, hence its classification as a zwitterionic species (Babić et al. 2007). This behavior of the molecule can foster a greater interaction with the silanol groups, which are more available in SBA-16. This can explain the lower release from SBA-16 than from HA/SBA-16.

Therefore, silica/hydroxyapatite nanocomposites can be successful employed as matrices to host ciprofloxacin, and the surface and structural properties of the material used are an important factor to control the amount of ciprofloxacin to be adsorbed and release.

6. Surface Functionalization of Nanoparticles

Studies related to the modifications in the surface of particles have demonstrated the influence that the functionalization can have in relation to the possible forms of interactions of the materials with the biological medium. The United States - Food and Drug Administration (FDA) in its report on nanotechnology (U.S. Food and Drug Administration 2007) highlights the importance of surface modification of nanoparticles (e.g., bonds of different chemical groups on the surface) in determining the biological interaction.

In some cases, characteristics such as the charge or position of the molecules on the surface of the functionalized materials may affect the particles toxicity more significantly than the surface area of these particles (Warheit et al. 2005). Lockmann et al. studied the performance of nanovesicles with different charges on the cells, and could verify in this experiment that the positively charged nanovesicles induced cerebral edema, whereas this behavior was not observed with the neutral nanovesicles nor with the negatively charged nanovesicles in low concentrations (Paul R. Lockman, Joanna M. Koziara, Russell J. Mumper 2004).

The surface modification of mesoporous silica materials with specific organic molecules has been the subject of several studies with the objective of obtaining diversity and functionality for the application of these materials (Gracielle Ferreira Andrade et al. 2013). In this way, the synthesis, modification and control of these materials in nanometric scale represent the access to new properties, increasing the possibilities of applications. These materials can be targeted to a specific type of function by undergoing chemical changes on their surface, in addition, these changes may provide a better interaction of the molecules absorbed in that material(El-Nahhal and El-Ashgar 2007).

Due to the high surface area and the presence of reactive groups (silanols) on their surface, the mesoporous silica materials can act as reservoirs for active principles. They have high capacity of absorption of molecules, being able to promote, for example, the protection of biological molecules against enzymes and phagocytic cells during absorption in the human body (Zhou, Wang, and Tan 2014). They can also serve as barriers against undesirable degradation or metabolization, thus providing, in the case of drugs as active principles, a dose maintenance within the range of therapeutic efficacy and ensuring, in the case of the molecules such as nucleic acids and proteins, the performance at the desired site.

Mesoporous matrices with organic groups anchored on the walls of their pores, used as a controlled drug release system, may offer different adsorption capacity and release of the drug molecules when comparing with unmodified materials (Manzano et al. 2008). Considering that in a carrier device the interactions between the molecules and the material are responsible for their absorption and release, as well as the fact that the interactions of the surface of the material with the biological medium can influence the release of the drug from this material, it is very important to study the influence of surface modifications more judiciously on these different systems.

6.1. Functionalization Process

Various types of ordered mesoporous materials, such as M41S, FSM 16, HMS, MSU and SBA, have been synthesized in the presence of ionic, neutral and nonionic surfactants (De et al. 2011). The functionalization or modification of these materials has played an important role in several technological aspects, such as the improvement of thermal/hydrothermal stability, the immobilization of organic molecules, the development of new catalysts, new adsorbents and, especially, applications in nanotechnology (Chong et al. 2004).

Therefore, several studies have been directed to confer chemical specificity to the mesoporous solids through the introduction of organic molecules. These materials can be prepared and modified with a wide variety of combinations of molecules, diversifying the properties of the material. The higher versatility introduced, coupled with the new properties, presents a great potential of applications, such as catalysis, immobilization of enzymes, adsorption of heavy metals, manufacture of controlled drug release systems, among others (Liu et al. 2003; Xue and Shi 2004).

The silica structure consists of SiO_4 tetrahedral units distributed randomly and linked by siloxane (Si-O-Si) bridges with dispersed silanol (Si-OH) groups, covering the entire surface, which can be modified. According to the arrangement of these silanols groups, they can be divided into isolated groups (or free silanols) in which the silicon atom has three bonds in the silica network structure and the fourth bond is associated with a single OH group; or bridged silanols, where two individual silane groups, attached to different silicon atoms, are close enough to form a hydrogen bond. The third type of silanol group, the geminated silane, consists of two hydroxyl groups that are bonded to a silicon atom and are very close to forming a hydrogen bond between each other (El-Nahhal and El-Ashgar 2007).

The silanol groups are derived from the condensation of silicic acid during the process of preparation of silica gel and give polar characteristics to the silica, being responsible for its adsorptive capacity. Due to these silanol groups, silica has a slightly acid character with characteristics of a Brönsted acid, and its acidic sites are responsible for the control of the surface reactivity; thus it is interesting that the silanol groups be free for possible interactions before affecting any reactions.

With the chemical modification of the silica surface, more versatility and more refined properties are obtained by combining the properties of the functionalizing agent related to the surface-bound species and the specific properties of silica (Rámila et al. 2003) in a neutral medium, typical of a healthy biological medium, silica has a negative charge. Thus, electrostatic adsorption from hydrogen interactions provided by hydroxyl groups of positively charged drugs is an attractive method for loading them into the mesoporous matrix. And the search for adsorption expansion of different molecules not only of positive charges, is carried out by the introduction of functional groups that frequently have as terminal group: amine groups (Mamaeva, Sahlgren, and Lindén 2013).

One way to explore the reactivity of the silane groups on the silica surface is the silylation reaction, where an alkoxysilane is chemically bound to the surface, which in turn changes its properties, and this process is called organofunctionalization (Arakaki and Airoldi 1999). The modification of the surface by alkoxysilanes is due to the fixation of the modifying agent onto the inorganic support, creating an organic-inorganic hybrid compound. The success of the reaction in a non-aqueous medium depends on the availability of silanol groups for forming a covalent bond with the silylating agent in a monodentate, bidentate or tridentate manner (Figure 7), where the most common are mono and bidentate (FARIAS, R. F., AIROLDI 2000).

Methods for the functionalization of silica-based mesoporous materials are amply described. Generally, organic-inorganic hybrids of molecular sieves can be prepared by two routes: (1) *in situ* functionalization during synthesis (co-condensation) or (2) post synthesis functionalization (Yiu and Wright 2005). The organic functionalization of silicates allows better control over surface properties, modification of the hydrophilic/ hydrophobic character of the surface, alteration of the surface reactivity, protection of the surface against chemical attack, and at the same time the stabilization of the materials for hydrolysis.

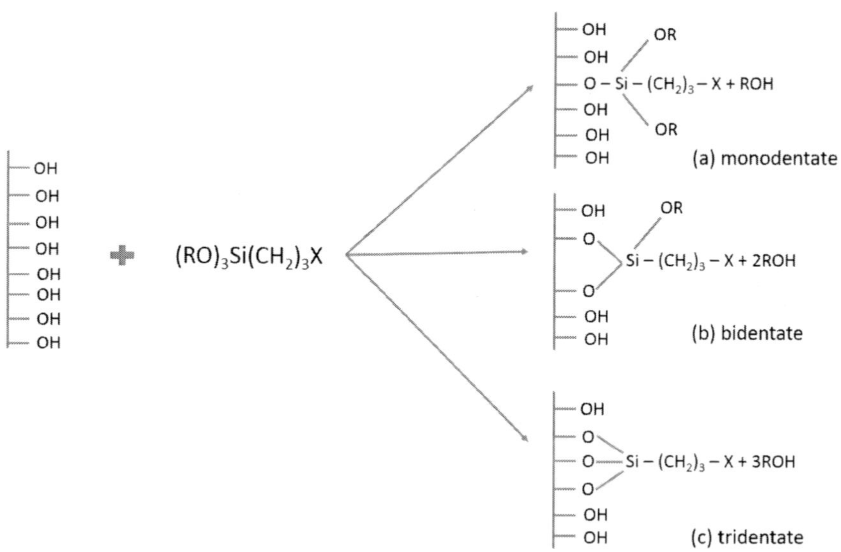

Figure 7. Different forms of organosilane anchoring on the surface of a support containing silanol groups: a) monodentate b) bidentate c) tridentate.

Behrens et al. (Ehlert et al. 2011) reported a sulfonated mesoporous silica film, used as an implant, with high capacity for the antibiotic ciprofloxacin. Additional layers of bis(trimethoxysilyl)hexane or dioctyltetramethyldisilazane were applied to delay the release and to prolong the effective antibacterial activity period. The results presented suggest that the development of drug-loaded mesopouros silica films as coating on medical implants is a promising approach to prevent bacterial implant infections during the most critical period after implantation. Moreover, the data presented by them showed that the release of ciprofloxacin can be successfully controlled by the application of organosiloxane layers.

There are several works with functionalization of silica and hydroxyapatite in the literature, with significant contributions by this group. Sousa and collaborators (Izquierdo-Barba et al. 2009) have performed a chemical modification of the SBA-15 mesoporous material with octadecyltrimethoxysilane in order to study its influence on the release rate of ibuprofen. Futhermore, Cipreste et al. described the synthesis of Hydroxyapatite (HA) nanorods and a route of functionalization of the HA surface with folic acid (folate). The results indicated that mesoporous hydroxyapatite nanorods, around 70 nm long, were successfully synthesized with pure crystalline phase and folate can be strongly linked to hydroxyapatite nanorod surfaces (Cipreste et al. 2016). Furthermore, Freitas et al. (Freitas et al. 2017) have prepared a multifunctional nanotheranostic system based on MCM-41 through post-synthesis functionalization of the mesoporous silica MCM-41 with the tumor-homing peptide CREKA and diethylenetriaminepentaacetic dianhydride (DTPA), a ligand for copper ions, which was activated in a nuclear reactor with the radionuclide ^{64}Cu. Additionally, the nanoparticles were loaded with the clinically approved anticancer drug methotrexate and the drug release kinetics profile was investigated. The results showed that the multifunctional silica-based theranostic system could serve as a platform for cancer targeted, controlled drug delivery and PET imaging to be applied in cancer therapy.

Recently, the synthesis of surface-functionalized mesoporous silica (SBA-16) and silica composed of calcium phosphate (SBA-16/HA) particles have been applied as efficient drug carriers (Gracielle Ferreira Andrade et al. 2017). The particles were synthesized, functionalized with 3-aminopropyltriethoxysilane (APTES) by post-synthesis grafting and loaded with the osteomyelitis antibiotic agent ciprofloxacin. The results revealed that the SBA-16APTES sample presents similar ciprofloxacin incorporation ratio (28.5% w/w) as compared to the SBA16/HAAPTES sample (30.6% w/w). The *in vitro* ciprofloxacin release behavior from SBA16APTES Cipro and SBA-16/HAAPTES Cipro samples was investigated as a function of time (Figure 8). The release profiles of SBA-16APTES Cipro and SBA-16/HAAPTES Cipro matrices exhibited an initial burst release effect and the maximum release achieved in 76h for the SBA-16APTES Cipro sample was approximately 53%, as compared to the SBA-16/HAAPTES Cipro samples, which reached 51%.

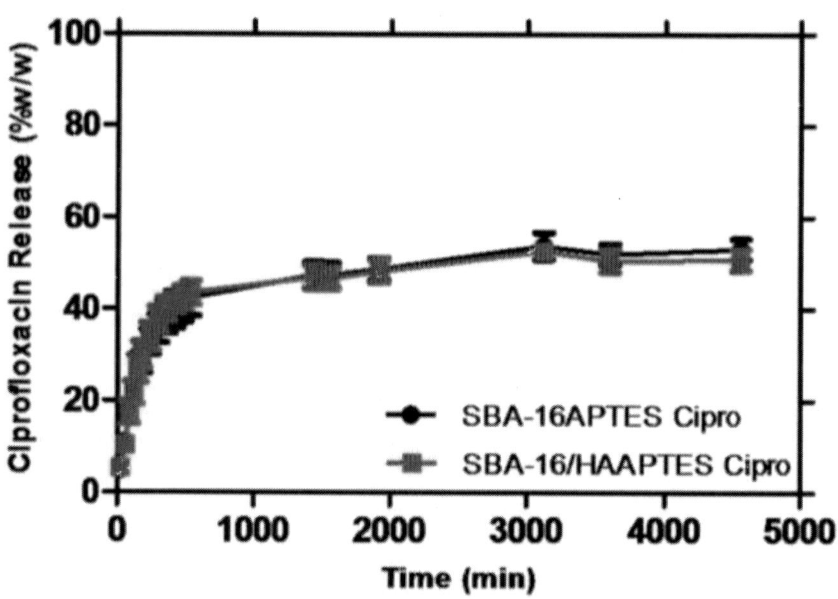

Figure 8. Release kinetic profiles of ciprofloxacin from SBA-16APTES Cipro and SBA-16/HAAPTES Cipro samples. Values expressed as mean ± SEM (Gracielle Ferreira Andrade et al. 2017).

Andrade et al. have previously assessed the behaviour of the system SBA-16 and SBA-16/HA without APTES during drug delivery process. Drug loading percentage inside the matrices showed a lower ratio of ciprofloxacin-incorporated than matrices functionalized with APTES. This result can be explained by the interaction of functional groups of ciprofloxacin molecule with amine groups through hydrogen bonding. These interactions could be more intense than the interaction of ciprofloxacin with the same matrices without functionalization, as described by Andrade (Gracielle Ferreira Andrade et al. 2017), and this could explain a larger incorporation and a smaller release.

7. Ciprofloxacin-Silica/Hydroxyapatite Bactericidal Efficiency

Osteomyelitis, an example of a bone disease that may be caused by the microorganisms *Staphylococcus aureus* and *Pseudomonas aeruginosa* (Devanand Venkatasubbu et al. 2011), has a highly complicated treatment with antimicrobial therapy. As antimicrobial treatments often involve a long course of therapy, satisfactory antibiotic exposure is needed to ensure the eradication of the microorganism (Devanand Venkatasubbu et al. 2011). However, an intensive and improper use of antibiotics can select resistant microorganisms and has seriously increased the frequency of resistance among human pathogens promoting favorable conditions for infections to emerge, advance and persist (Andersson and Hughes 2010; Capeletti et al. 2014a). Therefore, effective antimicrobial therapy is an essential component of most curative regimens for infectious diseases, including osteomyelitis (Fraimow 2009).

Ciprofloxacin, a broad-spectrum fluoroquinolone antibacterial agent, is potent against a wide range of Gram-positive and Gram-negative pathogenic bacteria, which are present in osteomyelitis (Redgrave, Sutton, and, Mark A. Webber 2014). The absorption of antibiotics carried out through the systemic route is small in bone tissue due to the limited blood circulation in these infected sites (H. W. Kim, Knowles, and Kim 2004). Thus, a high local drug dose cannot be achieved at the site of infection (Devanand Venkatasubbu et al. 2011). It is agreed that extended-release preparation is advantageous to improve patient compliance, as frequent administration can be reduced by maintaining a constant plasma drug concentration over a prolonged period of time (Blasi, Aliberti, and Tarsia 2007).

In the quest for this targeted and controlled release, manifold classes of antimicrobial nanoparticles (NPs) and nanosized carriers for antibiotics delivery have been established as efficient for treating infectious diseases (Huh and Kwon 2011a). Additionally, the possibility of encapsulated antimicrobial drugs inside nanostructures similar to silica nanoparticles has already been reported in the literature (Botequim et al. 2012).

Furthermore, the surface functionalization of these materials may influence the effectiveness against microorganisms. In a previous work, the biological activity of functionalized mesoporous silica/hydroxyapatite composite loaded with ciprofloxacin against susceptible bacteria. The antimicrobial activity of the particles was measured against, Gram-positive bacteria, as *Staphylococcus aureus* and *Bacillus cereus,* and Gram-negative bacteria as *Pseudomonas aeruginosa* and *Escherichia coli.*

SBA-16 and SBA-16/HA samples functionalized with 3-aminopropyltriethoxysilane containing ciprofloxacin presented a high antibacterial action against all microorganisms, especially when compared to the results obtained with pure ciprofloxacin, as can be seen in Table 1. SBA-16/HA and SBA-16APTES without ciprofloxacin showed significant antimicrobial activity against *E. coli*. SBA-16/HAAPTES and SBA-16 also had antimicrobial activity, although in a less significant way. These results indicate that the materials have antimicrobial activity (Gracielle Ferreira Andrade et al. 2017).

Table 1. *In vitro* growth inhibition of microorganism induced by compounds at the concentration of 250μg.mL^{-1}

Microorganism	*Staphylococcus aureus*	*Pseudomonas aeruginosa*	*Escherichia coli*	*Bacillus cereus*
Ciprofloxacin	76.4 ± 2.4	77.4 ± 2.1	88.3 ± 1.0	85.9 ± 1.3
Ampicillin	95.9 ± 0.3	93.3 ± 0.6	97.5 ± 0.4	93.6 ± 0.7
HA/SBA-16	22.1 ± 2.0	18.0 ± 2.5	83.4 ± 0.4	9.1 ± 2.5
HA/SBA-16APTES	9.9 ± 1.5	6.0 ± 0.9	26.8 ± 3.0	9.6 ± 1.4
HA/SBA-16 APTES Cipro	96.3 ± 0.8	86.3 ± 1.8	96.4 ± 0.6	89.1 ± 1.6
SBA-16	7.2 ± 1.6	3.0 ± 0.4	25.2 ± 2.3	0
SBA-16APTES	1.6 ± 0.7	0	77.0 ± 0.5	0
SBA-16APTES Cipro	93.3 ± 0.9	88.8 ± 1.2	95.6 ± 1.5	84.6 ± 2.8

Results are mean values of quintuplicate assays ± standard deviation (expressed as % inhibition).

Nanotechnology has been investigated as a promising alternative to the current antibiotic-based approaches, especially in delivery of antimicrobial drugs, in particular in overcoming antibiotics-resistant pathogens (Huh and Kwon 2011a). Capeletti et al. demonstrated the effective bactericidal activity of a noncomplex nanomaterial against susceptible and antibiotic-resistant bacteria without significant cytotoxicity, which was able to entrap tetracycline antibiotic into silica nanospheres. The results presented show nanoparticles with efficient antibacterial properties against susceptible and resistant bacteria with no significant toxicity to mammalian cells. On susceptible strains, the antibiotic action predominated as expected whereas the silica component of the nanoparticles was also highly effective on the resistant strains. Hence, this new strategy has become very attractive in clinical settings where susceptible and resistant strains often occur together (Capeletti et al. 2014b).

CONCLUSION

The present study reports the versatility of the nanocomposites, consisting of hydroxyapatite nanocrystals grown within mesoporous silica, which has as objective biological applications. The applicability of those systems as matrices for controlled drug delivery and also in regenerative bone tissue was studied. The results indicate that the ordered mesoporous silica and hydroxyapatite have the potential to encapsulate bioactive molecules, such as ciprofloxacin, for use in biomedicine.

The loading and release of ciprofloxacin from nanocomposites were discussed and the features of this release were measured. Moreover, this work demonstrated the usefulness of these bioceramics, covering the synthesis of the mesoporous silica/hydroxyapatite composite, the loading of ciprofloxacin drugs, and the evaluation of cell viability and composite bioactivity using stem cells. Furthermore, the pure silica and the composite matrices showed bioactivity which are of great relevance in the field of tissue engineering. The use of nanoparticles is a promising strategy in the design of effective antimicrobial agents against susceptible and antibiotic-resistant bacteria.

Acknowledgments

This work has been supported by CAPES, CNPq, FAPEMIG and CDTN (CNEN).

References

Andersson, Dan I, and Hughes, Diarmaid. 2010. "Antibiotic Resistance and Its Cost: Is It Possible to Reverse Resistance?" *Nature Reviews. Microbiology* 8 (4). Nature Publishing Group: 260–71. doi:10.1038/nrmicro2319.

Andrade, Gracielle F., Carvalho, Juliana L., Júnior, Armando S. C., Goes, Alfredo M., and Sousa, Edésia M. B. 2015. "Osteogenic Differentiation of Adipose-Derived Stem Cells in Mesoporous SBA-16 and SBA-16 Hydroxyapatite Scaffolds." *RSC Adv.* 5 (67): 54551–62. doi:10.1039/C5RA07330H.

Andrade, Gracielle Ferreira, Quintão Arantes Faria, Jerusa Araújo, Gomes, Dawidson Assis, Branco de Barros, André Luís, Fernandes, Renata Salgado, Soares Coelho, Amanda Cristina, Takahashi, Jacqueline Aparecida, da Silva Cunha, Armando, and Barros de Sousa, Edésia Martins. 2017. "Mesoporous Silica SBA-16/hydroxyapatite-Based Composite for Ciprofloxacin Delivery to Bacterial Bone Infection." *Journal of Sol-Gel Science and Technology*. doi:10.1007/s10971-017-4557-y.

Andrade, Gracielle Ferreira, Gomide, Viviane Silva, da Silva Júnior, Armando Cunha, Goes, Alfredo Miranda, and Barros de Sousa, Edésia Martins. 2014. "An in Situ Synthesis of Mesoporous SBA-16/hydroxyapatite for Ciprofloxacin Release: In Vitro Stability and Cytocompatibility Studies." *Journal of Materials Science. Materials in Medicine* 25 (11): 2527–40. doi:10.1007/s10856-014-5273-6.

Andrade, Gracielle Ferreira, Ferreira Soares, Daniel Crístian, dos Santos, Raquel Gouvêa, and Barros Sousa, Edésia Martins. 2013. "Mesoporous Silica SBA-16 Nanoparticles: Synthesis, Physicochemical Characterization, Release Profile, and in Vitro Cytocompatibility Studies." *Microporous and Mesoporous Materials* 168 (March). Elsevier Inc.: 102–10. doi:10.1016/j.micromeso.2012.09.034.

Arakaki, L. N. H., and Airoldi, Claudio. 1999. "The Relevant Role of the Silylating Agent in the Modification of Polymer Surfaces." *Quimica Nova*. doi:10.1590/S0100-40421999000200016.

Arcos, Daniel, and Vallet-Regí, María. 2010. "Sol-Gel Silica-Based Biomaterials and Bone Tissue Regeneration." *Acta Biomaterialia* 6 (8). Acta Materialia Inc.: 2874–88. doi:10.1016/j.actbio.2010.02.012.

———. 2013. "Bioceramics for Drug Delivery." *Acta Materialia* 61 (3): 890–911. doi:10.1016/j.actamat.2012.10.039.

Babić, Sandra, Horvat, Alka J. M., Mutavdžić Pavlović, Dragana, and Kaštelan-Macan, Marija. 2007. "Determination of pKa Values of Active Pharmaceutical Ingredients." *TrAC Trends in Analytical Chemistry* 26 (11): 1043–61. doi:10.1016/j.trac.2007.09.004.

Barbosa J., Barrón D., Jiménez-Lozano E. 1999. "Electrophoretic Behaviour of Quinolones in Capillary Electrophoresis. Effect of pH and Evaluation of Ionization Constants." *J Chromatogr A.* 839: 183–92.

Berridge, Michael V., Herst, Patries M., and Tan, An S.. 2005. "Tetrazolium Dyes as Tools in Cell Biology: New Insights into Their Cellular Reduction." *Biotechnology Annual Review* 11 (5): 127–52. doi:10.1016/S1387-2656(05)11004-7.

Best, S. M., Porter, A. E., Thian, E. S., and Huang, J. 2008. "Bioceramics: Past, Present and for the Future." *Journal of the European Ceramic Society* 28 (7): 1319–27. doi:10.1016/j.jeurceramsoc.2007.12.001.

Best, S., Sim, B., Kayser, M., and Downes, S. 1997. "The Dependence of Osteoblastic Response on Variations in the Chemical Composition and Physical Properties of Hydroxyapatite." *Journal of Materials Science. Materials in Medicine* 8 (2): 97–103. http://www.ncbi.nlm.nih.gov/pubmed/15348777.

Blasi, Francesco, Aliberti, Stefano, and Tarsia, Paolo. 2007. "Clinical Applications of Azithromycin Microspheres in Respiratory Tract Infections." *International Journal of Nanomedicine* 2 (4): 551–59.

Botequim, D., Maia, J., Lino, M. M. F., Lopes, L. M. F., Simões, P. N., Ilharco, L. M., and Ferreira, L. 2012. "Nanoparticles and Surfaces Presenting Antifungal, Antibacterial and Antiviral Properties." *Langmuir* 28 (20): 7646–56. doi:10.1021/la300948n.

Capeletti, Larissa Brentano, De Oliveira, Luciane Franca, De Almeida Gonçalves, Kaliandra, De Oliveira, Fernanda Affonso, Saito, Ângela, Kobarg, Jörg, Santos, João H. Z., and Cardoso, Mateus Borba. 2014a. *"Tailored Silica-Antibiotic Nanoparticles: Overcoming Bacterial Resistance with Low Cytotoxicity Tailored Silica-Antibiotic Nanoparticles: Overcoming Bacterial Resistance with Low Cytotoxicity."* doi:10.1021/la4046435.

———. 2014b. "Tailored Silica-Antibiotic Nanoparticles : Overcoming Bacterial Resistance with Low Cytotoxicity Tailored Silica-Antibiotic Nanoparticles : Overcoming Bacterial Resistance with Low Cytotoxicity." *Langmuir*. doi:10.1021/la4046435.

Cassidy, John W. 2015. "Nanotechnology in the Regeneration of Complex Tissues." *Bone Tissue Regen Insights* 5: 25–35. doi:10.4137/BTRI. S12331.Nanotechnology.

Chong, A. S. Maria, Zhao, X. S., Kustedjo, Angeline T., and Qiao, S. Z. 2004. "Functionalization of Large-Pore Mesoporous Silicas with Organosilanes by Direct Synthesis." *Microporous and Mesoporous Materials* 72: 33–42. doi:10.1016/j.micromeso.2004.04.015.

Ciesla, Ulrike, Schuth, Ferdi. 1999. "Ordered Mesoporous Materials." *Microporous and Mesoporous Materials* 27: 131–49.

Cipreste, Marcelo Fernandes, Gonzalez, Ismael, da Mata Martins, Thaís Maria, Goes, Alfredo Miranda, de Almeida Macedo, Waldemar Augusto, and Barros de Sousa, Edésia Martins. 2016. "Attaching Folic Acid on Hydroxyapatite Nanorod Surfaces: An Investigation of the HA–FA Interaction." *RSC Advances* 6 (80): 76390–400. doi:10.1039/ C6RA14068H.

Curtis, Adam, and Wilkinson, Chris. 2001. "Nantotechniques and Approaches in Biotechnology." *Trends in Biotechnology* 19 (3): 97–101. doi:10.1016/S0167-7799(00)01536-5.

Dasgupta, Sudip, Banerjee, Shashwat S., Bandyopadhyay, Amit, and Bose, Susmita. 2010. "Zn- and Mg-Doped Hydroxyapatite Nanoparticles for Controlled Release of Protein." *Langmuir* 26 (7): 4958–64. doi:10.1021/la903617e.

De, Andreza, de Souza, Karynne Cristina, Mohallem, Nelcy D. S., de Sousa, Ricardo Geraldo, and Barros de Sous, Edesia Martins. 2011. "Multifunctional Nanocomposites Based on Mesoporous Silica: Potential Applications in Biomedicine." In *Advances in Diverse Industrial Applications of Nanocomposites*, 177–202. InTech. doi:10.5772/14595.

Desevaux, Cyril. 2002. *"C Haracterization of Crosslinked High Amylose Starch Matrix Implants 2. In Vivo Release of Ciprofloxacin"* 82: 95–103.

Devanand Venkatasubbu, G., Ramasamy, S., Ramakrishnan, V., and Kumar, J. 2011. "Nanocrystalline Hydroxyapatite and Zinc-Doped Hydroxyapatite as Carrier Material for Controlled Delivery of

Ciprofloxacin." *3 Biotech* 1 (3): 173–86. doi:10.1007/s13205-011-0021-9.

Díaz, A., López, T., Manjarrez, J., Basaldella, E., Martínez-Blanes, J. M., and Odriozola, J. A. 2006. "Growth of Hydroxyapatite in a Biocompatible Mesoporous Ordered Silica." *Acta Biomaterialia* 2 (2): 173–79. doi:10.1016/j.actbio.2005.12.006.

Drakopoulos, Anargiros I., and Ioannou, Pinelopi C. 1997. "Spectrofluorimetric Study of the Acid-Base Equilibria and Complexation Behavior of the Fluoroquinolone Antibiotics Ofloxacin, Norfloxacin, Ciprofloxacin and Pefloxacin in Aqueous Solution." *Analytica Chimica Acta* 354: 197–204. doi:10.1016/S0003-2670(97)00465-0.

Ehlert, Nina, Badar, Muhammad, Christel, Anne, Lohmeier, Sven Jare, Luessenhop, Tammo, Stieve, Martin, Lenarz, Thomas, Mueller, Peter Paul, and Behrens, Peter. 2011. "Mesoporous Silica Coatings for Controlled Release of the Antibiotic Ciprofloxacin from Implants." *J. Mater. Chem.* 21 (3): 752–60. doi:10.1039/C0JM01487G.

El-Nahhal, Issa M., and El-Ashgar, Nizam M. 2007. "A Review on Polysiloxane-Immobilized Ligand Systems: Synthesis, Characterization and Applications." *Journal of Organometallic Chemistry* 692 (14): 2861–86. doi:10.1016/j.jorganchem.2007.03.009.

Farias, R. F., Airoldi, C. 2000. "Synthesis and Reactivity of Lamellar Silica." *Química Nova* 23 (1).

Florek, J., and Kleitz, F. n.d. "*4 Ordered Mesoporous Silica : Synthesis and Applications*."

Fraimow, Henry S. 2009. "Systemic Antimicrobial Therapy in Osteomyelitis." *Seminars in Plastic Surgery* 23 (212): 90–99. doi:10.1055/s-0029-1214161.

Freitas, Luiza Baptista de Oliveira, de Melo Corgosinho, Laura, Araújo Quintão Arantes Faria, Jerusa, dos Santos, Virgílio Mateus, Magalhães Resende, Jarbas, Leal, Alexandre Soares, Assis Gomes, Dawidson, and Barros de Sousa, Edésia Martins. 2017. "Multifunctional Mesoporous Silica Nanoparticles for Cancer-Targeted, Controlled Drug Delivery and Imaging." *Microporous and Mesoporous Materials* 242: 271–83. doi:10.1016/j.micromeso.2017.01.036.

Gong, Tao, Xie, Jing, Liao, Jinfeng, Zhang, Tao, Lin, Shiyu, and Lin, Yunfeng. 2015. "Nanomaterials and Bone Regeneration." *Bone Research* 3 (July). doi:10.1038/boneres.2015.29.

Hartmann, Martin. 2005. "Re V Iews Ordered Mesoporous Materials for Bioadsorption and Biocatalysis." *Chem. Mater.* 17: 4577–93.

Hench, Larry L. 1991. "Bioceramics: From Concept to Clinic." *Journal of the American Ceramic Society* 74 (7): 1487–1510. doi:10.1111/j.1151-2916.1991.tb07132.x.

———. 2006. "The Story of Bioglass." *Journal of Materials Science: Materials in Medicine* 17: 967–78. doi:10.1007/s10856-006-0432-z.

Huh, Ae Jung, and Kwon, Young Jik. 2011a. "'Nanoantibiotics': A New Paradigm for Treating Infectious Diseases Using Nanomaterials in the Antibiotics Resistant Era." *Journal of Controlled Release* 156 (2). Elsevier B.V.: 128–45. doi:10.1016/j.jconrel.2011.07.002.

———. 2011b. "'Nanoantibiotics': A New Paradigm for Treating Infectious Diseases Using Nanomaterials in the Antibiotics Resistant Era." *Journal of Controlled Release: Official Journal of the Controlled Release Society* 156 (2). Elsevier B.V.: 128–45. doi:10.1016/j.jconrel.2011.07.002.

Izquierdo-Barba, Isabel, Sousa, Edesia, Doadrio, Juan Carlos, Doadrio, Antonio Luis, Pariente, Joaquín Pérez, Martínez, Africa, Babonneau, Florence, and Vallet-Regí, María. 2009. "Influence of Mesoporous Structure Type on the Controlled Delivery of Drugs: Release of Ibuprofen from MCM-48, SBA-15 and Functionalized SBA-15." *Journal of Sol-Gel Science and Technology* 50 (3): 421–29. doi:10.1007/s10971-009-1932-3.

Juhasz, Judith A., and Best, Serena M. 2012. "Bioactive Ceramics: Processing, Structures and Properties." *Journal of Materials Science* 47 (2): 610–24. doi:10.1007/s10853-011-6063-x.

Khademhosseini, Ali, and Langer, Robert. 2016. "A Decade of Progress in Tissue Engineering." *Nature Protocols* 11 (10): 1775–81. doi:10.1038/nprot.2016.123.

Kim, Hae Won, Knowles, Jonathan C., and Kim, Hyoun Ee. 2004. "Hydroxyapatite/poly(??-Caprolactone) Composite Coatings on Hydroxyapatite Porous Bone Scaffold for Drug Delivery." *Biomaterials* 25 (7–8): 1279–87. doi:10.1016/j.biomaterials.2003.07.003.

Kim, Insoo, Kim, Tae Hyung, Ma, Kyungwan, Park, Eun Seok, Oh, Kyung Taek, Lee, Eun Seong, Lee, Kang Choon, and Youn, Yu Seok. 2011. "A 4-Arm Polyethylene Glycol Derivative Conjugated with Exendin-4 Peptide and Palmitylamine Having Dual-Function of Size-Increase and Albumin-Binding for Long Hypoglycemic Action." *Regulatory Peptides* 167 (2–3). Elsevier B.V.: 239–45. doi:10.1016/j.regpep.2011.02.008.

Kokubo, T., Kim, H. M., et al. 2000. "What Kinds of Materials Exhibit Bone-Bonding?" In *Bone Engineering*, edited by J. E. Davies, 190–94. Toronto.

Kokubo, Tadashi, Kim, Hyun Min, and Kawashita, Masakazu. 2003. "Novel Bioactive Materials with Different Mechanical Properties." *Biomaterials* 24: 2161–75. doi:10.1016/S0142-9612(03)00044-9.

Hench, L. L., Wilson, June. 1993. *An Introduction to Bioceramics*.

Langer, Robert, and Vacanti, Joseph P. 1993. "ARTICLES Tissue Engineering." *Science* 260 (15): 920–26.

Larry L. Hench, Xynos, Ionnis D. & Polak, Julia M. 2004. "Bioactive Glasses for in Situ Tissue Regeneration." *Journal of Biomaterials Science, Polymer Edition* 15 (4): 543–62. doi:10.1163/156856204323005352.

LeGeros, Racquel Zapanta. 2002. "Properties of Osteoconductive Biomaterials: Calcium Phosphates." *Clinical Orthopaedics and Related Research*, no. 395(February): 81–98.

Liu, Zhimin, Dong, Zexuan, Han, Buxing, Zhang, Jianling, Zhang, Jianming, Hou, Zhenshan, He, Jun, and Jiang, Tao. 2003. "Preparation of Mesoporous MCM-41/poly(acrylic Acid) Composites Using Supercritical CO2 as a Solvent." *Journal of Materials Chemistry* 13: 1373. doi:10.1039/b211818c.

Mäkinen, Tatu J., Veiranto, Minna, Lankinen, Petteri, Moritz, Niko, Jalava, Jari, Törmälä, Pertti, and Aro, Hannu T. 2005. "In Vitro and in Vivo Release of Ciprofloxacin from Osteoconductive Bone Defect Filler." *Journal of Antimicrobial Chemotherapy* 56 (6): 1063–68. doi:10.1093/jac/dki366.

Mamaeva, Veronika, Sahlgren, Cecilia, and Lindén, Mika. 2013. "Mesoporous Silica Nanoparticles in Medicine-Recent Advances." *Advanced Drug Delivery Reviews* 65 (5). Elsevier B.V.: 689–702. doi:10.1016/j.addr.2012.07.018.

Manzano, M., Aina, V., Areán, C. O., Balas, F., Cauda, V., Colilla, M., Delgado, M. R., and Vallet-Regí, M. 2008. "Studies on MCM-41 Mesoporous Silica for Drug Delivery: Effect of Particle Morphology and Amine Functionalization." *Chemical Engineering Journal* 137 (1): 30–37. doi:10.1016/j.cej.2007.07.078.

Mizuno, Hideaki, Kitada, Kunio, Nakai, Kenta, and Sarai, Akinori. 2009. "PrognoScan: A New Database for Meta-Analysis of the Prognostic Value of Genes." *BMC Medical Genomics* 2: 18. doi:10.1186/1755-8794-2-18.

Nayak, Amit Kumar, Bhattacharyya, Ajoy, and Kumar Sen, Kalyan. 2011. "In Vivo Ciprofloxacin Release from Hydroxyapatite-Based Bone Implants in Rabbit Tibia: A Preliminary Study." *ISRN Orthopedics* 2011: 1–4. doi:10.5402/2011/420549.

Nishio, K., Neo, M., Akiyama, H., Nishiguchi, S., Kim, H. M., Kokubo, T., and Nakamura, T. 2000. "The Effect of Alkali- and Heat-Treated Titanium and Apatite-Formed Titanium on Osteoblastic Differentiation of Bone Marrow Cells." *Journal of Biomedical Materials Research* 52 (4): 652–61. http://www.ncbi.nlm.nih.gov/pubmed/11033547.

Ohgushi, H., Dohi, Y., Tamai, S., and Tabata, S. 1993. "Osteogenic Differentiation of Marrow Stromal Stem Cells in Porous Hydroxyapatite Ceramics." *Journal of Biomedical Materials Research* 27 (11): 1401–7. doi:10.1002/jbm.820271107.

Overbeck, J. P., Winckler, S. T., Meffert, R., Törmälä, P., Spiegel, H. U., and Brug, E. 1995. "Penetration of Ciprofloxacin into Bone: A New Bioabsorbable Implant." *Journal of Investigative Surgery : The Official*

Journal of the Academy of Surgical Research 8 (3): 155–62. http://www.ncbi.nlm.nih.gov/pubmed/7547723.

Patzakis, Michael J., Holtom, Paul D. 2003. "Newer Methods of Antimicrobial Delivery for Bone and Joint Infections." *AAOS Instructional Course Lecture* 52: 745–50.

Paul R. Lockman, Koziara, Joanna M., Mumper, Russell J., and Allen. David D., 2004. "Nanoparticle Surface Charges Alter Blood–Brain Barrier Integrity and Permeability." *Journal of Drug Targeting* 12 (635–641).

Pereira, Marivalda M., and Hench, Larry L. 1996. "Mechanisms of Hydroxyapatite Formation on Porous Gel-Silica Substrates." *Journal of Sol-Gel Science and Technology* 7: 59–68. doi:10.1007/BF 00401884.

Pistos, Constantinos, Koutsopoulou, Maria, and Panderi, Irene. 2004. "A Validated Liquid Chromatographic Tandem Mass Spectrometric Method for the Determination of Mirtazapine and Demethylmirtazapine in Human Plasma: Application to a Pharmacokinetic Study." *Analytica Chimica Acta* 514: 15–26. doi:10.1016/j.aca.2004.03.042.

Rámila, A., Muñoz, B., Pérez-Pariente, J., and Vallet-Regí, M. 2003. "Mesoporous MCM-41 as Drug Host System." *Journal of Sol-Gel Science and Technology* 26: 1199–1202. doi:10.1023/A:10207643 19963.

Rang, H. P. E. Dale, M. M. 2001. *Farmacologia*. Edited by Guanabara Koogan. 4ª.

Redgrave, Liam S., Sutton, Sam B., and Piddock, Laura J. V., Webber, Mark A. 2014. "Fluoroquinolone Resistance: Mechanisms, Impact on Bacteria, and Role in Evolutionary Success." *Trends in Microbiology* 22 (8): 438–45. http://dx.doi.org/10.1016/j.tim.2014.04.007.

Ren, Jun, Panpan Hao, Wei Sun, Ruina Shi, and Shusen Liu. 2017. "Ordered Mesoporous Silica-Carbon-Supported Copper Catalyst as an Efficient and Stable Catalyst for Catalytic Oxidative Carbonylation." *Chemical Engineering Journal* 328. Elsevier B.V.: 673–82. doi:10.1016/j.cej.2017.07.101.

Sharma, Prabodh Chander, Jain, Ankit, Jain, Sandeep, Pahwa, Rakesh, and Yar, Mohammad Shahar. 2010. "Ciprofloxacin: Review on Developments in Synthetic, Analytical, and Medicinal Aspects." *Journal of Enzyme Inhibition and Medicinal Chemistry* 25 (4): 577–89. doi:10.3109/14756360903373350.

Shi, Xuetao, Wang, Yingjun, Wei, Kun, Ren, Li, and Lai, Chen. 2008. "Self-Assembly of Nanohydroxyapatite in Mesoporous Silica." *Journal of Materials Science: Materials in Medicine* 19: 2933–40. doi:10.1007/s10856-008-3424-3.

Shirtliff, J., Hench V. L. L., 2003. "Bioactive Materials for Tissue Engineering, Regeneration and Repair." *Expert Review of Medical Devices* 38: 4697 – 4707. doi:10.1586/17434440.2.3.303.

Shrivastava, Siddhartha, Bera, Tanmay, Roy, Arnab, Singh, Gajendra, Ramachandrarao, P., and Dash, Debabrata. 2007. "Characterization of Enhanced Antibacterial Effects of Novel Silver Nanoparticles." *Nanotechnology* 18 (22). doi:10.1088/0957-4484/18/22/225103.

Sousa, A., Souza, K. C., and Sousa, E. M. B. 2008. "Mesoporous Silica/apatite Nanocomposite: Special Synthesis Route to Control Local Drug Delivery." *Acta Biomaterialia* 4 (3): 671–79. doi:10.1016/j.actbio.2007.11.003.

Sousa, Andreza De, Maria, Daniel Andrada, De Sousa, Ricardo Geraldo, and Barros De Sousa, Edésia Martins. 2010. "Synthesis and Characterization of Mesoporous silica/poly(N- Isopropylacrylamide) Functional Hybrid Useful for Drug Delivery." *Journal of Materials Science* 45: 1478–86. doi:10.1007/s10853-009-4106-3.

Tang, Fangqiong, Li, Linlin, and Chen, Dong. 2012. "Mesoporous Silica Nanoparticles: Synthesis, Biocompatibility and Drug Delivery." *Advanced Materials* 24 (12): 1504–34. doi:10.1002/adma.201104763.

U.S. Food and Drug Administration. 2007. "A Report of the U.S. Food and Drug Administration Nanotechnology Task Force July 25, 2007." *USDA*.

Valente, F. L., Reis, E. C. C., Sep??lveda, R. V., Ochoa, C. C. R., Santos, L. C., Corsini, C. M., and Borges, A. P. B. 2016. "Hydroxyapatite, Polycaprolactone and Alendronate Composites for Bone Regeneration in Rabbits' Olecranon: Histological Features." *Arquivo Brasileiro de Medicina Veterinaria E Zootecnia* 68 (2): 543–47. doi:10.1590/1678-4162-8343.

Valerio, P., Guimarães, M. H. R., Pereira, M. M., Leite, M. F., and Goes, A. M. 2005. "Primary Osteoblast Cell Response to Sol-Gel Derived Bioactive Glass Foams." *Journal of Materials Science. Materials in Medicine* 16 (9): 851–56. doi:10.1007/s10856-005-3582-5.

Valerio, Patricia, Pereira, Marivalda M., Goes, Alfredo M., and Leite, M. Fatima. 2004. "The Effect of Ionic Products from Bioactive Glass Dissolution on Osteoblast Proliferation and Collagen Production." *Biomaterials* 25 (15): 2941–48. doi:10.1016/j.biomaterials.2003.09.086.

Vallet-Regí, María, and Balas, Francisco. 2008. "Silica Materials for Medical Applications." *The Open Biomedical Engineering Journal* 2: 1–9. doi:10.2174/1874120700802010001.

Vallet-Regí, María, Balas, Francisco, Colilla, Montserrat, and Manzano, Miguel. 2007. "Bioceramics and Pharmaceuticals: A Remarkable Synergy." *Solid State Sciences* 9: 768–76. doi:10.1016/j.solidstatesciences.2007.03.026.

Vallet-Regí, María, Ruiz-González, Luisa, Izquierdo-Barba, Isabel, and González-Calbet, José M. 2006. "Revisiting Silica Based Ordered Mesoporous Materials: Medical Applications." *Journal of Materials Chemistry* 16: 26. doi:10.1039/b509744d.

Vallet-Regi, M., Ragel, C. Victoria, Salinas, Antonio J., Vallet-Regí, María, and Ragel, C. Victoria. 2003. "Glasses with Medical Applications." *European Journal of Inorganic Chemistry*, 1029–42. doi:10.1002/ejic.200390134.

Warheit, D. B., Brock, W. J., Lee, K. P., Webb, T. R., and Reed, K. L.. 2005. "Comparative Pulmonary Toxicity Inhalation and Instillation Studies with Different TiO_2 Particle Formulations: Impact of Surface Treatments on Particle Toxicity." *Toxicological Sciences : An Official Journal of the Society of Toxicology* 88 (2): 514–24. doi:10.1093/toxsci/kfi331.

Williams, David Franklyn. 1987. "Definitions in Biomaterials." *Bulletin of the Medical Library Association* 68: 250.

Wu, C., and Chang, J. 2012. "Mesoporous Bioactive Glasses: Structure Characteristics, Drug/growth Factor Delivery and Bone Regeneration Application." *Interface Focus* 2 (March): 292–306. doi:10.1098/rsfs.2011.0121.

Xue, J. M., and Shi, M. 2004. "PLGA/mesoporous Silica Hybrid Structure for Controlled Drug Release." *Journal of Controlled Release* 98: 209–17. doi:10.1016/j.jconrel.2004.04.023.

Xynos, I. D., Edgar, A. J., Buttery, L. D., Hench, L. L., and Polak, J. M. 2000. "Ionic Products of Bioactive Glass Dissolution Increase Proliferation of Human Osteoblasts and Induce Insulin-like Growth Factor II mRNA Expression and Protein Synthesis." *Biochemical and Biophysical Research Communications* 276 (2): 461–65. doi:10.1006/bbrc.2000.3503.

Yiu, Humphrey H. P., and Wright, Paul A. 2005. "Enzymes Supported on Ordered Mesoporous Solids: A Special Case of an Inorganic–organic Hybrid." *Journal of Materials Chemistry* 15: 3690. doi:10.1039/b506090g.

Zhang, Hongliang, Pommier, Yves, Leo, Elisabetta, and Marchand, Christophe. 2010. "DNA Topoisomerases and Their Poisoning by Anticancer and Antibacterial Drugs." *Chemistry and Biology* 17 (5). Elsevier Ltd: 421–33. doi:10.1016/j.chembiol.2010.04.012.

Zhou, Panyu, Wang, Jing, and Tan, Honglue. 2014. "Siliceous Mesostructured Cellular Foams/Composite Biomaterials for Bone Regeneration." *International Journal of Nanomedicine* 9: 4795–4807.

Zuk, P. A., Zhu, M., Mizuno, H., Huang, J., Futrell, J. W., Katz, A. J., Benhaim, P., Lorenz, H. P., and Hedrick, M. H. 2001. "Multilineage Cells from Human Adipose Tissue: Implications for Cell-Based Therapies." *Tissue Engineering* 7 (2): 211–28. doi:10.1089/107632701300062859.

In: Ciprofloxacin
Editor: Mohamed Said Attia
ISBN: 978-1-53614-534-2

Chapter 3

DISTRIBUTION OF CIPROFLOXACIN IN THE PERIPHERIES

Janis Vella[1,*], Kevin Cassar[2], Lilian M. Azzopardi[1], Anthony Serracino-Inglott[1] and Godfrey LaFerla[2]
[1]Department of Pharmacy, Faculty of Medicine and Surgery, University of Malta, Msida, Malta
[2]Department of Surgery, Faculty of Medicine and Surgery, University of Malta, Msida, Malta

ABSTRACT

Peripheral Arterial Disease (PAD) is a highly prevalent atherosclerotic syndrome which leads to a substantial degree of morbidity and mortality. The number of patients who are suffering from chronic conditions such as PAD is increasing as the life expectancy of the general population is increasing. Foot infections in PAD patients who are also suffering from diabetes, can lead to gangrene necessitating amputation. Ciprofloxacin is an antibiotic which is commonly administered to treat diabetic foot infections. The aims of this study were to develop and validate high performance liquid chromatography (HPLC)

[*] email: janis.vella@um.edu.mt.

methods of analysis for high throughput screening in a clinical setting. The developed methods were used to determine the concentrations of ciprofloxacin in blood and tissue samples of patients suffering from PAD of varying degrees. The distribution of ciprofloxacin in the peripheries of patients was evaluated and a 3-predictor regression model in relation to such a distribution was developed to help predict whether ciprofloxacin reaches the infected area in concentrations which are high enough to treat the infection in PAD patients. Blood and tissue samples were collected from 50 patients (33 male; 17 female), who were admitted to hospital for debridement or amputation procedures. The majority of patients (n = 49) were suffering from diabetes. Thirty-five patients were suffering from severe PAD. It was found that the concentration of ciprofloxacin reaching the infected tissue was dependent on: the severity of PAD, the number of medications that the patient was taking and on the concentration of ciprofloxacin in plasma. The developed regression model was tested on a sample of 10 PAD patients. The calculated value for ciprofloxacin concentrations obtained using the regression model was compared to the concentration of ciprofloxacin that was determined by HPLC. The innovative HPLC methods which were developed and validated for the determination of ciprofloxacin in plasma and tissue can be effectively used for high throughput analysis in a clinical setting where results usually need to be attained in a short period of time for a large number of patient samples. The developed regression model can help predict and calculate a tailored individualized dose of ciprofloxacin for patients suffering from foot infections. This can lead to adequate dosing in these patients with less undesirable effects and better treatment outcomes, avoiding unwanted complications and achieving higher levels of therapeutic success in the process.

Keywords: peripheral arterial disease, ciprofloxacin, blood, tissue, high performance liquid chromatography

1. Introduction

Peripheral Arterial Disease (PAD) is an atherosclerotic syndrome which leads to a substantial degree of morbidity and mortality (Althouse et al., 2014). The number of patients who are suffering from chronic conditions such as PAD is increasing as the life expectancy of the general population is increasing. The highly prevalent disease carries with it a high risk of cardiovascular and cerebrovascular events (Biscetti et al., 2014). It is estimated that there are 200 million people suffering from PAD worldwide (Criqui and Aboyans, 2015).

1.1. Severity of PAD

PAD can be classified according to its extent or severity. Patients suffering from PAD may experience intermittent claudication, critical ischemia and acute limb ischemia. PAD can be asymptomatic in some patients. Asymptomatic PAD patients still have risks of increased cardiovascular events and death (Hardman et al., 2014).

1.2. Diagnosis of PAD

PAD can manifest itself differently in different people and there are various ways how such a condition can be diagnosed. Classification systems such as the Rutherford system or Fontaine system can be used to assess PAD severity (Mills et al., 2014). Spectral waveform analyses can be used for the diagnosis of PAD. The ankle-brachial pressure index (ABPI) is a commonly employed tool for diagnosing PAD (Tehan et al., 2017). The ABPI may be used to confirm the presence of PAD in addition to patient history and physical examination (Mao et al., 2017).

1.3 Risk factors for PAD

The factors which pose the greatest risk for an individual to develop PAD are diabetes and cigarette smoking. Other risk factors for PAD include advanced age, hypertension, dyslipidemia and gender (Mao et al., 2017). Elevated levels of C-reactive protein, apolipoprotein B, lipoprotein a, homocysteine and fibrinogen and increased plasma viscosity are other factors which contribute to a higher risk for development of PAD (Bérard et al., 2013; Ding et al., 2014).

1.4. Foot Ulcers

Patients suffering from PAD are at an increased risk of developing foot ulcers and infections, particularly if neuropathy is present (Armstrong et al., 2011). Hyperglycemia has a major role in the development and progression of neuropathy. Trauma to a neuropathic foot can lead to the development of an ulcer which can become infected. Diabetic patients who suffer from PAD are more prone to develop foot ulcers and infections which are one of the most feared complications and the major cause of hospitalization (Chu et al., 2015). Infected foot ulcers can easily lead to irreversible tissue damage (Tiwari et al., 2012). In the absence of an adequate blood supply, ulcers may eventually lead to gangrene. The presence of infection in these cases is a major risk factor for amputation.

Causative microorganisms for foot infections include *Staphylococcus aureus, Pseudomonas aeruginosa, Escherichia coli, Enterococcus* spp. and *Stapyhylococcus epidermidis,* among others. Management of these foot infections includes the choice of correct antibiotic therapy together with effective wound management. Aggressive wound debridement should be performed where necessary. Offloading can also help in the healing of neuropathic foot ulcers. The use of casts and perioperative shoes also aid in such a process (Park and Anand, 2015). In the presence of combined bone and soft tissue infections, amputations are often required (Kisozi et al., 2017).

1.5. Antibacterial Therapy

Treatment for foot infections with antibiotics varies, depending on the severity of infection and the individual's response to the antibiotics. When the ulcer is not infected, treatment with antibiotics is not indicated. Mild infections are usually treated using oral antibacterial therapy. Moderate to severe infections are usually treated intravenously initially and then treatment is switched to an oral equivalent when possible. Severe infections are treated intravenously. The length of treatment depends on the need for surgical debridement and on the extent of the infection. Among the types of antibacterial agents which are administered to treat foot infections are ciprofloxacin, clindamycin, piperacillin and tazobactam (Gemechu et al., 2013).

The efficacy of antibacterial agents can be determined by the concentration of agent reaching the tissue of interest. The concentration of the drug in the tissue is thought to change proportionally with that of the drug in the plasma. A decrease in blood flow can lead to impaired penetration of the antibiotic in the tissue. Delivery of antibiotics to ischemic tissue is less and concentrations needed to achieve a therapeutic effect are usually not achieved, regardless of appropriate plasma concentrations (Stein et al., 2007). It would therefore be necessary to quantify the amount of drug which actually reaches the infected tissue, to be able to determine whether the right therapeutic concentrations are being achieved in this compartment. Knowledge of drug levels in biological fluids such as plasma and tissue can help optimize pharmacotherapy.

The aims of this study were to develop and validate high performance liquid chromatography (HPLC) methods of analysis, for high throughput screening in a clinical setting. The developed methods were used to determine the concentration of ciprofloxacin in the blood and tissue samples of patients suffering from PAD of varying degrees. Factors influencing the distribution of ciprofloxacin in the peripheries of these patients were evaluated and a 3-predictor regression model was established, in relation to these factors. This regression model will help predict whether the antibiotic is reaching the infected area in concentrations which are high enough to treat the infection effectively.

2. Methods

The study consisted of two parts- development and validation of HPLC methods for the determination of ciprofloxacin in plasma and tissue, and application of these methods to determine the concentrations of ciprofloxacin in the plasma and tissue of patients suffering from PAD. Subsequently, the 3-predictor regression model was then established.

2.1. Development of HPLC Method for the Quantification of Ciprofloxacin in Plasma

2.1.1. Chemicals and Consumables

The chemicals and consumables used for this study were:

Ciprofloxacin standard: ≥98% purity (Sigma Aldrich), Ofloxcain standard: ≥98% purity (Sigma Aldrich), Sulfadimidine sodium standard: ≥98% purity (Sigma Aldrich), Disodium hydrogen phosphate: 99.5% purity (Schlarau), Acetonitrile: 99.6% purity (Fisher Scientific), Methanol: 99% purity (Fisher Scientific), Orthophosphoric acid: 88% purity (Fisher Scientific), HPLC-grade water (Fisher Scientific), Reversed phase ACE®C_{18} column (250 x 4.6mm; 5μm particle size) and Reversed phase Pursuit 5 C_{18} MetaGuard® guard column (10 x 4.6mm).

2.1.2. Instrumentation

A Varian® ProStar HPLC unit was used. This unit had an online degasser, column oven and UV-vis detector which was set at 277nm. A Star® 800 Module Interface Box was used to register signals which were then processed using Galaxie® Workstation software. Peak area mode was used for signal quantification. A XS104 Mettler Toledo® analytical balance was used to weigh analytes. A TurboVap® LV Automated Evaporation System was used to carry out solvent evaporations. Samples were introduced through a fixed sample loop with a volume of 50μl. Temperatures of analyses were maintained at 25°C. The flow rate was set at 1.5ml/min.

2.1.3. Choosing the Internal Standard

Ofloxacin was initially chosen as the internal standard for the analysis. When ofloxacin was analyzed together with ciprofloxacin using a mobile phase of phosphate buffer and acetonitrile, both analytes had similar retention times of around 3 minutes. Changing the amount of acetonitrile in the mobile phase can lead to a shift in analyte retention times (Vella et al., 2014). To provide better analytical resolution, the amount of acetonitrile in the mobile phase was decreased from 30% to 26%, 25%, 24% and 23%. This did not provide any considerable shift in the retention time of the analytes. The internal standard was subsequently changed to sulfadimidine sodium. Sulfadimidine sodium exhibits similar extraction and chromatographic behaviour as ciprofloxacin. It also absorbs UV radiation well at 277nm (Figure 1).

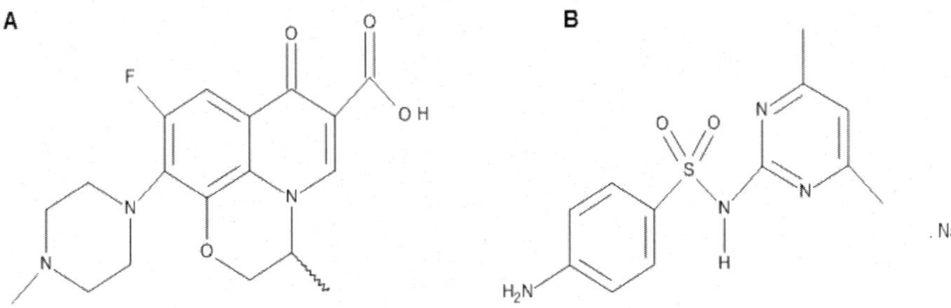

Figure 1. Ofloxacin (A) and Sulfadimidine sodium (B) were chosen as internal standards due to them both showing a significant amount of absorption at the same UV wavelength at which ciprofloxacin exhibits maximum absorption. This study is the first reported study documenting the use of sulfadimidine sodium as an internal standard for the chromatographic analysis of ciprofloxacin.

2.1.4. Preparation of Mobile Phase and Stock Solutions

The mobile phase which was used for analysis was prepared using a 0.02M phosphate buffer, at pH 2.7. The buffer was prepared using disodium hydrogen phosphate and orthophosphoric acid. This buffer was eluted with acetontrile to make up a mobile phase of phosphate buffer and acetonitrile 77:23 (v/v). All prepared solutions were stored in amber glass bottles.

Ciprofloxacin, being insoluble or slightly soluble in water (Bozkir et al., 2012; Mafra et al., 2012) was initially dissolved in methanol. During analysis of this solution following its storage for one week, 2 peaks were noted. Results attained were compared to previous analyses of the same solution after 1 week, where it was noted that the first peak which represented ciprofloxacin decreased in size whilst a new peak was observed at a later retention time. This second peak, which eluted after the peak for ciprofloxacin, could be due to an esterification reaction between ciprofloxacin and methanol, which lead to the formation of the methyl ester of ciprofloxacin during storage. This possible reaction has been previously documented (De Witte et al., 2007; Muchohi et al., 2011).

Due to this possible reaction occurring the stock solution was prepared using 0.2M hydrochloric acid. When solutions were analyzed, peak shouldering could be observed. Although previous studies have documented using hydrochloric acid to dissolve ciprofloxacin in (Muchohi et al., 2011), the low pH might have affected pH control during chromatography in this case. A 1mg/ml stock solution of ciprofloxacin was consequently prepared by dissolving ciprofloxacin in the mobile phase. A 1mg/ml stock solution of sulfadimidine sodium was prepared by dissolving sulfadimidine sodium in HPLC-grade water. A summary of the chromatographic conditions can be found in Table 1.

Table 1. Chromatographic parameters for the determination of ciprofloxacin in plasma

Instrumentation	Varian ProStar®
Stationary Phase	RP ACE C_{18} column (250x 4.6mm; 5μm particle size) at 25°C
Mobile Phase	0.02M phosphate buffer (pH 2.7) and acetonitrile 77:23 v/v. Flow rate 1.5ml/min
Uv Detector	277nm

2.2. Sample Preparation

Protein precipitation was chosen as the sample preparation technique for the analysis of ciprofloxacin. Protein precipitation was chosen as it involves the use of less volumes of organic solvent, which leads to less time needed for evaporating off this solvent to concentrate ciprofloxacin prior to analysis (Kataoka, 2003). Protein precipitation requires less sample preparation steps when compared to other techniques such as solid phase extraction, and this leads to less chances of errors. Protein precipitation is an efficient technique to use, when a large number of samples need to be analyzed at the same time (Hendriks, 2009). Since ciprofloxacin is polar in nature, it can be more efficiently separated by protein precipitation, rather than liquid-liquid extraction or solid phase extraction. Acetonitrile was chosen as the agent for precipitation. Protein precipitation using acetonitrile or methanol is a commonly-performed sample preparation technique for compounds such as ciprofloxacin (Garcia et al., 1999). Precipitation is better achieved using organic solvents having a lower polarity (Zhou, 2011). Acetonitrile is less polar than methanol and is therefore expected to precipitate plasma proteins better than methanol.

Drug-free human blood was centrifuged at 3,500g, using an Eppendorf Mini Spin® and the upper plasma layer was separated in tubes and spiked with ciprofloxacin and 30μl of the internal standard, sulfadimidine sodium (100μg/ml). One drop of 10M phosphate buffer (pH 2.7) was added and the tubes were vortex-mixed for 3 minutes using a Vortex Genie 2® (Model G560E).

To 400μl of this plasma, 500μl of ice-cold acetonitrile was added. This plasma-to-acetonitrile ratio was chosen as it resulted in adequate precipitation of plasma proteins. Published studies make use of equal, or close-to-equal volumes of acetonitrile and plasma for efficient separation (Weber et al., 1985; Khan and Khan 2005). When 1 ml of acetonitrile was added to 400μl of plasma protein, the formation of a cloudy supernatant could be observed following centrifugation. The addition of 1.5 volumes of acetonitrile to 1 volume of plasma is enough to remove 99.4% of the plasma proteins (Neckel et al., 2002). The use of greater volumes of organic solvent used for precipitation leads to increased assay time, due to more time needed for the organic layer to be evaporated off (Venn, 2005). Evaporation of the organic solvent from the sample should be as much as possible complete. The presence of organic solvent remaining in the sample can have an effect on chromatographic peak shape and retention time (Rossi and Sin, 2012).

The tubes were vortex-mixed for another 5 minutes. The samples were then centrifuged at 3,500g for 5 minutes. The supernatant was poured into 8ml silanized glass tubes. The glass tubes were silanized using dimethyldichlorosilane (DMDCS). An in-house procedure was used for the silanization of glass tubes, to prevent loss of ciprofloxacin through adsorption on the glass tubes (Vella et al., 2015). The DMDCS coating eliminates active sites on the glass tubes which could cause potential interactions between the contents and the glass. The silanized glass tubes were then placed in a Turbovap Concentrator®, with the water bath set at 50°C, for 20 minutes. The dried residue was then reconstituted with 100μl of the mobile phase and vortex-mixed for 3 minutes. Centrifugation was performed again at 3,500g, for 3 minutes and 50μl of the clear supernatant was injected into the HPLC unit.

2.3. Validation of HPLC Method for the Quantification of Ciprofloxacin in Plasma

Validation of the developed method for the analysis of ciprofloxacin in plasma was carried out, according to the International Conference on Harmonization (ICH) guidelines (ICH, 2005), to confirm suitability of the method. The method was validated for specificity, linearity, precision, accuracy, limit of quantification, limit of detection and stability.

2.3.1. Specificity

Five blank human plasma samples were analyzed to confirm specificity of the method.

2.3.2. Linearity

Seven different concentration standards were prepared from the stock solution of ciprofloxacin and analyzed. Peak area ratios of ciprofloxacin and sulfadimidine sodium were plotted against the concentration of ciprofloxacin in plasma and a calibration curve was set up. The concentration standards of ciprofloxacin ranged from 0.05 to 8μg/ml. This range includes the clinically relevant ciprofloxacin plasma concentration range (Hirata et al., 1989; Garelts et al., 1996).

2.3.3. Precision

Five replicates of each of the ciprofloxacin concentrations used for the calibration curve were analyzed on the same day to evaluate intra-day precision. One replicate of each concentration used for the calibration curve, was analyzed once for four consecutive days to evaluate inter-day precision. The percentage relative standard deviation (RSD) was used to express intra- and inter-day precision.

2.3.4. Accuracy

Three concentrations (0.5, 2 and 6μg/ml) of ciprofloxacin in plasma were analyzed in triplicate to assess recovery. Accuracy was expressed as the percentage recovery and was calculated as: measured value/theoretical value x 100.

2.3.5. Limit of Detection and Limit of Quantification

The limit of detection was the smallest concentration of ciprofloxacin in plasma which was analyzed and which gave a detector signal. Analyses for the limit of detection was performed in triplicate. The limit of quantification was the smallest concentration of ciprofloxacin in plasma which was analysed, gave a detector signal and could be quantified. Analyses for the limit of quantification was performed in triplicate.

2.3.6. Stability

The stability of ciprofloxacin in plasma was determined following the storage of samples of ciprofloxacin in plasma at -20°C. Three different concentrations (0.5, 2 and 8μg/ml) of ciprofloxacin in 4ml of plasma were stored. These concentrations were then analyzed in triplicate, after storing at -20°C for 1 week and 4 weeks respectively after leaving the plasma thaw for 2 hours, at 25°C.

2.4. Development of HPLC Method for the Quantification of Ciprofloxacin in Tissue

Method development for the quantification of ciprofloxacin in tissue, was carried out using pork tissue. Five hundred milligrams of pork tissue was accurately weighed and spiked with a known concentration of ciprofloxacin and sulfadimidine sodium. Since tissue can be considered as being a solid matrix, homogenization of this matrix had to be carried out prior to separating the analytes of interest from it.

2.4.1. Using Different Types of Tissue Homogenizer

Homogenization of tissue was attempted, using two types of homogenizers- a dounce hand-held glass homogenizer and an electric homogenizer (MSE®, UK). Use of both these types of homogenizers has been reported in literature (Buechler et al., 1984; Filigenzi et al., 2008; Sun et al., 2011). Five milliliters of pH 7.0 buffer was added to the 500mg of pork tissue. Such a ratio of 0.1g tissue per milliliter of liquid has been used for homogenisation in other reported studies (Yu and Cohen, 2004).

Reproducibility results for three concentration levels (0.5, 1.5 and 2μg/ml) were compared when using the two types of homogenizers. In each case, tissue was homogenized for 20 minutes. Each type of homogenization and analysis of the three concentration levels, was performed in triplicate, for both types of homogenizer.

2.4.2. Separation of Drugs from Tissue Homogenate and Analysis

Ciprofloxacin and sulfadimidine sodium were separated from the proteins in the tissue homogenate, using the same sample preparation technique as that used for plasma. Protein precipitation was carried out on 400μl of tissue homogenate, using 500μl of acetonitrile. Analysis was carried out using the same chromatographic conditions as described in Table 1.

2.4.3. Choosing the Type of Tissue Homogenizer

The type of tissue homogenizer was chosen based on reproducibility results attained when using the two types of homogenizers tested. Reproducibility results were assessed by comparing the ratios of the areas under the peaks for ciprofloxacin and sulfadimidine sodium. This was done in triplicate for all the three concentrations (0.5, 1.5 and 2μg/ml) of ciprofloxacin in tissue. Results were evaluated, by calculating the percentage RSD of the ratios of the areas under the peak for ciprofloxacin and sulfadimidine sodium. It was decided to carry out the method validation for the determination of ciprofloxacin in tissue using the electric tissue homogenizer, since better reproducibility was attained when using it (Table 2).

Table 2. Reproducibility results when using the Dounce and Electric Homogenizer

2μg/ml ciprofloxacin in tissue	Dounce Homogenizer	Electric Homogenizer
Average ratio of areas under the peak	0.44	0.97
Relative standard deviation	66.1%	2.38%
1.5μg/ml ciprofloxacin in tissue	Dounce Homogenizer	Electric Homogenizer
Average ratio of areas under the peak	1.05	0.80
Relative standard deviation	28.51%	8.37%
0.5μg/ml ciprofloxacin in tissue	Dounce Homogenizer	Electric Homogenizer
Average ratio of areas under the peak	0.07	0.26
Relative standard deviation	24.74%	2.25%

2.5. Validation of HPLC Method for the Quantification of Ciprofloxacin in Tissue

Validation of the developed method for the analysis of ciprofloxacin in tissue was carried out, according to the International Conference on Harmonization (ICH) guidelines (ICH, 2005) to confirm suitability of the method. The method was validated for specificity, linearity, precision, accuracy, limit of quantification, limit of detection and stability.

2.5.1. Specificity

Three blank human tissue samples were analysed to confirm specificity of the method.

2.5.2. Linearity

Six different concentration standards were prepared from the stock solution of ciprofloxacin and analyzed. Peak area ratios of ciprofloxacin and sulfadimidine sodium were plotted against the concentration of ciprofloxacin in tissue and a calibration curve was set up. The concentration standards of ciprofloxacin ranged from 0.05 to 2.5μg/ml. The ciprofloxacin concentrations used to set up the calibration curve were chosen according to the range of the concentrations of the maximum and minimum concentrations of ciprofloxacin found in tissue, which are reported in pharmacokinetic studies (Brunner et al., 1999; Müller et al., 1999).

2.5.3. Precision

Three replicates of each of the ciprofloxacin concentrations used for the calibration curve were analyzed on the same day to evaluate intra-day precision. One replicate of each concentration used for the calibration curve, was analyzed once for three consecutive days to evaluate inter-day precision. The percentage relative standard deviation (RSD) was used to express intra- and inter-day precision.

2.5.4. Accuracy

Three concentrations (0.5, 1.5 and 2.5μg/ml) of ciprofloxacin in tissue were analyzed in triplicate to assess recovery. Accuracy was expressed as the percentage recovery and was calculated as: measured value/theoretical value x 100.

2.5.5. Limit of Detection and Limit of Quantification

The limit of detection was the smallest concentration of ciprofloxacin in tissue which was analyzed and which gave a detector signal. Analyses for the limit of detection was performed in triplicate. The limit of quantification was the smallest concentration of ciprofloxacin in tissue which was analysed, gave a detector signal and could be quantified. Analyses for the limit of quantification was performed in triplicate.

2.5.6. Stability

The stability of ciprofloxacin in tissue was determined following the storage of samples of ciprofloxacin in tissue at -20°C. Two different concentrations (1 and 2μg/ml) of ciprofloxacin in tissue were stored. These concentrations were then analyzed in triplicate after 3 weeks and 6 weeks respectively after leaving the tissue samples thaw for 3 hours at 25°C.

2.6. Clinical Study

Following the development and validation of the methods for the determination of ciprofloxacin in plasma and tissue, the clinical study was undertaken, where blood and tissue samples were collected from patients suffering from varying degrees of PAD.

Necessary approvals including the University of Malta Research Ethics Committee approval were attained. The clinical part of the study took place at Mater Dei Hospital, Msida, Malta. Patients who were chosen to participate in the study were those undergoing debridement or minor amputation of the toes or feet who were due to receive intravenous ciprofloxacin prior to the procedure. Informed consent was obtained from all participants prior to recruitment.

2.6.1. Patient Profile Form

A patient profile form was filled in, following patient interviews and review of patient records. The form consisted of the following main sections:

- Patient number

- Date
- General social and demographic data
- Age, gender and weight
- Cigarette smoking habits
- Past medical history

In this section, information about diabetes, creatinine levels, presence or absence of neuropathy as well as previous history of resistant infections and seizures was listed. Co-morbidities or allergies that the patients were suffering from were included. A list of medications that the patient was taking was included in this section.

- Antibiotic administration

Information about the antibiotic/s used, the dose and the frequency of administration was documented.

- Wound characteristics

The location and type of lesion - whether it was an ulcer or gangrene were included. If gangrene was present, a distinction was made between wet and dry, with odour, pain or exudates. Any previous history of gangrene was noted. The severity of the wound infection- mild, moderate or severe - was included in this section.

2.6.2. Assessment of the Severity of PAD

The presence or absence and the severity of PAD was assessed by the vascular surgeon who was performing the debridement and amputation procedures. Measures to assess PAD were carried out using the Ankle Brachial Pressure Index (ABPI) and spectral waveform analysis. Results obtained from both methods were then used to assign the PAD severity (Table 3).

Table 3. Classification of Peripheral Arterial Disease

Classification of PAD		
Degree of PAD	ABPI Results	Spectral Waveform Analysis
Nil or borderline	0.91-1.29	Triphasic
Mild or moderate	0.51-0.90	Biphasic
Severe	0.0-0.50	Monophasic

2.6.3. Sampling and Storage of Blood and Tissue

A 200mg intravenous dose of ciprofloxacin was administered to the patient 30 minutes prior to the surgical intervention. A sample of total blood volume ranging between 3 to 5ml was collected from the patient by the anaesthetist present during the debridement or amputation procedure. The sample was collected 30 minutes after the administration of ciprofloxacin, at the end of the infusion. Blood was collected peripherally from the region of the cubital fossa and stored in a red-top Vaccutainer®. The tube containing the blood was centrifuged and the upper plasma layer was decanted and stored at -20°C until analysis.

Tissue samples were collected from the wound by the vascular surgeon who was performing the debridement or amputation procedure. The average debridement or amputation procedure took about 15 to 30 minutes to be completed. Each patient sample that was collected was rinsed with sterile saline and stored at -20°C until analysis.

Patient samples were then analyzed and the concentration of ciprofloxacin in each blood and tissue sample was determined using the developed and validated methods.

2.7. Data Analysis

Data from the patient profile form and the values for ciprofloxacin plasma and tissue concentrations were inputted into SPSS® statistics (version 22). Data was analysed for linear regressions and descriptive statistics.

Correlation of the covariates and fixed factors was carried out using the Kruskal Wallis test, the Spearman Correlation and the Chi-Squared test.

The distribution pattern for the values of ciprofloxacin in tissue in this group of patients was observed. Bivariate analysis was then carried out to correlate the values for the concentrations of ciprofloxacin in tissue with other factors which might influence these concentrations. Parameters which could affect the concentration of ciprofloxacin in the tissue of patients were determined using the parsimonious model.

The parameters which were considered for the model were gender, age, weight, smoking status, the type of diabetes, HbA1c levels, number of medications that the patient was taking, creatinine clearance, presence or absence of neuropathy, type of wound and PAD severity. Backward elimination was then carried out to exclude factors which were considered to be insignificant due to the large p-value attained. A 3-predictor regression model was developed.

2.8. Testing and Using the Developed Regression Model

Results from 10 of the patients which were included in the clinical study were randomly selected to test the developed regression model. The expected tissue concentration of ciprofloxacin was calculated using the data of the most significant 3 predictors included in the developed 3-predictor regression model. This calculated concentration value for ciprofloxacin was then compared with the already calculated ciprofloxacin tissue concentrations, which were previously determined using HPLC.

3. RESULTS

3.1. Validation of HPLC Method for the Quantification of Ciprofloxacin in Plasma

3.1.1. Specificity

Specificity was confirmed by the absence of peaks at the times when ciprofloxacin and sulfadimidine sodium usually elute (Figure 2).

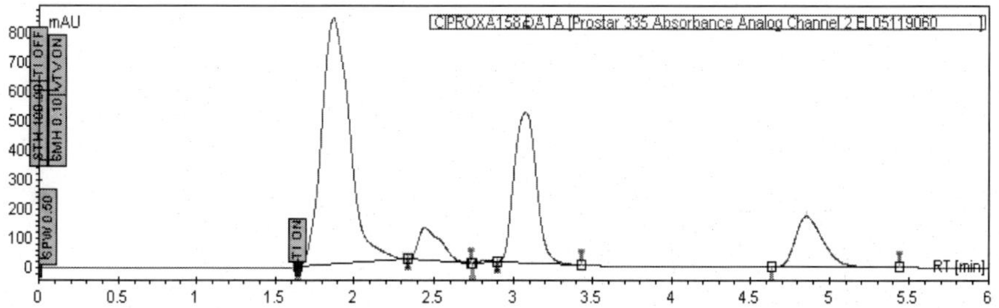

Figure 2. Chromatogram of ciprofloxacin (7µg/ml); retention time = 3.26 minutes and sulfadimidine sodium; retention time = 4.92 minutes in plasma.

3.1.2. Linearity

The linear equation y = mx+ c was used to perform least-squares analysis of the calibration data. The calibration curve for ciprofloxacin in plasma was linear in the concentration range of 0.05-8µg/ml. The average r value was of 0.999 (Figure 3).

3.1.3. Precision

The percentage RSD for the concentrations of ciprofloxacin in plasma in the intra-day study ranged between 0.05 and 8.94. The percentage RSD for the concentrations of ciprofloxacin in plasma in the inter-day study ranged between 1.00 and 12.04.

3.1.4. Accuracy

The recoveries of ciprofloxacin from plasma ranged from 90.00 to 96.11%.

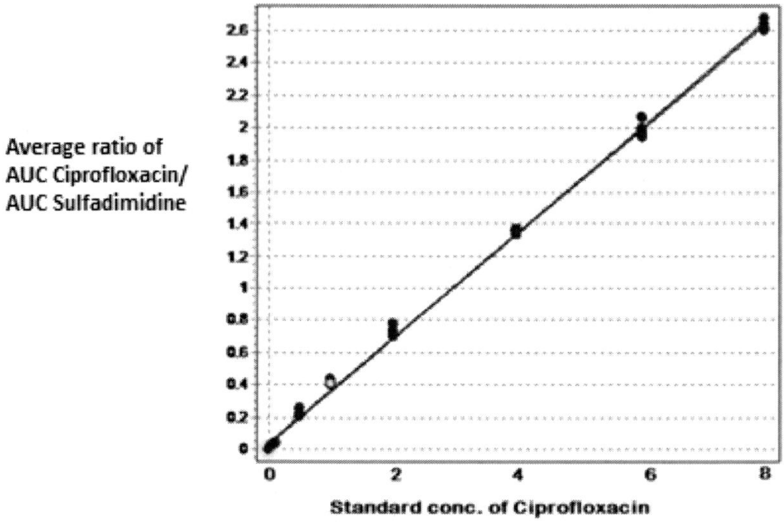

Figure 3. Calibration curve for ciprofloxacin in plasma (plot of ratio of areas under the peak vs standard concentration of ciprofloxacin in µg/ml).

3.1.5. Limit of Detection and Limit of Quantification

The limit of detection for the concentration of ciprofloxacin in plasma was found to be 0.1µg/ml and the limit of quantification for the concentration of ciprofloxacin in plasma was found to be 0.05µg/ml.

3.1.6. Stability

There was no significant change in the concentrations of ciprofloxacin in plasma which were determined following storage at -20°C when compared to the concentrations of ciprofloxacin in plasma which were determined following analysis immediately after the samples were prepared. When ciprofloxacin concentrations were analyzed in triplicate following storage after 1 week, percentage RSD values ranged from 0.51-3.18. When ciprofloxacin concentrations were analyzed in triplicate following storage after 4 weeks, percentage RSD values ranged from 0.47-2.08.

3.2. Validation of HPLC Method for the Quantification of Ciprofloxacin in Tissue

3.2.1. Specificity

Specificity was confirmed by the absence of peaks at the times when ciprofloxacin and sulfadimidine sodium usually elute.

3.2.2. Linearity

The linear equation y = mx+ c was used to perform least-squares analysis of the calibration data. The calibration curve for ciprofloxacin in tissue was linear in the concentration range of 0.05-2.5μg/ml. The average r value was of 0.993 (Figure 4).

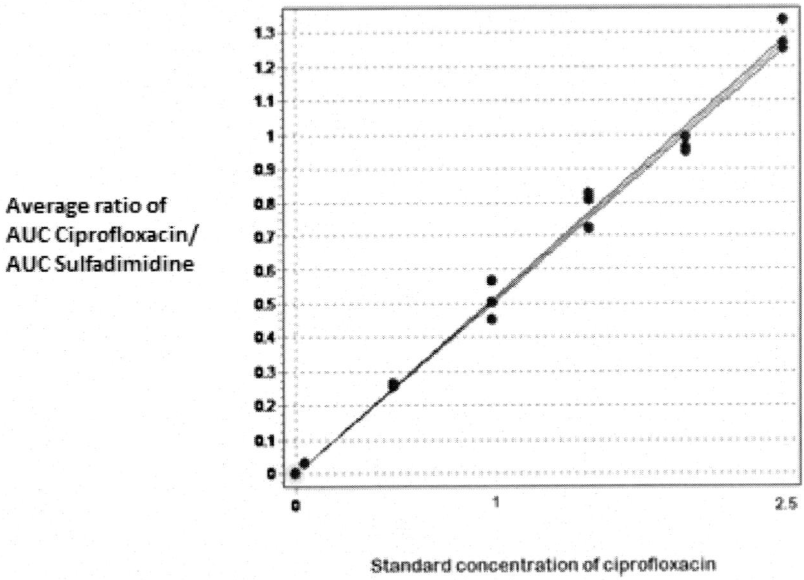

Figure 4. Calibration curve for ciprofloxacin in tissue (plot of ratio of areas under the peak vs standard concentration of ciprofloxacin in μg/ml).

3.2.3. Precision

The percentage RSD for the concentrations of ciprofloxacin in tissue in the intra-day study ranged between 1.18 and 8.26. The percentage RSD for the concentrations of ciprofloxacin in tissue in the inter-day study ranged between 2.46 and 10.15.

3.2.4. Accuracy

The recoveries of ciprofloxacin from tissue ranged from 94.00 to 106.00%.

3.2.5. Limit of Detection and Limit of Quantification

The limit of detection for ciprofloxacin in tissue and the limit of quantification for ciprofloxacin in tissue were both found to be 0.05µg/ml.

3.2.6. Stability

There was no significant change in the concentrations of ciprofloxacin in tissue which were determined following storage at -20°C when compared to the concentrations of ciprofloxacin following analysis immediately after the samples were prepared. When ciprofloxacin concentrations were analyzed in triplicate following storage after 3 weeks, percentage RSD values were 6.56 and 12.26. When ciprofloxacin concentrations were analyzed in triplicate following storage after 6 weeks, percentage RSD values were 3.57 and 6.08.

3.3. Concentrations of Ciprofloxacin

The concentration of ciprofloxacin determined in the plasma of patients (Figure 5) was higher than that which was determined in the tissue of patients at the time of sampling. The average concentration of ciprofloxacin in patient tissue was 0.28µg/ml (range 0.00-2.06µg/ml) and that in patient plasma was of 2.14µg/ml (0.00-8.00µg/ml).

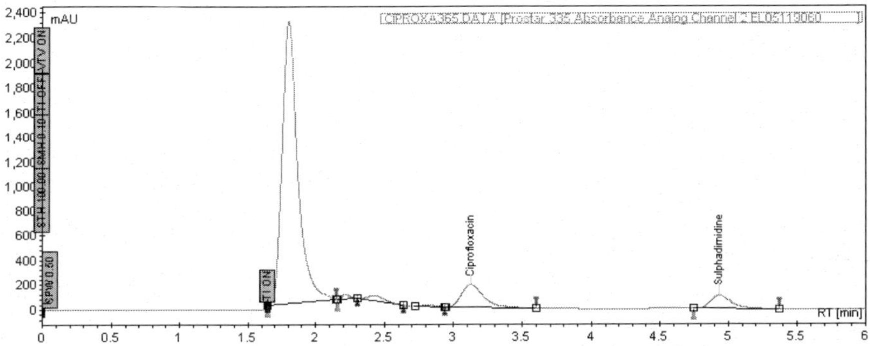

Figure 5. Chromatogram of ciprofloxacin (5.26μg/ml); retention time = 3.13 minutes and sulfdimidine sodium; retention time = 4.94 minutes in the plasma of a patient suffering from PAD.

3.4. Patient Characteristics

A total of 50 patients were included in the study. Thirty three patients were male and 17 patients were female. The patients' age ranged from 28 to 92 years, with a mean age of 68 years. The patients' weight ranged from 59 to 165kg with a mean weight of 80kg. The majority of the patients (n = 38) claimed that they never smoked cigarettes. Eight patients claimed that they are non-smokers but had smoked in the past 10 years. Four patients claimed to still be smoking at the time of the study.

The average HbA1c level for this group of patients was 8% (range: 5-14%). The majority of the patients (n = 35) were suffering from Type 2 diabetes. One patient was not a diabetic. The average rate of creatinine clearance for patients included in the study, was that of 68ml/minute (range: 10-177 ml/minute). The majority of the patients (n = 44) included in the study were suffering from neuropathy. Forty four patients did not have any history of resistant infections.

The number of medications taken per patient ranged from 1 to 18 different types of medication, with an average of 10 types of medication taken per patient. The majority of patients (n = 39) did not suffer from drug allergies. Those who had drug allergies (n = 11) were not allergic to ciprofloxacin. The most common types of co-morbidities in this group of patients were diabetes, hypertension, ischemic heart disease and congestive heart failure (Table 4).

Thirty patients had an ulcer and 20 patients were suffering from gangrene. Twelve of the patients suffering from gangrene had wet gangrene whilst the remaining 8 were suffering from dry gangrene. Nineteen patients had a previous history of gangrene. The majority of patients (n = 44) underwent surgery involving amputation. The other 6 patients had debridement of a wound.

Thirty four patients were suffering from severe PAD. Thirteen patients had mild to moderate PAD. Three patients had no PAD or borderline PAD. Twenty male patients and 14 female patients were suffering from severe PAD. Twelve male patients and 1 female patient were suffering from mild/moderate PAD. One male patient and 2 female patients had nil/borderline PAD.

The largest number of patients (n = 23) suffering from severe PAD had Type 2 diabetes. Eleven patients suffering from severe PAD had Type 1 diabetes. Three patients suffering from mild/moderate PAD had Type 1 diabetes. One patient who had nil/borderline PAD did not have diabetes.

Table 4. The most common patient comorbidities (N = 50)

Comorbidity	No. of patients
Diabetes mellitus	49
Hypertension	40
Ischemic heart disease	29
Congestive heart disease	16
Renal impairment	9
Hypercholesterolemia	7
Hyperlipidemia	5
Hypothyroidism	4
Prostatic hyperplasia	3
Cataracts	3
Gout	2
Anxiety and depression	2

3.5. Pharmacokinetic Model

Three predictors were included in the parsimonious model for determining the expected ciprofloxacin tissue concentration: (i) severity of PAD (ii) number of medications that the patient was taking (iii) ciprofloxacin plasma concentration. The best predictor of the three was the severity of PAD followed by the number of medications and ciprofloxacin concentration in plasma.

The regression coefficient of 1.3416 for nil/borderline PAD indicated that the concentration in tissue for the group of patients having nil/borderline PAD was expected to be 1.3416 units higher compared with the group of patients suffering from severe PAD. The regression coefficient of 0.215 for mild/moderate PAD indicated that the concentration of ciprofloxacin in tissue in the group of patients suffering from mild/moderate PAD was 0.215 units higher compared with the group of patients suffering from severe PAD given that the other effects were kept constant.

The regression model relating the concentration of ciprofloxacin in the tissue of patients to the severity of PAD, the number of medications that the patient was taking and plasma ciprofloxacin concentration is:

$$Expected\ C_{tissue} = 0.2366 + 1.3416\ (PAD_1) + 0.215\ (PAD_2) - 0.0093\ (Meds) + 0.0175C_{plasma}$$

where:

C_{tissue} = ciprofloxacin tissue concentration in μg/g

PAD_1 = 1 for patients with nil/borderline PAD; PAD_1 = 0 for patients with mild/moderate or severe PAD

PAD_2 = 1 for patients with mild/moderate PAD; PAD_2 = 0 for patients with mild/borderline or severe PAD

Meds = number of medications that the patient was taking

C_{plasma} = concentration of ciprofloxacin in plasma in μg/g.

3.6. Testing the Developed Regression Model

Values for the concentration of ciprofloxacin in tissue which were determined by HPLC analysis were comparable to those attained by the regression model and any differences between the values were not significant. The average results for the concentration of ciprofloxacin in tissue calculated by HPLC and by the regression model were 0.125μg/ml (±0.007), 0.12μg/ml (±0.014), 0.11μg/ml (±0.000), 0.115μg/ml (±0.007), 0.125 μg/ml (±0.021), 0.11μg/ml (±0.000), 0.18μg/ml (±0.000), 0.345μg/ml (±0.035), 0.345μg/ml (±0.007) and 0.335μg/ml (±0.007) (Table 5) (Vella et al., 2015).

Table 5. Testing the regression model

Patient code	Number of medications	[Ciprofloxacin in plasma] (μg/ml)	Severity of PAD	[Ciprofloxacin] in tissue calculated by model (μg/ml)	[Ciprofloxacin] in tissue calculated by HPLC (μg/ml)
3.	10	2.07	Severe	0.12	0.13
7.	13	1.78	Severe	0.11	0.13
12.	7	3.41	Severe	0.11	0.11
15.	9	1.95	Severe	0.12	0.11
21.	9	0.99	Severe	0.14	0.11
25.	10	1.95	Severe	0.11	0.11
26.	3	1.60	Severe	0.18	0.18
28.	7	3.96	Mild/moderate	0.32	0.37
40.	7	2.80	Mild/moderate	0.34	0.35
43.	12	0.10	Mild/moderate	0.34	0.33

DISCUSSION

The findings of this study are consistent with those made in previous pharmacokinetic studies where ciprofloxacin plasma concentrations are higher than those in tissue after 30 to 60 minutes from administration (Licitra et al., 1987; Brunner et al., 1999; Brunner et al., 2002).

The tissue concentrations of ciprofloxacin were lower in patients suffering from severe PAD. The reason for this is probably due to poor peripheral perfusion in patients suffering from more severe forms of the disease preventing larger concentrations of ciprofloxacin from reaching the site of interest. Dose adjustment is necessary to help achieve concentrations of the antibacterial drug which are higher than the minimum inhibitory concentration against most bacteria causing the infection.

Patients who were receiving a greater number of medications to treat their comorbidities, had lower tissue concentrations of ciprofloxacin. Ciprofloxacin is excreted mostly unchanged, and only about 10-20% of the administered dose is metabolized (Wilson and Grüneberg, 1997; Anadón et al., 2001). Ciprofloxacin is an inhibitor of CYP1A2 and affects the metabolism of other drugs being metabolized by the same enzyme (Zhang et al., 2008). It is unlikely that drug interactions, due to enzyme metabolism and competitive inhibition are the reason for lower tissue concentrations of ciprofloxacin.

A possible reason why ciprofloxacin concentrations are lower in the tissue of patients taking a greater number of medications, could be due to the comorbidities present in this group of patients. The most common comorbidities in this group of patients were diabetes, hypertension, ischemic heart disease and congestive heart failure (Table 4). These four conditions may cause rarefaction, which is a consequence of vascular remodeling. Rarefaction is related to vessel damage and inflammation and peripheral resistance, which can be with or without structural changes (Nusz et al., 2003; Hoenig et al., 2008; Gilbert, 2013; Gonzalez et al., 2013).

The predicted values of ciprofloxacin tissue concentrations which were estimated using the parsimonious regression model were very similar to the ciprofloxacin concentrations determined when using HPLC. This demonstrates that the model developed can be effectively applied in a clinical setting when trying to predict the concentration of ciprofloxacin which reaches the affected tissue and hence identifying patients who may be at risk of infection due to inadequate levels of ciprofloxacin reaching the site of infection. This will help determine whether the concentration of ciprofloxacin at the site of interest lies above the minimum inhibitory concentration against the bacteria causing the infection. Knowledge of the concentration of ciprofloxacin in plasma, the severity of PAD, if present and the number of medications that the patient is taking to treat any comorbidities can help determine the concentration of ciprofloxacin in the tissue. This knowledge can support the clinical team in the successful treatment of the infection.

Conclusion

The developed and validated methods for the determination of ciprofloxacin in patient plasma and tissue are adequate for high throughput analysis in the clinical setting due to the short run time (less than 6 minutes) and the need for small sample volumes (400μl). The methods are simple to use, have good accuracy and precision and high sensitivity and selectivity.

The developed parsimonious model can be effectively applied in a clinical setting, to help predict the concentration of ciprofloxacin which is likely to reach the affected tissue. This can help in the administration of an appropriate individualized dose of ciprofloxacin, possibly decreasing the occurrence of complications and reducing the need for surgical interventions.

References

Althouse, Andrew D, Abbott, J Dawn, Forker, Alan D, Bertolet, Marianne, Barinas-Mitchell, Emma, Thurston, Rebecca C. 2014. Risk factors for incident peripheral arterial disease in type 2 diabetes: results from the bypass angioplasty revascularization investigation in type 2 diabetes (BARI 2D) trial. *Diabetes Care* 37: 1346-52.

Anadón, Arturo, Martínez-Larrañga, Maria Rosa, Iturbe, Javier, Martínez, Maria A, Díaz, Maria J. Frejo Maria T et al., 2001. Pharmacokinetics and residues of ciprofloxacin and its metabolites in broiler chickens. *Res Vet Sci* 71: 101-9.

Armstrong, David, G, Cohen, Kelman, Courric, Stephane, Bharara, Manish, Marston, William. 2011. Diabetic foot ulcers and vascular insufficiency: our population has changed, but our methods have not. *J Diabetes Sci Technol* 5: 1591-5.

Bérard, Annie M, Bedel, Aurelie, Le Trequesser, Remi, Freyburger, Genevieve, Nurden, Alan, Colomer, Sylvie. 2013. Novel risk factors for premature peripheral arterial occlusive disease in non-diabetic patients: a case-control study. *PLoS One*. 8: e37882.

Biscetti, Federico, Porreca, Carlo F, Bertucci, Flavio, Straface, Giuseppe, Santoliquido, Angelo, Tondi, Paolo et al., 2014. TNFRSF11B gene polymorphisms increased risk of peripheral arterial occlusive disease and critical limb ischemia in patient with type 2 diabetes. *Acta Diabetol*. 51: 1025-32.

Bozkir, Asuman, Denli, Zeynep F, Basaran, Bemin. 2012. Effect of hydroxypropyl-β-cyclodextrin on the solubility, stability and in vitro release of ciprofloxacin for ocular drug delivery. *Acta Pol Pharm.* 69: 719-24.

Brunner, Martin, Hollenstein, Ursula, Delacher, Simon, Jäger, Dorothea, Schmid, Rainer, Lackner, Edith et al., 1999. Distribution and antimicrobial activity of ciprofloxacin in human soft tissues. *Antimicrob Agents Chemother*. 43:1307-9.

Brunner, Martin, Staβ, Heino, Möller, Jan-Georg, Schrolnberger, Claudia, Erovic, Boban, Hollenstein, Ursula et al., 2002. Target site concentrations of ciprofloxacin after single intravenous and oral doses. *Antimicrob Agents Chemother*. 46: 3724-30.

Buechler, Kenneth F, Beynen, Anton C, Geelen, Math J. 1984. Studies on the assay, activity and sedimentation behaviour of acetyl-CoA carboxylase from isolated hepatocytes incubated with insulin or glucagon. *Biochem J*. 221: 869-74.

Chu, Yuejie, Wang, Chao, Zhang, Jinghang, Wang, Penghua, Xu, Jun, Ding, Min. 2015. Can We Stop Antibiotic Therapy When Signs and Symptoms Have Resolved in Diabetic Foot Infection Patients? *Int J Low Extrem Wounds*. 14: 277-83.

Criqui, Michael H, Aboyans, Victor. 2015. Epidemiology of Peripheral Arterial Disease. *Circ Res*. 116:1509-26.

De Witte, Bavo, Dewulf, Jo, Demeestere, Kristol, De Ruyck, Michael, Van Langenhove, Herman. 2007. Critical points in the analysis of ciprofloxacin by high-performance liquid chromatography. *J Chromatogr A*. 1140: 126-30.

Ding, Shimei, Qu, Wei, Dang, Shuangsuo, Xie, Xuan, Xu, Jing, Wang, Yuhuan. 2014. Serum nesfatin-1 is reduced in Type 2 diabetes mellitus patients with peripheral arterial disease. *Med SciMonit*. 4:987-91.

Filigenzi, Michael S, Puschner, Birgit, Aston, Linda S, Poppenga, Robert H. 2008. Diagnostic determination of melamine and related compounds in kidney tissue by liquid chromatography/tandem mass spectrometry. *J Agric. Food Chem*. 56: 7593-9.

Garcia, MA, Solans, C, Aramayona, JJ, Rueda, S, Bregante, MA, de Jong, A. 1999. Simultaneous determination of enrofloxacin and its primary metabolite, ciprofloxacin, in plasma by HPLC with fluorescence detection. *Biomed. Chromatogr*. 13: 350-3.

Garrelts, James C, Jost, Gary, Kowalsky, Steven F, Krol, George J, Lettieri, John T. 1996. Ciprofloxacin pharmacokinetics in burn patients. *Antimicrob Agents Chemother*. 40:1153-6.

Gemechu, Fassil W, Seemant, Fnu, Curley, Catherine A. 2013. Diabetic foot infections. *Am Fam Physician*. 88: 177-84.

Gilbert, Richard E. 2013. Endothelial loss and repair in the vascular complications of diabetes. *Circ J*. 77:849-56.

Gonzalez-Quesada, Carlos, Cavalera, Michele, Biernacka, Anna, Kong Ping, Lee Dong-Wook, Saxena Amit, et al., 2013. Thrombospondin-1 induction in the diabetic myocardium stabilizes the cardiac matrix, while promoting vascular rarefaction through angiopoietin-2 upregulation. *Circ Res*. 113:1131-44.

Hardman, Rulon L, Jazaeri, Omid, Yi J, Smith M, Gupta, Rajan. 2014. Overview of classification systems in Peripheral Arterial Disease. *Semin Intervent Radiol.* 31: 378-88.

Hendriks, Gert. 2009. Theoretical models in LC based bioanalytical method development. *J Pharm Biomed Anal.* 49: 1-10.

Hiarata, Cheryl A, Guay, David R, Awni, Walid M, Stein, Daniel J, Peterson, Phillip K. 1989. Steady-state pharmacokinetics of intravenous and oral ciprofloxacin in elderly patients. *Antimicrob Agents Chemother.* 33: 1927-31.

Hoenig, Michel R, Bianchi, Cesario, Rosenzweig, Anthony, Sellke, Frank W. 2008. The cardiac microvasculature in hypertension, cardiac hypertrophy and diastolic heart failure. *Curr Vasc Pharmacol.* 6: 292-300.

International Conference on Harmonisation (ICH). Validation of analytical procedures: text and methodology Q2(R1) [Online] 2005 Nov [cited 2018 January 11]. *ICH.* Available from: URL: http://www.ich.org/fileadmin/Public_Web_Site/ICH_Products/Guidelines/Quality/Q2_R1/Step4/Q2_R1__Guideline.pdf.

Kataoka, Hiroyuki. 2003. New trends in sample preparation for clinical and pharmaceutical analysis. *Trends Analyt Chem.* 22: 232-4.

Khan, Khalid M, Khan, Farid M. 2005. Extraction and separation of ciprofloxacin by HPLC from human plasma. *Int Chem Pharm Med J.* 2: 267-70.

Kisozi, Twaha, Mutebi, Edris, Kisekka, Musubire, Lhatoo, Samden, Sajatovic, Martha, Kaddumukasa, Mark. 2017. Prevalence, severity and factors associated with peripheral neuropathy among newly diagnosed diabetic patients attending Mulago hospital: a cross-sectional study. *Afr Health Sci.* 17: 463-73.

Licitra, Carmelo M, Brooks, Robert G, Sieger, Barry E. 1987. Clinical efficacy and levels of ciprofloxacin in tissue in patients with soft tissue infection. *Antimicrob Agents Chemother.* 31: 805-7.

Mafra, Luis, Santos, Sergio M, Siegel, Renee, Alves, Ines, Paz, Filipe A, Dudenko, Dmytro et al., 2012. Packing interactions in hydrated and anhydrous forms of the antibiotic ciprofloxacin: a solid- state NMR, X-ray diffraction, and computer simulation study. *J Am Chem Soc*. 134: 71-4.

Mao, Yong, Huang, Yixiang, Yu, Haining, Xu, Peng, Yu, Guangping, Yu, Jinming et al., 2017. Incidence of peripheral arterial disease and its association with pulse pressure: a prospective cohort study. *Front Endocrinol*. 8: 333.

Mills, Joseph L, Conte, Michael S, Armstrong, David G, Pomposelli, Frank B, Schanzer, Andres, Sidawy, Anton N et al., 2014. The society for vascular surgery lower extremity threatened limb classification system: risk stratification based on wound, ischemia and foot infection (WIfI). *J Vasc Surg*. 59: 220-34.

Muchohi, Simon N, Thuo, Nahashon, Karisa, Japhet, Muturi, Alex, Kokwaro, Gilbert, Maitland, Kathryn. 2011. Determination of ciprofloxacin in human plasma using high-performance liquid chromatography coupled with fluorescence detection: application to a population pharmacokinetics study in children with severe malnutrition. *J Chromatogr B Analyt Technol Biomed Life Sci*. 879: 146-52.

Müller, Markus, Brunner, Martin, Hollenstein, Ursula, Jouhadar, Christian, Schmid, Rainer, Minar, Erich et al., 1999. Penetration of ciprofloxacin into the interstitial space of inflamed foot lesions in non-insulin-dependent diabetes mellitus patients. *Antimicrob Agents Chemother*. 43: 2056-8.

Neckel, Ulrike, Johkhadara, Christian, Frossard, Martin, Jägerc, Walter, Müller, Markus, Mayer, Bernhard X. 2002. Simultaneous determination of levofloxacin and ciprofloxacin in microdialysates and plasma by high-performance liquid chromatography. *Anal Chim Acta*. 463: 199-206.

Nusz, David J, White, David C, Dai, Qunsheng, Pippen, Anne M, Thompson, Micheal A, Walton, G Brant. 2003. Vascular rarefaction in peripheral skeletal muscle after experimental heart failure. *Am J Physiol Heart Circ Physiol*. 285(4): 1554-62.

Park, Tae H, Anand, Ashish. 2015. Management of diabetic foot: brief synopsis for busy orthopedist. *J Clin Orthop Trauma*. 6: 24-9.

Rossi, David T, Sinz, Michael. 2012. *Mass spectrometry in drug discovery*. 1st ed. New York: Marcel Dekker Inc.

Stein, Gary E, Schooley, Sharon, Peloquin, Charles A, Missavage, Anne, Havlicheck, Daniel H. 2007. Linezolid tissue penetration and serum activity against strains of methicillin-resistant *Staphylococcus auerus* with reduced vancomycin susceptibility in diabetic patients with foot infections. *J AntimicrobChemother*. 60: 819-23.

Sun, Feng, Ong, Jasmine C, Yu, Qiang, Chan, Eli. 2011. Quantification of 3-deazaneplanocin A, a novel epigenetic anticancer agent, in rat biosamples by hydrophilic interaction liquid chromatography-tandem mass spectrometric detection. *J Chromatogr B Analyt Technol Biomed Life Sci*. 879: 285-90.

Tehan, Peta E, Barwick, Alex L, Sebastian, Mathew, Chuter, Vivienne H. 2017. Diagnostic accuracy of resting systolic toe pressure for diagnosis of peripheral arterial disease in people with and without diabetes: a cross-sectional retrospective case-control study. *J Foot Ankle Res*. 10:58.

Tiwari, Shalbha, Pratyush, Daliparthy D, Dwivedi, Awanridra, Gupta, Sunjit K, Rai, Madhukar, Singh, Surya K. 2012. Microbiological and clinical characteristics of diabetic foot infections in northern India. *J Infect Dev Ctries*. 6:329-32.

Vella, Janis, Mifsud, Martina, Sammut-Bartolo, Nicolette, Ferrito, Victor, Serracino-Inglott, Anthony, Azzopardi, Lilian M. 2014. The combined effects of pH and acetonitrile composition on the separation of two lincosamide antibiotics. *Asian J Pharm Clin Res*. 7:96-100.

Vella, Janis, Busuttil, Francesca, Sammut-Bartolo, Nicolette, Sammut, Carmel, Ferrito, Victor, Serracino-Inglott, Anthony. 2015. A simple HPLC-UV method for the determination of ciprofloxacin in human plasma. *J. Chromatogr B Analyt Technol Biomed Life Sci*. 989:80-5.

Vella, Janis, Vella, Maria, Cassar, Kevin, Camilleri, Liberato, Serracino-Inglott, Anthony, Azzopardi, Lilian M et al., 2016. Factors affecting penetration of ciprofloxacin in lower extremity ischaemic tissues. *Int J Low Extrem Wounds*. 15: 126-31.

Venn, Richard F. 2005. *Principles and practice of bioanalysis*, 2nd edition. London: Taylor and Francis.

Weber, Alan, Chaffin, Donald, Smith, Arnold, Opheim, Kent E. 1985. Quantitation of ciprofloxacin in body fluids by high-pressure liquid chromatography. *Antimicrob Agents Chemother.* 27: 531-4.

Wilson, AP, Grüneberg, RN. 1997. *Ciprofloxacin: 10 years of clinical experience.* Oxford: Maxim Medical.

Yu Chongwoo, Cohen Lucinda H. 2004. Tissue sample preparation- not the same old grind. *LC GC Eur.* 17: 1-6.

Zhang, Li, Wei, Min-ji, Zhao, Cai-yun, Qi, Hui-min. 2008. Determination of the inhibitory potential of 6 fluoroquinolones on CYP1A2 and CYP2C9 in human liver microsomes. *Acta Pharmacol Sin.* 29: 1507-14.

Zhou, Michael. 2011. *Regulated bioanalytical laboratories: technical and regulatory aspects from global perspectives.* 1st ed. New Jersey: Wiley.

In: Ciprofloxacin
Editor: Mohamed Said Attia
ISBN: 978-1-53614-534-2

Chapter 4

CIPROFLOXACIN AND BACTERIAL PATHOGENS: CORRELATION TO MICROBIAL RESISTANCE

Neveen M. Saleh[1]*, PhD, Mohamed M. Abd-Almouty, PhD and Mona I. Mabrouk, PhD
Department of Microbiology,
National Organization for Drug Control and Research,
Giza, Egypt

ABSTRACT

Ciprofloxacin is a second-generation quinolone that has expanded Gram-negative activity and atypical pathogen coverage, but with limited Gram-positive activity. Ciprofloxacin for many years was considered as a drug choice for the treatment of different bacterial infection due to pharmacokinetics advantages. However, broad application of ciprofloxacin has been followed by the emergence of resistance using

* Corresponding Author Email: salehneveen@yahoo.com.

different mechanisms. Since ciprofloxacin is central to the management of severe infections; emerging resistance to this antibiotic is a paramount concern. More recently, outbreaks of ciprofloxacin-resistant bacterial infections were reported in many countries as United States, Taiwan, Egypt, and Japan. Bacterial resistance to ciprofloxacin is usually mediated by mutations in bacterial enzymes that are DNA gyrase (*gyrA* and *gyrB*) and topoisomerase IV (*parC* and *parE*) genes, as well as by active efflux alongside outer membrane proteins modification. Plasmid-mediated resistance to quinolones in Gram-negative bacteria has also been described.

Keywords: bacterial infection, ciprofloxacin activity, resistance mechanism

LIST OF ACRONYMS

A.	*Acinetobacter baumannii*
ABC	ATP-Binding Cassette
CoNS	Coagulase-Negative *Staphylococci*
H.	*Haemophilus*
IM	Inner membrane
K.	*Klebsiella*
LPS	Lipopolysaccharide
EP	Efflux pump
MAR	Major Facilitator Superfamily Resistance
MDR	Multi-Drug Resistant
MSSA	Methicillin-Sensitive *S. aureus*
MRSA	Methicillin-Resistant *S. aureus*
M.	*Mycobacteria*
MATE	Multidrug and Toxic Compound Extrusion
NGNB	Non-fermenting Gram-negative bacilli
P.	*Pseudomonas*
PG	Peptidoglycan
OMP	*Outer Membrane Proteins*
QRD	Quinolone Resistance Determining Region

ORF	Open Reading Frame
S.	*Streptococcus*
SMR	Small Multidrug Resistance
RND	Resistance Nodulation Division
VAP	Ventilator-Associated Pneumonia

INTRODUCTION

Ciprofloxacin belongs to a class of antibiotics known as quinolones. The active ingredient of ciprofloxacin works by killing the bacteria that cause gastrointestinal infections (travelers' diarrhea), urinary infections and other infections, thereby producing symptoms such as diarrhea, pain, and fever. It kills the bacteria by stopping a bacterial enzyme called DNA-gyrase from working. This enzyme is involved in replicating and repairing the genetic material (DNA) of the bacteria. If it doesn't work, the bacteria can't repair themselves or reproduce. This kills the bacteria and clears up the infection. A quinolone antibiotic is a member of a large group of broad-spectrum bactericides that have a bicyclic core structure related to the compound 4-quinolone (Norris and Mandell 1988). They are used in human and veterinary medicine for the treatment of bacterial infections. Nearly, all quinolone antibiotics in modern use are fluoroquinolone as ciprofloxacin, which contains a fluorine atom in their chemical structure and is effective against both Gram-negative and Gram-positive bacteria. Ciprofloxacin, one of the most widely used antibiotics worldwide and is a prescription-only medicine.

Fluoroquinolone, since the mid-1980s, have become a major group of synthetic antibiotics with activities against many pathogenic microorganisms starting from *Enterobacteriaceae* and opportunists such as *Pseudomonas aeruginosa* to the Gram-positive pathogens including *streptococc*i and *staphylococci*. In some areas such as pyelonephritis, gonorrhoea, enteric fevers, oral management of osteomyelitis, and *P. aeruginosa* infections, they have become drugs of choice, often replacing parenteral therapy with cephalosporins and aminoglycosides. However, bacterial resistance has appeared not only in predictable species such as staphylococci and *P. aeruginosa* but also among organisms such as *Escherichia coli,* which was initially thought unlikely to be compromised.

Ciprofloxacin Spectrum of Activity

Therapy of an infection must often be started before the causative microbe is identified. The spectrum of activity of the drug and knowledge of potentially resistant micro-organisms is therefore important. Ciprofloxacin is a second-generation fluoroquinolone with a broad spectrum of activity that usually results in the death of the bacteria (bactericidal). Its spectrum of activity includes most strains of bacterial pathogens responsible for respiratory, urinary tract, gastrointestinal, and abdominal infections, including Gram-positive and Gram-negative pathogens.

Ciprofloxacin Activity against Gram-Positive Isolates

Streptococcus pneumonia is an encapsulated Gram-positive bacterium often found in the nasopharynx of healthy children and adults as part of the normal flora. However, in certain instances, it can cause invasive diseases such as meningitis, bacteremia, bacteremic pneumonia and mucosal infections including otitis media and pneumonia (Deng et al. 2013). Ciprofloxacin demonstrated moderate activity against *S. pneumoniae* especially penicillin sensitive *S. pneumoniae* (Garrison 2003; Goldstein and Citron 1992; Hasegawa et al. 2006; Ho et al. 1999; Niki et al. 2011).

Streptococcus pyogenes, also known as group A streptococcus, is most commonly associated with mild, self-resolving infections of the skin and oropharynx. However, dissemination of the bacteria to normally sterile sites within the body can lead to a variety of invasive conditions that are associated with high morbidity and mortality (Reglinski and Sriskandan

2015). Ciprofloxacin showed variable activity against *S. pyogenes* strains (Orscheln et al. 2005; Van heirstraeten et al. 2012; Yan et al. 2008).

Staphylococcus aureus is one of the most frequently isolated bacterial pathogens in human clinics. Infections caused by this bacterium may affect any organ, and resistant strains have a significant participation in nosocomial infections (Prévost 2013). The activity of ciprofloxacin is only modest against methicillin-sensitive *S. aureus* (MSSA) (Bauernfeind 1997; Cormican and Jones 1997). However; clinically significant resistance to ciprofloxacin has developed for *S. aureus* especially methicillin-resistant *S. aureus* [MRSA] (Gilbert et al. 2001; Daum et al. 1990; Picazo et al. 2010; Niki et al. 2011) which correlates with the rapid loss of the clinical utility of ciprofloxacin for *S. aureus* infections.

Coagulase-Negative Staphylococci (CoNS) as typical opportunists, represent one of the major nosocomial pathogens, having a substantial impact on human life and health. They are particularly associated with the use of indwelling or implanted foreign bodies, which are indispensable in modern medicine (Becker, Heilmann, and Peters 2014). Data suggest that ciprofloxacin may not be useful for the treatment of severe infection caused by CoNS, since the rates of ciprofloxacin resistance in CoNS are very high (Fajardo Olivares et al. 2011; Olivares et al. 2010),

Enterococcus faecalis and *Enterococcus faecium* are among the leading causative agents of nosocomial infections and are infamous for their resistance to many antibiotics (Paganelli, Willems, and Leavis 2012). Ciprofloxacin offer only decreased clinically important activity against enterococcal strains as it showed poorer activity against both *Enterococcus* species especially against vancomycin-resistant *Enterococcus spp.* (Hidalgo et al. 2008; Itokazu et al. 1996; Hardy et al. 2000).

Ciprofloxacin Activity against Gram-Negative Isolates

Enterobacteriaceae

The *Enterobacteriaceae* is a family of Gram-negative bacilli that are responsible for a broad range of infections in humans and animals. Among notable genera are *Escherichia, Salmonella, Enterobacter, Klebsiella, Citrobacter, Shigella, Morganella, Proteus,* and *Serratia* (Paterson 2012). One of the strong points of ciprofloxacin lay in its excellent activity against most species of *Enterobacteriaceae* such as *E. coli, Klebsiella pnumoniae, K. oxytoca, Proteus mirabilis P. vulgaris, Enterobacter cloacae, Enterobacter aerogenes, Citrobacter fruendii, Citrobacter koseri, Morganella morganii*, and *Serratia spp.* (Keepers et al. 2017; Sutherland and Nicolau 2015; Bouchillon et al. 2013; Lockhart et al. 2007; Rhomberg and Jones 2007; Sutherland, Verastegui, and Nicolau 2016; Hackel et al. 2015).

Salmonella and *Shigella* cause a well-characterized spectrum of disease in humans, ranging from asymptomatic carriage to hemorrhagic colitis and fatal typhoidal fever. These pathogens are responsible for millions of cases of food-borne illness in the U.S. each year, with substantial costs measured in hospitalizations and lost productivity (Dekker and Frank 2015). WHO diarrhea guidelines focus on rehydration, and the provision of zinc and they specifically address Shigella infections by recommending ciprofloxacin be given to children with dysentery (Tickell et al. 2017). Antimicrobial resistance has emerged in *Salmonella enterica*, to the traditional first-line drugs chloramphenicol, ampicillin, and trimethoprim-sulfamethoxazole (Mirza, Beeching, and Hart 1996). In response to the development and spread of MDR *Salmonella serovar* Typhi, the use of ciprofloxacin was recommended as an alternative for the treatment of typhoid fever (Parry and Threlfall 2008; Rowe, Ward, and Threlfall 1997). Although resistance to ciprofloxacin has been reported in many studies all over the world (Yoo et al. 2004; Aarestrup et al. 2003); the prevalence of fluoroquinolone-resistant isolates in United States found to be low (Crump et al. 2011).

Nonfermentative Gram-Negative Rods

Pseudomonas aeruginosa is a Gram-negative bacillus found widely in nature, in soil and water. Classified as an opportunistic pathogen, *P.*

aeruginosa causes disease infrequently in normal hosts but is a major cause of infection in patients with underlying conditions (Prince 2012). Ciprofloxacin is generally active against *P. aeruginosa* strains, however resistance to it is now common (Karlowsky et al. 2003; Keepers et al. 2017; Sutherland and Nicolau 2015; Bouchillon et al. 2013; Lockhart et al. 2007; Rhomberg and Jones 2007; Sutherland, Verastegui, and Nicolau 2016; Hackel et al. 2015).

Acinetobacter baumannii (*A. baumannii*) is an example of an opportunistic pathogen which is generally harmless to healthy individuals but can cause serious infections such as ventilator-associated pneumonia (VAP), wound infections and bacteraemias in critically ill hospital patients (James 2011). Activity against *A. baumannii* appears to vary considerably with a significant number of strains is now resistant to ciprofloxacin (Karlowsky et al. 2003; Hackel et al. 2015).

Nonfermenting Gram-negative bacilli (NFGNB) other than *P. aeruginosa* and *A. baumannii* have emerged as important healthcare-associated pathogens. The importance of isolation of non-fermenters such as *Stenotrophomonas maltophilia and Burkholderia cepacia*has increased in last decade after more and more reports are correlating them with either infection outbreaks in hospitals, or healthcare-associated infections (McGowan 2006). Many strains of NFGNB being susceptible to ciprofloxacin while others being resistant (Chawla, Vishwanath, and Munim 2013; Rhomberg and Jones 2007).

Ciprofloxacin Activity against Gram-Negative Coccobacilli

Haemophilus influenzae is a Gram-negative coccobacillus frequently isolated from the sputum of individuals with influenza pneumonia (High, Fan, and Schwartzman 2015). It is among the most common causes of bacterial meningitis and other invasive infections in infants and young children throughout the world (Steinhoff, Cherian, and Schlaudecker 2011). Ciprofloxacin has strong antibacterial activity against most *H.*

influenza strains (Biedenbach et al. 2012; Melo-Cristino and Serrano 2006; Hasegawa et al. 2006).

M. catarrhalis is a mucosal pathogen, causing infections of the upper respiratory tract in young children and the lower respiratory tract in adults with chronic lung disease. *M. catarrhalis* is the third most common cause of otitis media in children (after *Haemophilus influenzae* and *Streptococcus pneumoniae) (Cooke and Slack 2017)*. Many studies reported a potent activity of ciprofloxacin against *M. catarrhalis* strains (Hsu et al. 2012; Gupta, Arora, and Kundra 2011; Pingault et al. 2010; Biedenbach et al. 2012).

Ciprofloxacin Activity against Anaerobic Bacteria

Infections caused by anaerobic bacteria are common, arise from the sites where they are normal flora (endogenous) and can be serious or life-threatening. Anaerobic bacteria are fastidious, difficult to isolate, and often overlooked (Brook and Long 2012). Ciprofloxacin has not, so far, been considered the drug of choice for anaerobic infections since the activity of it was only marginal (Appelbaum 1999; Stein and Goldstein 2006). It was reported that ciprofloxacin lacked *in vitro* potency against many important anaerobic bacteria such as *Bacteroides spp., Clostridium spp., Propionibacterium acnes, Peptococcus spp., Fusobacterium spp., and prevotella spp.* (Fernandes et al. 1986; Goldstein and Citron 1992).

Ciprofloxacin Activity against Mycobacteria

Mycobacterial diseases often require prolonged therapy with multidrug regimens. Fluoroquinolone have excellent bactericidal activity against many mycobacterial species, including most strains of *Mycobacterium tuberculosis* complex and *M. fortuitum*, and some strains of *M. kansasii*, *M. avium-intracellulare* complex, and *M. leprae*. In addition; fluoroquinolones achieve effective serum, tissue, and intracellular levels following oral administration; and produce few adverse effects. These properties have led to the increasing use of fluoroquinolones including ciprofloxacin for the treatment of mycobacterial infections especially tuberculosis and leprosy (Alangaden and Lerner 1997; Jacobs 1995; Castro, Navarro, and Biot 2013). Ciprofloxacin is especially most active against rapidly growing mycobacteria (i.e., *M. fortuitum*) (Kawahara, Tada, and Nagare 2001).

Ciprofloxacin Activity against *Bacillus anthracis*

Bacillus anthracis, a Gram-Positive, rod-shaped, aerobic, immobile, capsulated, spore-forming bacterium belonging to the family *Bacillacae;* is the causative agent of anthrax (Pontieri 2016; Constable et al. 2017). Although the vegetative form of *B. anthracis* is not very robust, the spores persist in the environment for decades, easily withstand cold temperatures, and even survive in dried and salted hides (Constable et al. 2017). Because of the mortality associated with inhalational anthrax, two or more antimicrobial agents predicted to be effective are recommended; ciprofloxacin or doxycycline should be used for initial intravenous therapy until antimicrobial susceptibility results are known (CDC 2001). For cutaneous anthrax, ciprofloxacin and doxycycline also are first-line therapy (CDC 2001). Many studies reported that ciprofloxacin has potent activity against *B. anthracis* (Jones et al. 2003; Mohammed et al. 2002; Ortatatli et al. 2012; Kreizinger et al. 2016).

Ciprofloxacin Clinical Indications

The licensed uses for ciprofloxacin in the United States are quite limited, and it is to be considered as a drug of the final resort when all other antibiotics have failed (Sharma et al. 2010). Ciprofloxacin is the only fluoroquinolone agent approved for Gram-negative bone and joint infections. It is also the primary fluoroquinolone approved for gastrointestinal infections, including infectious diarrhea (when therapy is warranted) and typhoid fever (Bolon 2011).

Ciprofloxacin is approved for treatment of the following:

* In adult patients

- Urinary Tract Infections caused by *Escherichia coli, Klebsiella pneumoniae, Enterobacter cloacae, Serratia marcescens, Proteus mirabilis, Providencia rettgeri, Morganella morganii, Citrobacter diversus, Citrobacter freundii, Pseudomonas aeruginosa*, methicillin-susceptible *Staphylococcus epidermidis, Staphylococcus saprophyticus, or Enterococcus faecalis*.
- Acute Uncomplicated Cystitis in females caused by *Escherichia coli or Staphylococcus saprophyticus*.
- Chronic Bacterial Prostatitis caused by *Escherichia coli or Proteus mirabilis.*
- Lower Respiratory Tract Infections caused by *Escherichia coli, Klebsiella pneumoniae, Enterobacter cloacae, Proteus mirabilis, Pseudomonas aeruginosa, Haemophilus influenzae, Haemophilus parainfluenzae,* or penicillin-susceptible *Streptococcus pneumoniae.* Also, *Moraxella catarrhalis* for the treatment of acute exacerbations of chronic bronchitis

NOTE: Although effective in clinical trials, ciprofloxacin is not a drug of first choice in the treatment of presumed or confirmed pneumonia secondary to *Streptococcus pneumoniae*.

- Acute Sinusitis caused by *Haemophilus influenzae, penicillin-susceptible Streptococcus pneumoniae,* or *Moraxella catarrhalis*.
- Skin and Skin Structure Infections caused by *Escherichia coli, Klebsiella pneumoniae Enterobacter cloacae, Proteus mirabilis, Proteus vulgaris, Providencia stuartii, Morganella morganii, Citrobacter freundii, Pseudomonas aeruginosa*, methicillin-

susceptible *Staphylococcus aureus*, methicillin-susceptible *Staphylococcus epidermidis*, or *Streptococcus pyogenes*.

- Bone and Joint Infections caused by *Enterobacter cloacae, Serratia marcescens,* or *Pseudomonas aeruginosa.*
- Complicated Intra-Abdominal Infections (used in combination with metronidazole) caused by *Escherichia coli, Pseudomonas aeruginosa, Proteus mirabilis, Klebsiella pneumoniae,* or *Bacteroides fragilis.*
- Infectious Diarrhea caused by *Escherichia coli* (enterotoxigenic strains), *Campylobacter jejuni, Shigella boydii, Shigella dysenteriae, Shigella flexneri or Shigella sonnei* when antibacterial therapy is indicated
- Typhoid Fever (Enteric Fever) caused by *Salmonella* enterica serovar Typhi

NOTE: The efficacy of ciprofloxacin in the eradication of the chronic typhoid carrier state has not been demonstrated.

* In pediatric patients (1 to 17 years of age)

- Complicated Urinary Tract Infections and Pyelonephritis due to *Escherichia coli*

NOTE: Although effective in clinical trials, ciprofloxacin is not a drug of first choice in the pediatric population due to an increased incidence of adverse events compared to controls, including events related to joints and/or surrounding tissues

* Adult and Pediatric Patients

- Inhalational anthrax (post-exposure): To reduce the incidence or progression of disease following exposure to aerosolized *Bacillus anthracis.*

Bacterial Resistance Mechanism

Bacterial Replication

Bacterial chromosome is composed of a single, double-stranded DNA circle greater than 1000 µm that undergo tertiary folding and compaction to decrease its volume to suit inside a bacterial cell and that is accomplished by several approaches: (1) macromolecular crowding created by the high concentration of solutes in the cytoplasm, (2) long-range DNA folding into 50–80 topologically independent domains, (3) negative DNA supercoiling, (4) the existence of small DNA is bending proteins.

DNA synthesis occurs at a rate of 50 000 bp/min/ replication fork and for replication to occur efficiently, the DNA strands must separate, and tangles, precatenates (crossovers), knots and catenates (intermolecular links) must be removed from the bacterial chromosome. However, bacteria produce enzymes called DNA topoisomerase that control and modulate the topology of the chromosomal DNA to facilitate replication, recombination, and expression. Two of these enzymes, DNA gyrase, and DNA topoisomerase IV, are targets of the fluoroquinolone (Drlica and Zhao 1997a) and both have different physiological functions, despite they have mechanistic and structural similarities (Champoux 2001; Gentry and Osheroff 2013; Levine, Hiasa, and Marians 1998; Pommier et al. 2010).

Bacterial DNA Topoisomerases II

The DNA cleavage and ligation reactions, which contains the core of enzyme function, use a non-canonical two-metal-ion mechanism (Schmidt et al. 2010; Deweese and Osheroff 2010; Pitts et al. 2011). Gyrase and topoisomerase IV generate staggered cuts in the DNA backbone that are 4 bp apart and on opposite strands (leaving a 5′-overhang). To maintain genomic integrity during this process, the enzyme form covalent bonds between active site tyrosine residues and the generated 5′-DNA termini (2,4-5,9) union. These covalent enzyme-cleaved DNA complexes are known as "cleavage complexes."

DNA Gyrase

DNA gyrase is a tetramer comprise two subunits A and two B, encoded by the gyrA (100-kilodalton Protein) and gyrB (90-kilodalton protein) genes, respectively Figure 1. This essential bacterial enzyme, discovered in 1976 in Escherichia coli by Gellert and co-workers (Gellert 1981), contains gyrA and gyrB are detected at 48 and 83 min, on the E. coli genome, but in some bacteria they are adjacent to each other and oriA; this configuration is known as the fluoroquinolone resistance determining region (QRDR) (Tillotson, Dorrian, and Blondeau 1997; Wiedemann and Heisig 1994). GyrA contains the active site tyrosine residue where gyrB contains the ATPase domain and the TOPRIM domain, which binds the divalent metal ions involved in DNA cleavage and ligation. DNA gyrase is the only of type II topoisomerase that introducing negative supercoil into DNA, responsible for removing topological stress arising from the translocation of transcription and replication complexes along DNA (Figure 2). In addition, gyrase to set the superhelical density of the bacterial chromosome should be work in conjunction with the ω protein (a type I topoisomerase) (Levine, Hiasa, and Marians 1998; Champoux 2001; Pommier et al. 2010; Gentry and Osheroff 2013).

Topoisomerase IV

Topoisomerase IV is a homolog of DNA gyrase, comprising four subunits, two of both C and E, encoded by means of parC and parE genes, and GrlA and GrlB in Gram-negative and in Gram-positive bacteria, respectively (Figure 1). The topoisomerase IV locus was described in 1990 (Andriole 2005) and a number of fluoroquinolone resistance markers had already been described and mapped to this locus. In *Staphylococcus aureus*, the flq locus, now called as grlA, is equivalent to parC in different bacteria that includes S*treptococcus pneumoniae*.

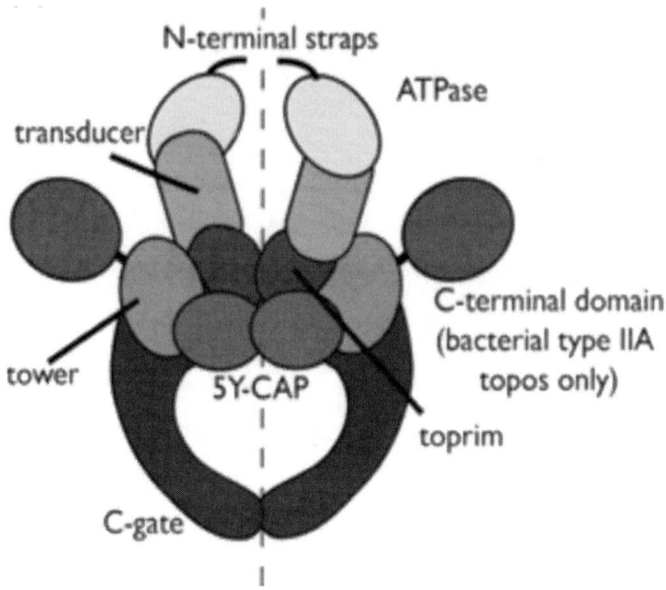

Figure. 1. DNA gyrase and Topoisomerase IV structure (Schoeffler and Berger 2005).

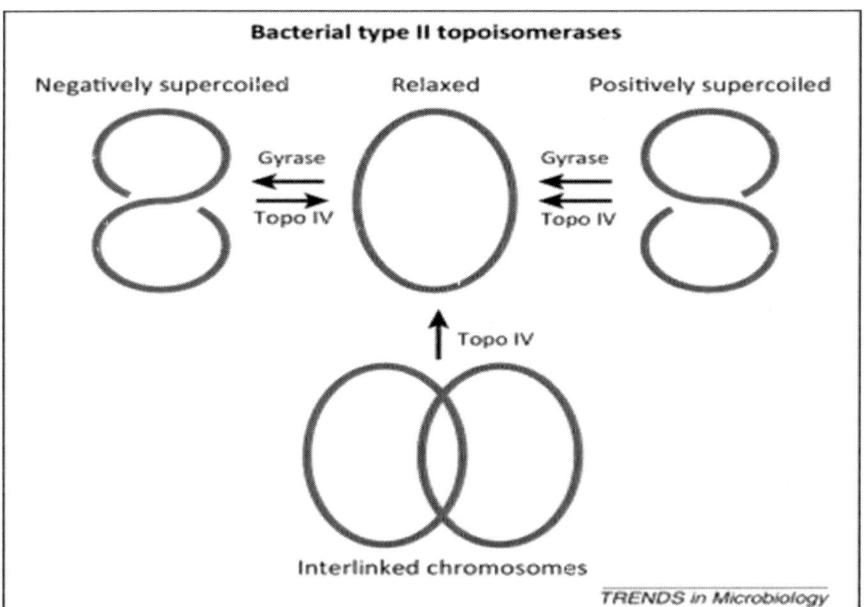

Figure 2. Bacterial type II topoisomerase (Gyrase and topoisomerase IV) function showing supercoiled action (Figure adapted from (Schoeffler and Berger 2005).

In *E. coli*, the nfxD locus is now parE. The reaction mechanism of topoisomerase IV is similar to that of gyrase but topoisomerase IV binds to DNA crossovers rather than wrapping DNA. Similarly, Topoisomerase IV is involved in decatenation, the unlinking of replicated daughter chromosomes and is removing knots that acquire within the bacterial chromosome as a result of fundamental cellular approaches Figure 2 (Zechiedrich et al. 2000; Deibler, Rahmati, and Zechiedrich 2001; Pommier et al. 2010; Levine, Hiasa, and Marians 1998; Champoux 2001).

Mechanism of Enzyme Action

Gyrase and topoisomerase IV modulate the topological state of DNA via wrapping DNA into a positive supercoil and then passing an intact double helix through a temporary double-stranded break that they generate in a separate segment of DNA. This technique is an ATP -dependent process. In the presence of ATP, the system is driven forward, increasing supercoiling, however, in the absence of ATP, the process is driven back again, relaxing the DNA. Preserving the DNA chromosome wound into loops allows the movement of replication forks (Aldred, Kerns, and Oshero 2014; Hooper 2001).

This topoisomerization process results in introduction (or removal) of DNA supercoils, thus affecting the negative supercoiling of DNA necessary to initiate DNA replication and remove positive supercoils that accumulate before an advancing replication fork, in case of gyrase where, in case of topoisomerase IV, the process results in separation of the interlocking of daughter DNA strands that arise during replication which facilitates the segregation of daughter DNA molecules into daughter cells Figure 3.

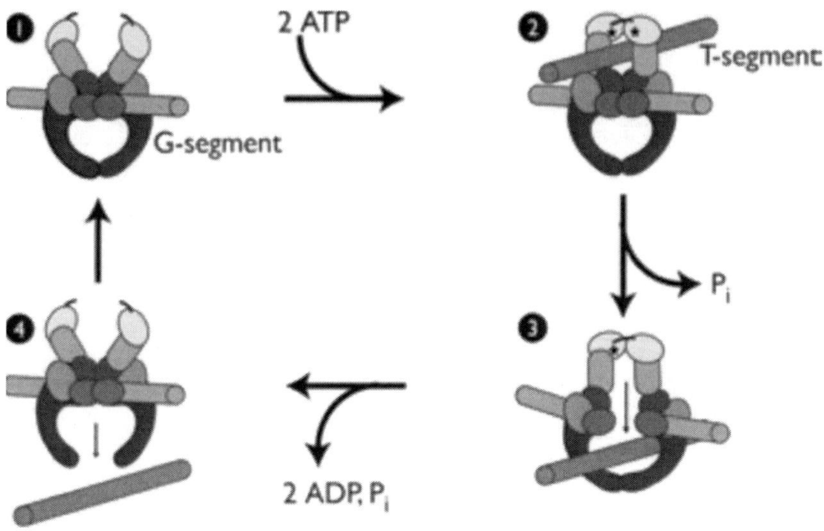

Figure 3. Modle for DNA gyrase mechanism of action showing supercoiling cycle figure provided by (Schoeffler and Berger 2005).

Mechanism of Drug Action

Ciprofloxacin, likely other fluoroquinolone antibiotics, directly inhibit bacterial DNA synthesis. Bacterial enzymes, type II topoisomerases, gyrase and topoisomerase IV, are the cellular targets for fluoroquinolone action (Anderson and Osheroff 2001; Drlica et al. 2009; Hooper 1999; Hooper 2001; Drlica et al. 2008). Ciprofloxacin mechanism of action onsets by interfering with bacterial DNA replication and transcription through inhibition of DNA gyrase/topoisomerase II and DNA topoisomerase IV (Drlica and Zhao 1997b; Oliphant and Green 2002).

Inhibition occurs by interaction of the fluoroquinolones with complexes that formed as a result of DNA and either of the two target enzymes with the formation of quinolone-enzyme-DNA complexes Figure 3. and thus, the generation of oxidative free radicals as singlet oxygen (1O2) and superoxide anion (O2-), and the subsequent cellular death (Chen et al. 1996; Umezawa et al. 1997; Hooper 2001).

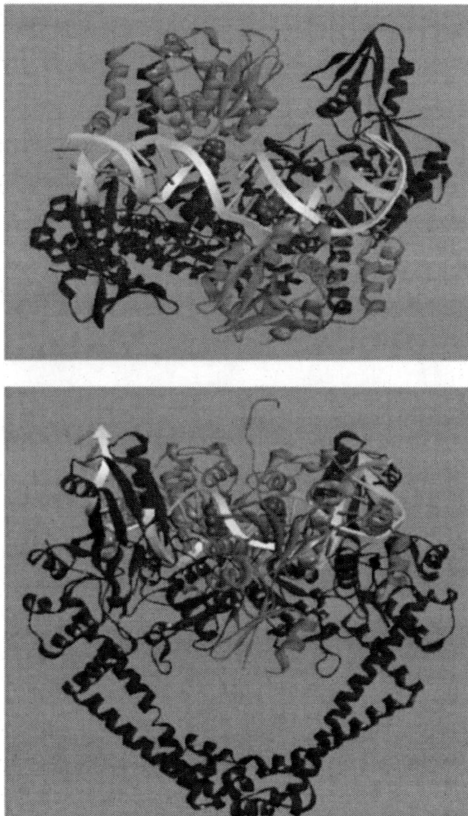

Figure 4. Crystal structure of a moxifloxacin-stabilized *Acinetobacter baumannii* topoisomerase IV−DNA cleavage complex. The catalytic core of the enzyme is shown. Moxifloxacin is colored red; the topoisomerase IV A and B subunits are colored blue and green, respectively, and DNA is colored yellow. The top panel is a top view of the cleavage complex showing two quinolone molecules intercalating 4 bp apart at the sites of DNA cleavage. The bottom panel is a front view (rotated by 90° from the top view) of the cleavage complex. Protein Data Bank accession 2XKK was visualized using Discovery Studio 3.5 Visualizer (Accelrys Software Inc.) (Wohlkonig, et al., 2010).

Additionally, in both topoisomerization reaction, the drug appears to trap the enzyme on DNA with forming a physical barrier the replication fork movement (Hiasa, Yousef, and Marians 1996), RNA polymerase (Willmott et al. 1994), and DNA helicase (Shea and Hiasa 1999). The collision of the replication fork with these trapped complexes triggers other poorly defined events within the cell that ultimately result in cell death Figure 4 (Hooper 1999; Hooper and Wolfson 1993).

The main target for Gram-negative bacterial inhibition was DNA gyrase, and in Gram-Positive bacterial activity corresponds with inhibition of DNA IV topoisomerase (Hooper 2000), in addition, Pan and co-works (Pan et al. 1996) as stated that DNA gyrase was the primary targets for fluoroquinolone but surprising, genetic studies in Streptococcus pneumonia found that topoisomerase IV, rather than gyrase, was the primary cellular target for ciprofloxacin.

Mechanism of Ciprofloxacin Resistance

During the past decades, attention has been given to bacterial resistance of bacteria to fluoroquinolone antibiotics especially ciprofloxacin. A resistance of fluoroquinolone described multiple mechanisms and significant clinical impact.

Mutations may occur rapidly during therapy with ciprofloxacin, which may be the most significant factor limiting the use of these group of antimicrobials. Mutations in Gram-negative and Gram-positive bacteria cause ciprofloxacin resistance by one or two basic main mechanistic categories, i) alterations in the drug target, and ii) alterations in the permeation of the drug to reach its target by modification in outer membrane proteins (OMP) and/or overexpression of efflux pump of antibiotics from cells. Fluoroquinolone/quinolone-modifying or-degrading enzymes haven't been reported as a mechanism of fluoroquinolone resistance Figure 5 (Hooper and Wolfson 1993; Hooper 1999; Hawkey 2003).

Target Enzymes Mutation

The most extensively studied resistance mechanism was alterations in target enzymes, which are localized to specific domains of each subunit. Spontaneous mutations in the genes, encoding the enzyme subunits, resulted from these alterations and thus can exist in small numbers (1 in

106 to 1 in 109 cells) in large bacterial populations. In gyrA and parC subunits of topoisomerase enzymes in resistant bacteria, the resistance occurs due to changes in amino acids, particularly in certain regions of each enzyme subunit called the fluoroquinolone-resistance-determining-region (QRDR), which make the enzyme less sensitive to inhibition by fluoroquinolone (Aldred, Kerns, and Oshero 2014). This region in the amino terminus has the active site, a tyrosine that is covalently linked to the broken DNA strand during enzyme action and the changes of amino acid reduce the affinity of the enzyme-DNA complex with a fluoroquinolone (Willmott and Maxwell 1993).

One of the common resistance mutations in GyrA, the change of serine at position 83 to tryptophan, causes reduced binding of quinolone to the gyrase-DNA complex that changes stated in *E. coli*, *Pseudomonas aeruginosa* and *Salmonella* sp. (Willmott and Maxwell 1993).

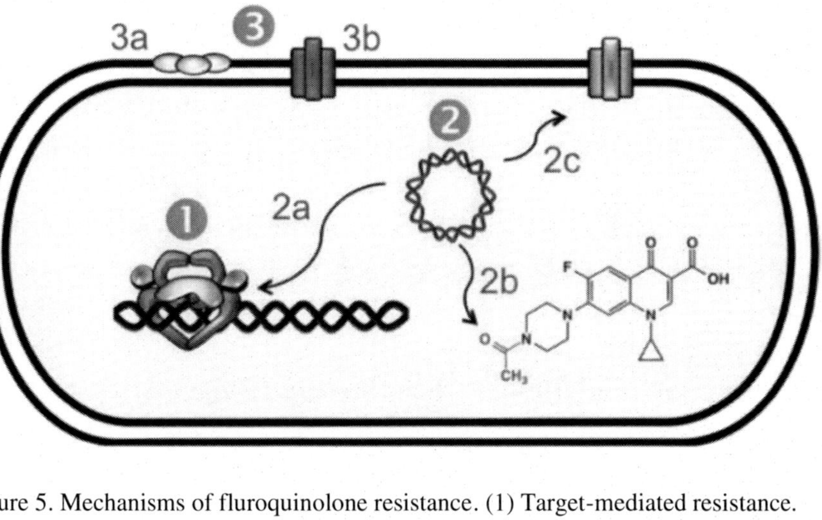

Figure 5. Mechanisms of fluroquinolone resistance. (1) Target-mediated resistance. Mutations in gyrase and topoisomerase IV weaken quinolone−enzyme interactions. (2) Plasmid-mediated resistance. (2a) Qnr proteins (yellow) decrease topoisomerase−DNA binding and protect enzyme− DNA complexes from quinolones. (2b) Aac(6′)-Ib-cr is an aminoglycoside acetyltransferase that acetylates the free nitrogen on the C7 ring of ciprofloxacin and norfloxacin, decreasing their effectiveness. (2c) Plasmid-encoded efflux pumps decrease the concentration of fluoroquinolone in the cell. (3) Chromosome-mediated resistance. (3a) Underexpression of porins in Gram-negative species decreases drug uptake. (3b) Overexpression of chromosome-encoded efflux pumps decreases drug retention in the cell. Adapted from reference Aldred et al. 2014.

Additionally, if amino acid changes present in gyrB and parE subunits of resistant bacteria are usually localized to the mid-portion of the subunit in a domain involved in interactions with their complementary subunits, mutations in these subunits are much less common than those in gyrA or parC. Studying the crystal structure of yeast topoisomerase II, which related to DNA gyrase and topoisomerase IV, had suggested that this resistance-determining domain was not in proximity to the resistance-determining domains of gyrA and parC (Berger et al. 1996). However, the structure of enzyme conformations suggested that the resistance-determining regions of both subunits might be in proximity during certain parts of the enzyme catalytic cycle, perhaps defining an enzyme conformation to which fluoroquinolone bind (Berger 1998).

In Gram-positive bacteria, as staphylococci and streptococci, mutations in parC are observed frequently in resistant isolates, and single transitions in parC sound to be sufficient to produce clinical resistance but without full resistance (Bast et al. 2000; Schmitz et al. 1998; Piddock et al. 2002) However, additional target mutations in such parC mutants will achieve enough clinical resistance (Hooper 2002) where resistance mutations that transform the structure of the gyrB and parE subunits are less popular than those altering the structure of gyrA and parC subunits. The level of resistance of a point enzyme can increase as other amino acids are changed by additional mutations (Fournier and Hooper 1998).

Decreased Accumulation of Ciprofloxacin Inside the Bacterial Cell

In the bacterial cell, both enzymes, DNA gyrase and topoisomerase IV, are in the cytoplasm, ciprofloxacin must traverse the peptidoglycan layer and the cell membrane of Gram-positive bacteria to reach its targets by simple diffusion and outer membrane layer of Gram-negative bacteria (Ng et al. 1994).

The antibiotic resistance caused by reduced accumulation was shown to require the presence and enhanced expression of endogenous efflux systems that actively pump drug from the cytoplasm and in Gram-negative bacteria is associated with reductions in porins but measurements of diffusion rates suggest that porin reductions alone are generally not sufficient to account for resistance (Nikaido and Thanassi 1993).

Efflux Pumps

The cell envelops of bacteria is considered as an initial formidable barrier, which provides a protection for bacteria against the external environment. Efflux pumps are endogenous efflux systems of proteins nature, inserted into cytoplasmic membrane, and these pumps have physiological functions as transporters with the responsibility for transport of a substance in and out of the cytoplasm. The main role of efflux pump is to be the removal of toxic substances from the cell and its membrane (I. T. Paulsen, Brown, and Skurray 1996). Among the array of efflux pumps found in bacteria, are the multi-drug resistance efflux pumps (MDR) that typically found in most, if not all, bacteria, including wild-type bacteria susceptible to antibiotics (Putman et al. 2000; Paulsen et al. 1996). The efflux pumps are stimulated by either the proton gradient across the cell membrane or by ATP hydrolysis.

In Gram-positive and Gram-negative bacteria, these systems typically have structural features of three components: 1) the efflux pump located in the cytoplasmic membrane, 2) an outer membrane protein, and a 3) membrane fusion protein thought to link both (Murakami et al. 2002) (Figure 6). To date, at least six major groups of active drug efflux pump transporters have been identified in bacteria: ATP-binding cassette (ABC), a major facilitator superfamily resistance, (MFS), small multidrug resistance (SMR), multi-antimicrobial resistance nodulation division (RND), and multidrug and toxic compound extrusion (MATE) (Lomovskaya et al. 2001; Nakayama et al. 2003).

The AcrAB-TolC system in *Salmonella* comprises the cytoplasmic membrane localized AcrB and the accessory protein AcrA, linking AcrB with the outer membrane protein (OMP) TolC (Elkins and Nikaido 2003). The overexpression of AcrAB-tolC is mediated by the transcriptional activators MarA and SoxS, which are regulated by MarR and SoxR proteins (Miller and Sulavik 1996; Rosner and Slonczewski 1994; Webber and Piddock 2001).

Resistance in most cases of bacteria can occur as a result of increased expression of these pumps that have been associated with low levels of fluoroquinolone resistance through increase transcription of the structural gene for the pump either from effects on the gene promoter or from alterations in other regulatory proteins that affect pump components expression (Hooper 2002). Although fluoroquinolone is synthetic antimicrobial agents, many of them are substrates for a range of efflux systems. The conditions under which there is physiologically increased expression of these systems are unknown (Figure 7).

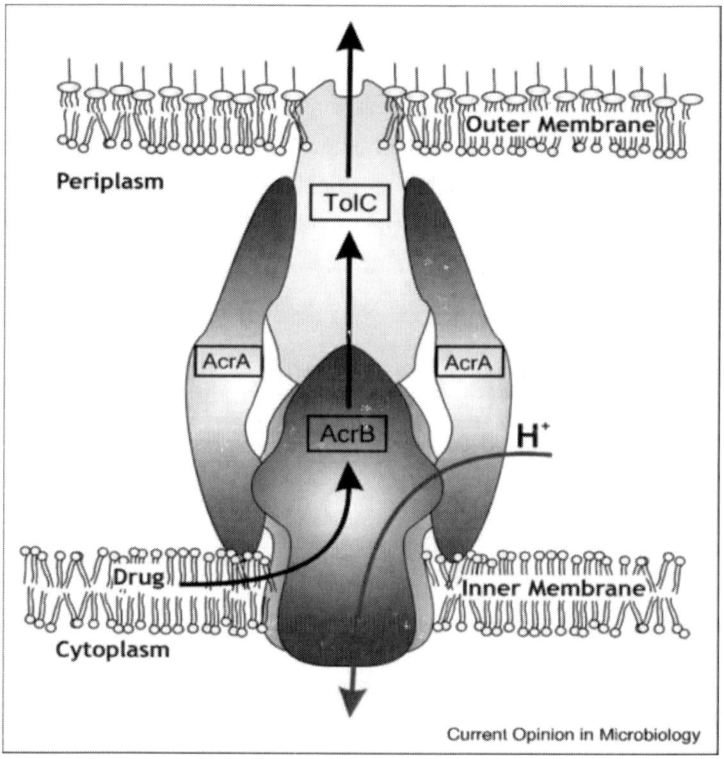

Figure 6. Schematic diagram of the RND system (AcrAb/TolC) of multidrug efflux pump AcrB are situated in the inner membrane and function in a complex with two other proteins, an outer membrane channel (TolC), and a periplasmic adaptor protein (AcrA). Figure adapted from (Pos, 2009).

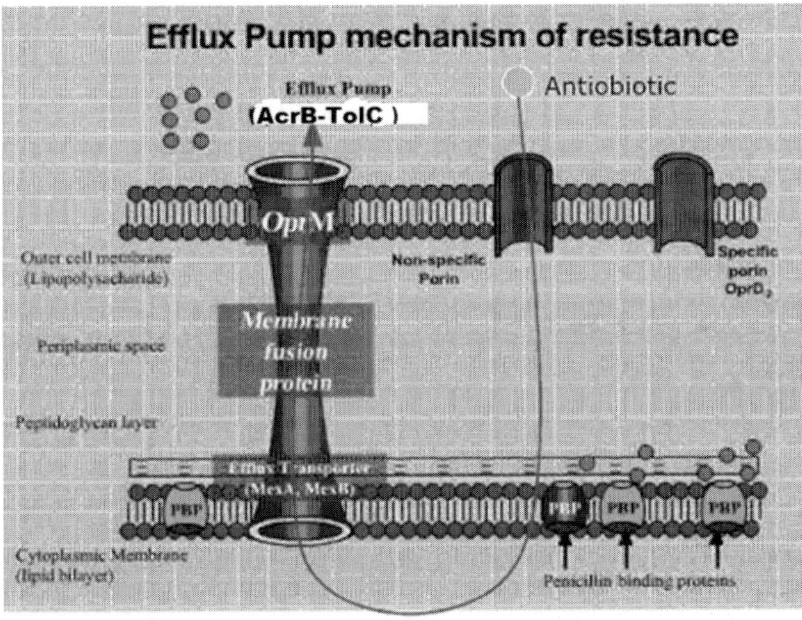

Figure 7. Efflux Pump Mechanism of antibiotic resistance. Figure adapted from Bailey et al. 2008; Piddock 1994).

Among pathogenic bacteria, *Escherichia coli, Campylobacter jejuni, P. aeruginosa, Salmonella sp., Acinetobacter baumennii, S. aureus, and Streptococcus pneumonia,* and others have been most extensively examined for efflux systems causing fluoroquinolone resistance with various types of MDR efflux pumps (Table1) (Jumbe et al. 2006; Kaatz, Seo, and Ruble 1993; Lin, Michel, and Zhang 2002; Morita et al. 2001; (Paulsen et al. 2001; Piddock et al. 2000; Ling et al. 2003). In *E. coli*, fluoroquinolone are extruded out of cells by over-expressed tripartite MDR pumps of the RND family (Tseng et al. 1999) as AcrAB-TolC, and other Enterobacteriaceae family such as *Salmonella enterica, Enterobacter aerogenes, Proteus mirabilis, and K. pneumoniae* (Mazzariol et al. 2002; Okusu, Ma, and Nikaido 1996; Piddock et al. 2000; Pradel and Pagès 2002; Visalli et al. 2003). Recently, AdeABC efflux pump in Acinetobacter that has regulated by the two-component system (AdeR-AdeS): AdeS is a sensor kinase and AdeR is a response regulator, was characterized for ciprofloxacin and other antibiotics resistance.

The overexpression of AdeABC efflux pump can be done by either the insertion sequence (IS) Aba-1 upstream of the adeABA operon or by the point mutation in AdeSR (Ardebili, Lari, and Talebi 2014; Magnet, Courvalin, and Lambert 2001; Marchand et al. 2004; Mugnier, Poirel, and Nordmann 2009).

P. aeruginosa have four identified such efflux systems, each differing by which fluoroquinolone are preferred substrates (Köhler et al. 1997; Nikaido 1998b; Nikaido 1998a; Poole 2000) such as MexAB-OprM (Poole, Heinrichs, and Neshat 1993), MexCD-OprJ (Poole et al. 1996) and MexEF-OprN (Köhler et al. 1997) that hat contribute to fluoroquinolone resistance in clinical settings (Fukuda et al. 1990; Fukuda et al. 1995; Cho et al. 1999; Jalal and Wretlind 1998; Hirai et al. 1987; Jakics et al. 1992).

On the other hand, Masuda et al. 1999; Srikumar et al. 2000 declared that the particularly well-studied efflux pump in *P. aeruginosa*, is the MexAB-OprM, of RND family is the only one that is created constitutively (Poole, Tetro, et al. 1996) and consequently contributes to intrinsic resistance have been associated in fluoroquinolone resistance within the clinical setting.

The interplay of two resistance mechanisms (gene mutation and overexpression of efflux pump) may coexist in a single bacterial cell, and such resistance has been correlated with highly fluoroquinolone-resistant clinical isolates of many Gram-negative and Gram-positive bacteria (Cho et al. 1999; Jalal and Wretlind 1998; Everett et al. 1996; Guerin et al. 2000), *P. aeruginosa* (Lomovskaya et al. 1999), *E. coli* (Oethinger et al. 2000) and S. aureus (Kaatz and Seo 1997), The combined resistance was much higher than that conferred by each of the mechanisms when present single. In *P. aeruginosa* single-step gyrase and efflux mutants conferred similar from 4- to 8-fold with developments in fluoroquinolone resistance (Lomovskaya et al. 1999). Deletion of mexAB-oprM from strains overproducing the corresponding pump resulted in a 64- fold increase in susceptibility, also regardless of the presence of target mutations, indicating that the fold reduction in MIC due to inhibition of the pump(s) depends particularly on the level of pump expression.

Additionally, Abouzeed et al. 2008 have described the role of the AcrAB-TolC efflux system as a significant cause of high-level resistance to fluoroquinolone in *Salmonella enterica* serovar Typhimurium DT204 and an essential mechanism for multidrug resistance (MDR) in serovar Typhimurium DT104 (Baucheron et al. 2004; 2002).

On the other hand, fluoroquinolone resistance mediated by efflux, in Gram-positive bacteria, has been recognized in various species such as *S. aureus, S. pneumoniae*, the viridans group streptococci, enteroccocci, and *Bacillus subtilis* (Table 1). Studies showed that MDR efflux pumps involved in resistance to fluoroquinolone belong to the MF family (Saier et al., 1999a). In *Staphylococcus aureus*, NorA (Neyfakh et al., 1993; Ng et al., 1994; Yoshida et al., 1990b) as well as additional genes that encode other pumps such as NorB, and NorC have been described (Fournier, Aras, and Hooper 2000; E. Ng, Trucksis, and Hooper 1994; Truong-Bolduc, Strahilevitz, and Hooper 2006) In addition, multidrug-resistance transporters of Gram-negative bacteria, antimicrobial efflux transporters of Gram-positive bacteria driving via the energy of the proton motive force to export antimicrobials from the cell (Pao, Paulsen, and Saier 1998; I. T. Paulsen, Brown, and Skurray 1996). The transcriptional regulators MgrA and NorG and the ArlRS two-component regulatory system controlled staphylococcal efflux pumps expression (Fournier, Aras, and Hooper 2000; I. T. Paulsen 2003). Moreover, MgrA and ArlRS regulate expression of several other genes, that responsible for capsule biosynthesis and autolysin production, therefore linking efflux pump expression to coordinate other principles cellular metabolic activities. Mutations in MgrA and NorG and the overexpression of those proteins from plasmids could control the pump expression patterns as well as can variously cause resistance to a fluoroquinolone and other antibiotics.

Wild-type cells of *S. aureus* have weakly expressed NorA gene, that important for low-level resistance to fluoroquinolone (Kaatz and Seo 1995), but to mediate resistance to fluoroquinolone, mutational upregulation of norA gene expression have been informed that appearing in a concomitant increase of the NorA efflux pump production (Kaatz, Seo, and Ruble 1993). However, mutations in the norA promoter seemed to explain the upregulation in the gene expression of fluoroquinolone-resistant strains (Kaatz and Seo 1997; Kaatz, Seo, and Foster 1999; Kaatz, Seo, and Ruble 1993; (Ng, Trucksis, and Hooper 1994), even though expand norA expression in such strains can occur independently of norA promoter mutations (Kaatz and Seo 1997). In fact, efflux-mediated fluoroquinolone resistance was identified in different *S. aureus* clinical strains that lacked mutations within the norA promoter, although norA expression itself become no longer assessed (Mun˜oz-Bellido et al. 1999). Consequently, additional loci absolutely impact on norA expression and may be the site of mutation in these strains. Consistent with this, fluoroquinolone resistance increase induction of norA gene expression in an *in vitro*-selected fluoroquinolone-resistant mutant lacking mutations in norA or indeed the flanking DNA (Kaatz and Seo 1995). Despite the fact that a regulator of norA gene expression has yet to be proved, an open reading frame, dubbed ORF A (Kaatz, Seo, and Ruble 1993) or norR (Paulsen et al. 1996), has been suggested upstream of norA whose product is homologous to the TetR repressor (Paulsen et al. 1996). Recently, a two-component regulatory system, ArlR-ArlS, was demonstrated to alter expression of norA, possible via an unidentified 18-kDa protein which interacts with the norA promoter (Fournier, Aras, and Hooper 2000).

NorA of *S. aureus* has homologues in *S. pneumonia*, PmrA were established in *Streptococcus pneumonia* (Gill, Brenwald, and Wise 1999) and the probability of efflux pumps existence in these organisms has recently been examined (L. J. V. Piddock et al. 1998; L. J. Piddock, Jin, and Everett 1997; Brenwald, Gill, and Wise 1998). The presence of an alternative reserpine-sensitive efflux pump in *S. pneumonia* has recently been presented (L. J. Piddock et al. 2002) and thirty-four ciprofloxacin-resistant (MIC $\geq$ 2 mg/L) clinical isolates of *S. pneumonia* have been represented for susceptibility and mutations in parC/E and gyrA/B.

Despite fluoroquinolone resistance in *S. pneumonia* is typically associated to mutations in gyrA or parC (Fukuda and Hiramatsu 1999; Munoz and Campa 1996), efflux-mediated resistance appears to be ordinary prevalent, occurring in 45% of 273 fluoroquinolone-resistant clinical isolates according to Brenwald et al. 1998. Confirming the involvement of PmrA gene in fluoroquinolone resistance, the sensitivity of isolates to fluoroquinolone has been restored with gene inactivation, suggesting that PmrA-mediated fluoroquinolone resistance relies upon increased pmrA expression. However, fluoroquinolone resistance due to efflux has currently been defined in the viridians group streptococci, sometimes in combination with mutations in *parC* (Ferrandiz et al. 1999).

Gram-positive bacteria are the most resistant to fluoroquinolone. Two genes encoding homologue of NorA had been recognized in *Bacillus subtilis*, Bmr (Neyfakh 1992; Neyfakh, Bidnenko, and Chen 1991) and Blt (Ahmed et al. 1995) transporters, that capable of accommodate fluoroquinolone especially ciprofloxacin and many molecules as dyes and energy inhibitors (Ahmed et al. 1995; Neyfakh 1992). Bmr is expressed constitutively, with null mutants exhibiting stronger susceptibility to fluoroquinolone and other agents (Ahmed et al. 1994; Neyfakh, Bidnenko, and Chen 1991), and fluoroquinolone-MDR happens because of gene amplification (Neyfakh, Bidnenko, and Chen 1991). In comparison, inactivation of blt has no effect on the resistance of wild-type *B. subtilis*, and Blt contributes to FQMDR only in mutant strains displaying increased expression of the blt gene (Ahmed et al. 1995). The bmr gene is undoubtedly regulated via the product of a gene, bmrR, in response to Bmr pump substrates which bind to the BmrR protein (Ahmed et al. 1994). The blt gene is also undoubtedly regulated, with the aid of the product of the bltR gene, although substrates of the Blt efflux pump do not induce blt expression or bind to the BltR protein (Ahmed et al. 1995). So far, the product of a gene mta has also been regulated both bmr and blt expression by acting on their respective promoters (Baranova, Danchin, and Neyfakh 1999).

Permeability of Outer Membrane Proteins (Porins) Alteration

The cellular accumulation of fluoroquinolone uptake is regulated via the opposing movements of diffusion-mediated drug uptake and pump-mediated efflux. In contrast to Gram-positive species, the outer membrane of Gram-negative bacteria poses an additional barrier that drugs must cross to get in the cell. Consequently, drug influx in Gram-negative species is promoted by protein channels with a beta-barrel structure called "porins" (Mitscher 2005; Robicsek, Jacoby, and Hooper 2006; Strahilevitz et al. 2009; Martinez-Martinez et al. 2003; Jacoby 2005).

Gram-negative bacterial cell wall usually has two membranous systems (Figure 8) first: the inner one (IM), termed the plasma membrane, is an internal trilamellar structure bound the bacterial protoplasm and form a phospholipids bilayer. The second layer is an outer membrane (OM) also presents a trilamellar structure (with two electron dense leaflets, outer and inner) and consists of proteins, having receptors, porins, which known as protein channel and responsible for drug influx in Gram-negative species, and an asymmetric distribution of lipids. This membrane blocks opposition against toxic compounds, such as antibiotics, whose targets are largely beyond this surface layer (Blair et al. 2015). The outer leaflet of outer membrane has consisted primarily of lipopolysaccharide (LPS) projecting outside and the inner one containing phospholipids and lipoproteins (Chatterjee and Chaudhuri 2012; Kamio and Nikaido 1967)

The LPS layer has three exceptional layers: (i) lipid-A, (ii) the core polysaccharide forming the inner and the outer cores, and (iii) the O-specific polysaccharide chains (Figure 8) projecting outward. The lipid part of LPS serves as the lipid anchor and is generally comprised of fatty acids, sugars, and phosphate groups. Both membranes, IM and OM, are separated through periplasm called a gel-like layer.

Such a layer has a thin layer (4-nm thick) of peptidoglycan (PG) which is attached to each of OM and IM through different protein-protein interactions also other proteins including the so-called resident "housekeeping" proteins and enzymes, the resident and temporary components of secretory pathways.

Pseudomonas aeruginosa has three lipoproteins, Oprl, OprL, and OprF, which join the OM with the PG layer, while wild-type Salmonella spp. have specific domains in the envelop that improve interactions between the outer membrane protein (Omp) and the peptidoglycan layer (PG) also interactions between the Omp and the inner membrane protein (IMP) respecting the PG (Deatherage et al. 2009). Such protein-protein interactions involving the PG supply the required strength and stability to the bacterial envelope or rather the surface arrangements of bacteria (Figure 9).

The OM carries the unique trimeric proteins referred to as porins, which are channel-forming proteins, allow small molecules (\600 daltons) to cross through periplasmic space. Once in the periplasm, proteins within the plasma membrane allow the pass of molecules into the cytoplasm. Accordingly, there are two pathways that antibiotics can take through the outer membrane depending on protonation-deprotonation states of the drug: a lipid-mediated pathway for hydrophobic fluoroquinolone, and general diffusion porins for hydrophilic one (Delcour 2010), because of the ciprofloxacin's small size with charge characteristics allow them to pass the outer membrane through porin proteins, that form general diffusion channels; moreover, they also appear to cross the cytoplasmic membrane via diffusion (Hooper 1999).

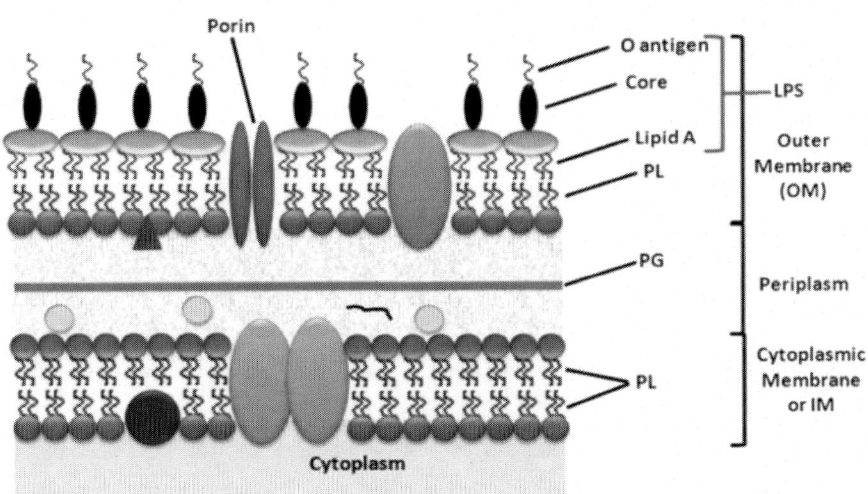

Figure 8. Schematic diagram of the outer membrane (OM), cytoplasmic or IM, and the intermediate periplasmic layer containing the peptidoglycan (PG). The IM consists of the two phospholipid (PL) leaflets and different lipoproteins. The outer membrane consists of two leaflets, the inner leaflet being composed of one phospholipid layer and the outer leaflet of lipid-A, core polysaccharide, and the O-antigen polysaccharide chains projecting outward. Figure adapted from (Chatterjee and Chaudhuri 2012).

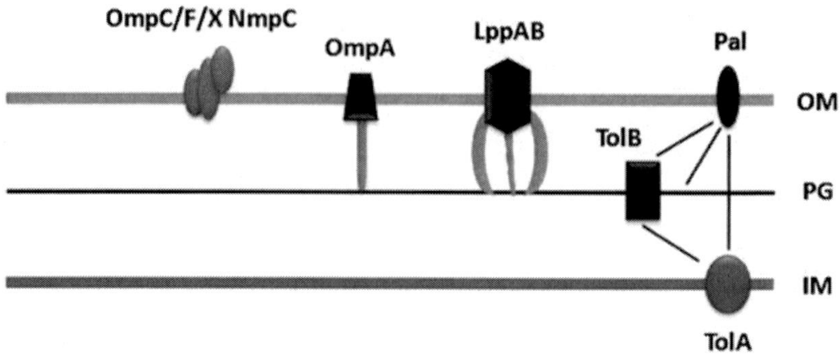

Figure 9. Proteins interconnecting different layers of the cell envelope. Integral OM proteins OmpC, OmpF, OmpX, and NmpC normally do not connect to other layers of the envelope. Lpp and OmpA form an interconnection between PG and OM, whereas Pal of the OM, Tol B of the PG, and Tol A of the IM form interconnections between the different components of the envelope. The thinner straight line represents covalent interaction; the thicker straight line or the curved lines represent noncovalent interactions. Figure adapted from (Chatterjee and Chaudhuri 2012).

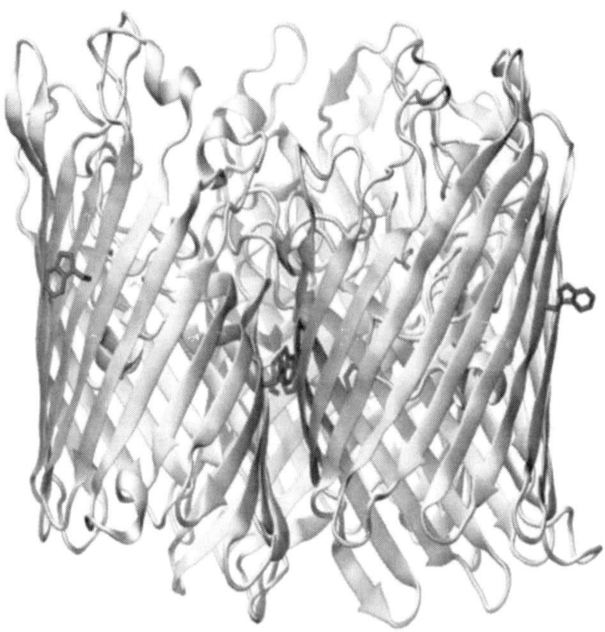

Figure 10. The structure of the OmpF homotrimer in ribbon representation, with the fluorescent tryptophan residues highlighted in red. The center of the homotrimer (the inter-subunit region) is not a channel and is completely hydrophobic, contributing to the exceptionally high stability of the trimer. Figure adapted from (Mizuno, Chou, and Inouye 1983).

The most abundant two outer membrane porins have been characterized in *Escherichia coli* and *Salmonella* sp., are OmpF (Figure 10) and OmpC (Overbeeke and Lugtenberg 1980), both are highly homolog (Mizuno, Chou, and Inouye 1983) and both show a homotrimeric structure, with each monomer forming a separate channel (Cowan et al. 1992; Basle et al. 2006) with special focus on OmpF because of its well understood structural and functional properties relative to any other major porins.

Bacteria have advanced strategies to resist antibiotics by modifications of entry pathways, which comprise loss of outer membrane porins or alterations of the lipopolysaccharide (LPS) that somewhat responsible for modification of antibiotic potency or uptake of antibiotics (Cohen, McMurry, and Levy 1988; Rajyaguru and Muszynski 1997; Blair et al. 2015) which act synergistically with overexpression Efflux pump.

Nikaido 1998b provided low-level resistance to fluoroquinolone relates to entry into the bacterial cell and characterized by regulations in nature and amount of porins, mainly architectural modification in OmpF with mutational changes in regulatory genes (marA, soxS, robA), which influence the action of several efflux pumps. The interaction of both alterations in cell envelope restricting the ingress of antimicrobials and active efflux is complicated (Hawkey 2003).

Table 2. Porins related to antibiotic resistance in Gram-negative bacteria

Species	Porin	Reference
Pseudomonas aeruginosa	OprD	(Dubois et al. 2001)
Escherichia coli	OmpC OmpF	(Tavio et al. 1999)
Klebsiella pneumoniae	OmpK35	(Chen et al. 2003)
Salmonella enterica	OmpF	(Rushdy et al. 2013)
Acinetobacter baumannii	CarO	(Limansky et al. 2002)

Pseudomonas aeruginosa is well-studied Gram-negative bacteria for reducing permeability, *Pseudomonas aeruginosa* has four fundamental (OprF, OprP, OprB, OprD) and two minor (OprC, OprE) outer membrane proteins act as porins (Bellido et al. 1992; Hancock, Siehnel, and Martin 1990; Wylie and Worobec 1995) Table 2. Alteration of porin size or loss of porin proteins involved in the uptake of antimicrobial agents, as proven for anti-pseudomonal antibiotics (Yoneyama, Yamani, and Nakae 1995), has been shown to result in an increase in bacterial resistance (Achouak, Heulin, and Pages 2001), Antibiotic resistance has been associated in Ps. aeruginosa, with a deficient in both OprF and OprD (Gimeno et al. 1996; Dubois et al. 2001). Additionally, changes in porins of Enterobacter aerogenes has been related with a decrease in outer membrane permeability with multi-drug resistance emergence (Charrel et al. 1996; Chevalier et al. 2000; De et al. 2001), indeed though that alteration is probably reversible with the removal of the selective pressure (Bornet et al. 2000).

Loss of OmpF has been determined to be amongst one of the resistance mechanisms evaluated by *E. coli* (Tavio et al. 1999) and *Salmonella enterica* against fluoroquinolone (Rushdy et al. 2013). Porin deficiency associated with the evolution of bacterial resistance might only show a minor role, alike as other mechanisms might account for major of the observed multi-drug resistance (James and Reeves 1996; Weindorf, Schmidt, and Martin 1998). In clinical isolates of other Gram-negative bacteria, like *Acinetobacter baumannii*, reduction in porin expression jointly with the action of a class D beta-lactamase, has likewise been shown in carbapenem resistance (Bou et al. 2000).

CONCLUSION

Improper use of agents from this important class of antibiotics will worsen current problems with antibiotic resistance. Increasing the medical application of fluoroquinolone especially ciprofloxacin, increasing the arising of resistance issues. The molecular techniques are the prevailing technique to the study of quinolone resistance, simultaneously with the availability of agents with novel structures, a better understanding of the mechanisms of action and resistance are emerging. Two major resistance mechanisms are assumed to be the most powerful: mutations in the primary target (topoisomerase) and overexpression of multidrug efflux pumps and/or alteration of outer membrane proteins (porins). Chromosomal mutations occur in the gyrA and gyrB genes, which code for the A and B subunits of DNA gyrase and in parC and parE, which code for the C and E subunits of topoisomerase IV.

REFERENCES

Aarestrup, Frank Møller, Wiuff, Camilla, Mølbak, Kåre and Threlfall, E. John 2003. "Is It Time to Change Fluoroquinolone Breakpoints for Salmonella Spp.? [1]." *Antimicrobial Agents and Chemotherapy*. doi:10.1128/AAC.47.2.827-829.2003.

Alangaden, G. J., and Lerner, S. A. 1997. "The Clinical Use of Fluoroquinolones for the Treatment of Mycobacterial Diseases." *Clinical Infectious Diseases: An Official Publication of the Infectious Diseases Society of America* 25 (5): 1213–21.

Aldred, Katie J., Kerns, Robert J. and Oshero, Neil. 2014. *"Mechanism of Quinolone Action and Resistance."*

Appelbaum, Peter C. 1999. "Quinolone Activity against Anaerobes." In *Drugs*, 58:60–64. doi:10.2165/00003495-199958002-00012.

Bailey, A. M., Paulsen, I. T. and Piddock, L. J. V. 2008. "RamA Confers Multidrug Resistance in Salmonella Enterica via Increased Expression of acrB, Which Is Inhibited by Chlorpromazine." *Antimicrobial Agents and Chemotherapy* 52: 3604–11.

Bauernfeind, A. 1997. "Comparison of the Antibacterial Activities of the Quinolones Bay 12-8039, Gatifloxacin (AM 1155), Trovafloxacin, Clinafloxacin, Levofloxacin and Ciprofloxacin." *Journal of Antimicrobial Chemotherapy* 40 (5): 639–51. doi:Doi 10.1093/Jac/40.5.639.

Becker, Karsten, Christine Heilmann, and Georg Peters. 2014. "Coagulase-Negative Staphylococci." *Clinical Microbiology Reviews*. doi:10.1128/CMR.00109-13.

Biedenbach, Douglas J., Farrell, David J., Flamm, Robert K., Liverman, Lisa C., McIntyre, Gail and Jones, Ronald N. 2012. "Activity of JNJ-Q2, a New Fluoroquinolone, Tested against Contemporary Pathogens Isolated from Patients with Community-Acquired Bacterial Pneumonia." *International Journal of Antimicrobial Agents* 39 (4): 321–25. doi:10.1016/j.ijantimicag.2011.11.016.

Bolon, Maureen K. 2011. "The Newer Fluoroquinolones." *Medical Clinics of North America*. doi:10.1016/j.mcna.2011.03.006.

Bouchillon, Sam K., Badal, Robert E., Hoban, Daryl J. and Hawser, Stephen P. 2013. "Antimicrobial Susceptibility of Inpatient Urinary Tract Isolates of Gram-Negative Bacilli in the United States: Results from the Study for Monitoring Antimicrobial Resistance Trends (SMART) Program: 2009-2011." *Clinical Therapeutics* 35 (6): 872–77. doi:10.1016/j.clinthera.2013.03.022.

Brook, Itzhak, and Long, Sarah S. 2012. "187 - Anaerobic Bacteria: Classification, Normal Flora, and Clinical Concepts." In *Principles and Practice of Pediatric Infectious Diseases (Fourth Edition)*, edited by Sarah S Long, Fourth Edi, 958–66.e3. London: Content Repository Only! doi:https://doi.org/10.1016/B978-1-4377-2702-9.00189-6.

Castro, William, Navarro, Maribel and Biot, Christophe. 2013. "Medicinal Potential of Ciprofloxacin and Its Derivatives." *Future Medicinal Chemistry* 5 (1): 81–96. doi:10.4155/fmc.12.181.

CDC. 2001. "Update: Investigation of Bioterrorism-Related Anthrax and Interim Guidelines for Exposure Management and Antimicrobial Therapy, October 2001." *MMWR Morb. Mortal. Wkly. Rep.* 50 (42): 909–19. http://www.ncbi.nlm.nih.gov/entrez/query.fcgi?cmd=Retrieve{&}db=PubMed{&}dopt=Citation{&}list{_}uids=11699843.

Chatterjee, S. N., and Chaudhuri, Keya. 2012. "Gram-Negative Bacteria: The Cell Membranes." In *Outer Membrane Vesicles of Bacteria*, 15–34. SpringerBriefs in Microbiology.

Chawla, Kiran, Vishwanath, Shashidhar and Munim, Frenil C. 2013. "Nonfermenting Gram-Negative Bacilli Other than Pseudomonas Aeruginosa and Acinetobacter Spp. Causing Respiratory Tract Infections in a Tertiary Care Center." *Journal of Global Infectious Diseases*. India. doi:10.4103/0974-777X.121996.

Chen, F. J., Lauderdale, T. L., Ho, M. and Lo, H. J. 2003. "The Roles of Mutations in gyrA, parC, and ompK35 in Fluoroquinolone Resistance in Klebsiella Pneumoniae." *Microbial Drug Resistant* 9: 265–71.

Constable, Peter D., Hinchcliff, Kenneth W., Done, Stanley H. and Grünberg, Walter. eds. 2017. "21 - Systemic and Multi-Organ Diseases." In *Veterinary Medicine (Eleventh Edition)*, Eleventh E, 2002–2214. W.B. Saunders. doi:https://doi.org/10.1016/B978-0-7020-5246-0.00021-8.

Cooke, Fiona J., and Slack, Mary P. E. 2017. "Gram-Negative Coccobacilli." In *Infectious Diseases (Fourth Edition)*, edited by Jonathan Cohen, William G Powderly, and Steven M Opal, Fourth Edi, 1611–27.e1. Elsevier. doi:https://doi.org/10.1016/B978-0-7020-6285-8.00183-0.

Cormican, M. G., and Jones, R. N. 1997. "Antimicrobial Activity and Spectrum of LB20304, a Novel Fluoronaphthyridone." *Antimicrobial Agents and Chemotherapy* 41 (1): 204–11.

Crump, John A., Medalla, Felicita M., Joyce, Kevin W., Krueger, Amy L., Hoekstra, R. Michael, Whichard, Jean M. and Barzilay, Ezra J. 2011. "Antimicrobial Resistance among Invasive Nontyphoidal Salmonella Enterica Isolates in the United States: National Antimicrobial Resistance Monitoring System, 1996 to 2007." *Antimicrobial Agents and Chemotherapy* 55 (3): 1148–54. doi:10.1128/AAC.01333-10.

Daum, T. E., Schaberg, D. R., Terpenning, M. S., Sottile, W. S. and Kauffman, C. A. 1990. "Increasing Resistance of Staphylococcus Aureus to Ciprofloxacin." *Antimicrobial Agents and Chemotherapy* 34 (9): 1862–63. doi:10.1128/AAC.34.9.1862.

Dekker, John P., and Frank, Karen M. 2015. "Salmonella, Shigella, and Yersinia." *Clinics in Laboratory Medicine*. doi:10.1016/j.cll.2015.02.002.

Deng, Xianding, Church, Deirdre, Vanderkooi, Otto G., Low, Donald E., and Pillai, Dylan R. 2013. "Streptococcus Pneumoniae Infection: A Canadian Perspective." *Expert Review of Anti-Infective Therapy* 11 (8). Taylor {&} Francis: 781–91. doi:10.1586/14787210.2013.814831.

Dubois, V., Arpin, C., Melon, M. and et al. 2001. "Nosocomial Outbreak due to a Multiresistant Strain of Pseudomonas Aeruginosa, P12: Efficacy of Cefepime-Amikacin Therapy and Analysis of Beta-Lactam Resistance." *Journal of Clinical Microbiology.* 39: 2072–78.

Fajardo Olivares, Miguel, Orozco, Rocío Hidalgo, Rodríguez Garrido, Saray, Rodríguez-Vidigal, Francisco Félix, Tomé, Araceli Vera and Marcos, Manuel Robles. 2011. "Activity of Vancomycin, Ciprofloxacin, Daptomycin, and Linezolid against Coagulase-Negative Staphylococci Bacteremia." *Revista Española de Quimioterapia : Publicación Oficial de La Sociedad Española de Quimioterapia* 24 (2): 74–78.

Fernandes, Prabhavathi B., Shipkowitz, Nathan, Bower, Robert R.,. Jarvis, Kenneth P., Weisz, Jonina and Chu, Daniel T. W. 1986. "In-Vitro and in-Vivo Potency of Five New Fluoroquinolones against Anaerobic Bacteria." *Journal of Antimicrobial Chemotherapy* 18 (6): 693–701. doi:10.1093/jac/18.6.693.

Garrison, Mark W. 2003. "Comparative Antimicrobial Activity of Levofloxacin and Ciprofloxacin against Streptococcus Pneumoniae." *Journal of Antimicrobial Chemotherapy* 52 (3): 503–6. doi:10.1093/jac/dkg380.

Gilbert, D. N., Kohlhepp, S. J., Slama, K. A., Grunkemeier, G., Lewis, G., Dworkin, R. J., Slaughter, S. E. and Leggett, J. E. 2001. "Phenotypic Resistance of Staphylococcus Aureus, Selected Enterobacteriaceae, and Pseudomonas Aeruginosa after Single and Multiple In Vitro Exposures to Ciprofloxacin, Levofloxacin, and Trovafloxacin." *Antimicrobial Agents and Chemotherapy.* doi:10.1128/AAC.45.3.883-892.2001.

Goldstein, E. J., and Citron, D. M. 1992. "Comparative Activity of Ciprofloxacin, Ofloxacin, Sparfloxacin, Temafloxacin, CI-960, CI-

990, and WIN 57273 against Anaerobic Bacteria." *Antimicrobial Agents and Chemotherapy*.

Gupta, Naveen, Arora, Shamma and Kundra, Shailja. 2011. "Moraxella Catarrhalis as a Respiratory Pathogen." *Indian Journal of Pathology & Microbiology* 54 (4): 769–71. doi:10.4103/0377-4929.91496.

Hackel, M. A., Badal, R. E., Bouchillon, S. K., Biedenbach, D. J. and Hoban, D. J. 2015. "Resistance Rates of Intra-Abdominal Isolates from Intensive Care Units and Non-Intensive Care Units in the United States: The Study for Monitoring Antimicrobial Resistance Trends 2010-2012." *Surgical Infections* 16 (3): 298–304. doi:10.1089/sur.2014.060.

Hardy, Dwight, Amsterdam, Daniel, Mandell, Lionel A. and Rotstein, Coleman. 2000. "Comparative In Vitro Activities of Ciprofloxacin, Gemifloxacin, Grepafloxacin, Moxifloxacin, Ofloxacin, Sparfloxacin, Trovafloxacin, and Other Antimicrobial Agents against Bloodstream Isolates of Gram-Positive Cocci." *Antimicrobial Agents and Chemotherapy*.

Hasegawa, Miyuki, Sato, Yumie, Kanayama, Akiko, Matsuzaki, Kaoru, Muraoka, Hiroe, Amano, Ayako, Saika, Takeshi and Kobayashi, Intetsu 2006. "Antibacterial Activity of Tosufloxacin against Major Organisms Detected from Patients with Respiratory or Otorhinological Infections: Comparison with the Results Obtained from Organisms Isolated about 10 Years Ago." *Journal of Infection and Chemotherapy* 12 (3): 152–56. doi:10.1007/s10156-006-0434-2.

Hidalgo, Marylin, Reyes, Jinnethe, Cardenas, Ana Maria, Diaz, Lorena, Rincon, Sandra, Vanegas, Natasha, Diaz, Paula Lucia, Castaneda, Elizabeth and Arias, Cesar A. 2008. "Resistance Profiles to Fluoroquinolones in Clinical Isolates of Gram Positive Cocci." *BIOMEDICA* 28 (2): 284–94.

High, Nicola J., Fan, Feinan and Schwartzman, Joseph D. 2015. "Chapter 97 - Haemophilus Influenzae." In *Molecular Medical Microbiology (Second Edition)*, edited by Yi-Wei Tang, Max Sussman, Dongyou Liu, Ian Poxton, and Joseph Schwartzman, Second Edi, 1709–28.

Boston: Academic Press. doi:https://doi.org/10.1016/B978-0-12-397169-2.00097-4.

Ho, P. L., Que, T. L., Tsang, D. N., Ng, T. K., Chow, K. H. and Seto, W. H. 1999. "Emergence of Fluoroquinolone Resistance among Multiply Resistant Strains of Streptococcus Pneumoniae in Hong Kong." *Antimicrobial Agents and Chemotherapy* 43 (5): 1310–13. http://www.pubmedcentral.nih.gov/articlerender.fcgi?artid=89269{&}tool=pmcentrez{&}rendertype=abstract.

Hooper, D. C. 1999. "Mode of Action of Fluoroquinolones." *Drugs* 58: (suppl 2):6–10.

Hooper, D. C. and Wolfson, J. S. 1993. "Mechanisms of Quinolone Action and Bacterial Killing." In *Quinolone Antimicrobial Agents.*, 2d ed., 53–57. Washington, D.C.: American Society for Microbiology.

Hooper, D. C. 1999. "Mechanisms of Quinolone Resistance." *Drug Resistance Updates* 2: 38–55.

Hsu, Shih Fen, Lin, Yi Tsung, Chen, Te Li, Siu, L. K., Hsueh, Po Ren, Huang, Shih Tse and Fung, Chang Phone. 2012. "Antimicrobial Resistance of Moraxella Catarrhalis Isolates in Taiwan." *Journal of Microbiology, Immunology and Infection* 45 (2): 134–40. doi:10.1016/j.jmii.2011.09.004.

Itokazu, Gail S., Nathan, Catherine, Hariharan, Radhika, Kastman, Jay R., Kabins, Sherwin A. and Weinstein, Robert A. 1996. "The Comparative in Vitro Activity of Clinafloxacin and Other Antimicrobials against Vancomycin-Susceptible and Vancomycin-Resistant Enterococci." *Chemotherapy* 42 (4): 235–39. doi:10.1159/000239449.

Jacobs, Michael R. 1995. "Activity of Quinolones against Mycobacteria." *Drugs* 49 (2): 67–75. doi:10.2165/00003495-199500492-00011.

James, R. 2011. "13 - Infection Prevention and Control and the Role of Medical Textiles." In *Handbook of Medical Textiles*, edited by V T Bartels, 297–315. Woodhead Publishing Series in Textiles. Woodhead Publishing. doi:https://doi.org/10.1533/9780857093691.3.297.

Jones, M. E., Goguen, J., Critchley, I. A., Draghi, D. C., Karlowsky, J. A., Sahm, D. F., Porschen, R., Patra, G. and DelVecchio, V. G. 2003. "Antibiotic Susceptibility of Isolates of Bacillus Anthracis, a Bacterial

Pathogen with the Potential to Be Used in Biowarfare." *Clinical Microbiology and Infection* 9 (9): 984–86. doi:10.1046/j.1469-0691.2003.00775.x.

Karlowsky, James A., Draghi, Deborah C., Jones, Mark E., Thornsberry, Clyde, Friedland, Ian R. and Sahm, Daniel F. 2003. "Surveillance for Antimicrobial Susceptibility among Clinical Isolates of Pseudomonas Aeruginosa and Acinetobacter Baumannii from Hospitalized Patients in the United States, 1998 to 2001." *Antimicrobial Agents and Chemotherapy*. doi:10.1128/AAC.47.5.1681-1688.2003.

Kawahara, S., Tada, A. and Nagare, H. 2001. "Comparison of in Vitro Antimicrobial Activities of Ofloxacin, Levofloxacin, Ciprofloxacin, and Sparfloxacin against Various Mycobacteria." *Kekkaku* 76 (4): 357–62.

Keepers, Tiffany R., Gomez, Marcela, Celeri, Chris, Krause, Kevin M., Biek, Donald and Critchley, Ian. 2017. "Fosfomycin and Comparator Activity Against Select Enterobacteriaceae, Pseudomonas, and Enterococcus Urinary Tract Infection Isolates from the United States in 2012." *Infectious Diseases and Therapy*. Cheshire. doi:10.1007/s40121-017-0150-5.

Kreizinger, Zsuzsa, Sulyok, Kinga Mária, Makrai, László, Rónai, Zsuzsanna, Fodor, László, Jánosi, Szilárd and Gyuranecz, Miklós. 2016. "Antimicrobial Susceptibility of Bacillus Anthracis Strains from Hungary." *Acta Veterinaria Hungarica* 64 (2): 141–47. doi:10.1556/004.2016.015.

Limansky, Adriana S., Limansky, Adriana S., Viale, Alejandro M. and Viale, Alejandro M. 2002. "Loss of a 29-Kilodalton Outer Membrane Protein in." *Society* 40 (12): 4776–78. doi:10.1128/JCM.40.12.4776.

Lockhart, Shawn R., Abramson, Murray A., Beekmann, Susan E., Gallagher, Gale, Riedel, Stefan, Diekema, Daniel J., Quinn, John P. and Doern, Gary V. 2007. "Antimicrobial Resistance among Gram-Negative Bacilli Causing Infections in Intensive Care Unit Patients in the United States between 1993 and 2004." *Journal of Clinical Microbiology* 45 (10): 3352–59. doi:10.1128/JCM.01284-07.

McGowan, John E. 2006. "Resistance in Nonfermenting Gram-Negative Bacteria: Multidrug Resistance to the Maximum." *American Journal of Infection Control* 34 (5 SUPPL.). doi:10.1016/j.ajic.2006.05.226.

Melo-Cristino, J., and Serrano, Nuno. 2006. "The Viriato Study: Update of Antimicrobial Susceptibility Data of Bacterial Pathogens from Community-Acquired Respiratory Tract Infections in Portugal in 2001 and 2002." *Revista Portuguesa de Pneumologia* 9: 293–310. doi:10.1016/S2173-5115(06)70385-2.

Mirza, S. H., Beeching, N. J. and Hart, C. A. 1996. "Multi-Drug Resistant Typhoid: A Global Problem." *Journal of Medical Microbiology* 44 (5): 317–19. doi:10.1099/00222615-44-5-317.

Mizuno, T., Chou, M. Y. and Inouye, M. 1983. "A Comparative Study on the Genes for Three Porins of the Escherichia Coli Outer Membrane: DNA Sequence of the Osmoregulated ompC Gene." *J. Biol. Chem.* 258: 6932–40.

Mohammed, M. Jasmine, Marston, Chung K., Popovic, Tanja, Weyant, Robbin S. and Tenover, Fred C. 2002. "Antimicrobial Susceptibility Testing of Bacillus Anthracis: Comparison of Results Obtained by Using the National Committee for Clinical Laboratory Standards Broth Microdilution Reference and Etest Agar Gradient Diffusion Methods." *Journal of Clinical Microbiology* 40 (6): 1902–7. doi:10.1128/JCM.40.6.1902-1907.2002.

Niki, Yoshihito, Hanaki, Hideaki, Matsumoto, Tetsuya, Yagisawa, Morimasa, Kohno, Shigeru, Aoki, Nobuki, Watanabe, Akira. et al. 2011. "Nationwide Surveillance of Bacterial Respiratory Pathogens Conducted by the Japanese Society of Chemotherapy in 2008: General View of the Pathogens' Antibacterial Susceptibility." *Journal of Infection and Chemotherapy* 17 (4): 510–23. doi:10.1007/s10156-011-0214-5.

Norris, S., and Mandell, G. L. 1988. *The Quinolones: History and Overview.* Edited by VT. Andriole. London.: Academic Press Ltd.

Olivares, M. F., Orozco, R., Gutierrez, S. R., Eseverri, E. G., Vidigal, F. F. R. and Marcos, M. R. 2010. "Activity of Daptomycin, Ciprofloxacin, Clindamycin and Cotrimoxazole against Coagulase-Negative

Staphylococcus Strains with Diminished Susceptibility to Vancomycin." *Revista Espanola De Quimioterapia* 23 (2): 81–86.

Orscheln, Rachel C., Johnson, Dwight R., Olson, Stephen M., Presti, Rachel M., Martin, Judith M., Kaplan, Edward L. and Storch, Gregory A. 2005. "Intrinsic Reduced Susceptibility of Serotype 6 Streptococcus Pyogenes to Fluoroquinolone Antibiotics." *The Journal of Infectious Diseases* 191 (8): 1272–79. doi:10.1086/428856.

Ortatatli, Mesut, Karagoz, Alper, Percin, Duygu, Kenar, Levent, Kilic, Selcuk and Durmaz, Riza. 2012. "Antimicrobial Susceptibility and Molecular Subtyping of 55 Turkish Bacillus Anthracis Strains Using 25-Loci Multiple-Locus VNTR Analysis." *Comparative Immunology, Microbiology and Infectious Diseases* 35 (4): 355–61. doi:10.1016/j.cimid.2012.02.005.

Paganelli, Fernanda L., Willems, Rob J. and Leavis, Helen L. 2012. "Optimizing Future Treatment of Enterococcal Infections: Attacking the Biofilm?" *Trends in Microbiology*. doi:10.1016/j.tim.2011.11.001.

Parry, Christopher M., and Threlfall, E. J. 2008. "Antimicrobial Resistance in Typhoidal and Nontyphoidal Salmonellae." *Current Opinion in Infectious Diseases*. doi:10.1097/QCO.0b013e32830f453a.

Paterson, David L. 2012. "313 - Infections Due to Other Members of the Enterobacteriaceae, Including Management of Multidrug-Resistant Strains." In *Goldman's Cecil Medicine (Twenty-Fourth Edition)*, edited by Lee Goldman and Andrew I Schafer, Twenty-Fou, 1874–77. Philadelphia: W. B. Saunders. doi:https://doi.org/10.1016/B978-1-4377-1604-7.00313-4.

Picazo, Juan J., Betriu, Carmen, Rodríguez-Avial, Iciar, Culebras, Esther, López, Fátima and Gómez, María. 2010. "[Comparative Activity of Daptomycin against Clinical Isolates of Methicillin-Resistant Staphylococcus Aureus and Coagulase-Negative Staphylococci]." *Enfermedades Infecciosas Y Microbiolog{í}a Cl{í}nica* 28 (1): 13–16. doi:10.1016/j.eimc.2008.09.012.

Piddock, L. J. V. 1994. "New Quinolones and Gram Positive Bacteria." *Antimicrob Agents Chemother* 38: 163–69.

Pingault, Nevada M., Bowman, Jacinta M., Lehmann, Deborah and Riley, Thomas V. 2010. "Antimicrobial Susceptibility of Moraxella Catarrhalis Isolated from Children in KalgoorlieBoulder, Western Australia." *Pathology* 42 (3): 273–79. doi:10.3109/0031302 1003631270.

Pontieri, Eugenio. 2016. "Chapter 2 - Bacillus Cereus Group Diagnostics: Chromogenic Media and Molecular Tools." In *The Diverse Faces of Bacillus Cereus*, edited by Vincenzo Savini, 15–33. Academic Press. doi:https://doi.org/10.1016/B978-0-12-801474-5.00002-5.

Pos, K. M. 2009. "Trinity Revealed: Stoichiometric Complex Assembly of a Bacterial Multidrug Efflux Pump." *Proc Natl Acad Sci U S A* 106: 6893–94.

Prévost, Gilles. 2013. "Chapter 562 - Exfoliative Toxins – Staphylococcal Epidermolysins." In *Handbook of Proteolytic Enzymes*, edited by Neil D Rawlings and Guy Salvesen, 2539–43. Academic Press. doi:https://doi.org/10.1016/B978-0-12-382219-2.00562-7.

Prince, Alice S. 2012. "155 - Pseudomonas Aeruginosa." In *Principles and Practice of Pediatric Infectious Diseases (Fourth Edition)*, edited by Sarah S Long, Fourth Edi, 842–46.e2. London: Content Repository Only! doi:https://doi.org/10.1016/B978-1-4377-2702-9.00157-4.

Reglinski, Mark, and Sriskandan, Shiranee. 2015. "Chapter 38 - *Streptococcus Pyogenes*." In *Molecular Medical Microbiology (Second Edition)*, edited by Yi-Wei Tang, Max Sussman, Dongyou Liu, Ian Poxton, and Joseph Schwartzman, Second Edi, 675–716. Boston: Academic Press. doi:https://doi.org/10.1016/B978-0-12-397169-2.00038-X.

Rhomberg, Paul R., and Jones, Ronald N. 2007. "Contemporary Activity of Meropenem and Comparator Broad-Spectrum Agents: MYSTIC Program Report from the United States Component (2005)." *Diagnostic Microbiology and Infectious Disease* 57 (2): 207–15. doi:10.1016/j.diagmicrobio.2006.07.009.

Rowe, B., Ward, L. R. and Threlfall, E. J. 1997. "Multidrug-Resistant Salmonella Typhi: A Worldwide Epidemic." *Clinical Infectious Diseases : An Official Publication of the Infectious Diseases Society of*

America 24 (table 1): S106–9. doi:10.1093/clinids/24. Supplement_1.S106.

Rushdy, A. A., Mabrouk, M. I., Abu-Sef, F. A. H., Kheiralla, Z. H., All, S. M. A. and Saleh, N. M. 2013. "Contribution of Different Mechanisms to the Resistance to Fluoroquinolones in Clinical Isolates of Salmonella Enterica." *Brazilian Journal of Infectious Diseases* 17 (4): 431–37. doi:10.1016/j.bjid.2012.11.012.

Schoeffler, A. J., and Berger, J. M. 2005. "Recent Advances in Understanding Structure-Function Relationships in the Type II Topoisomerase Mechanism." *Biochemical Society Transactions* 33: 1465–70.

Sharma, Prabodh Chander, Jain, Ankit, Jain, Sandeep, Pahwa, Rakesh and Yar, Mohammad Shahar. 2010. "Ciprofloxacin: Review on Developments in Synthetic, Analytical, and Medicinal Aspects." *Journal of Enzyme Inhibition and Medicinal Chemistry*. doi:10.3109/14756360903373350.

Stein, G. E., and Goldstein, E. J. C. 2006. "Fluoroquinolones and Anaerobes." *Clinical Infectious Diseases* 42 (11): 1598–1607. doi:10.1086/503907.

Steinhoff, Mark C., Cherian, Thomas and Schlaudecker, Elizabeth P. 2011. "{CHAPTER} 27 - Haemophilus Influenzae." In *Tropical Infectious Diseases: Principles, Pathogens and Practice (Third Edition)*, edited by Richard L Guerrant, David H Walker, and Peter F Weller, Third Edit, 193–95. Edinburgh: W.B. Saunders. doi:https://doi.org/10.1016/B978-0-7020-3935-5.00027-6.

Sutherland, Christina A., and Nicolau, David P. 2015. "Susceptibility Profile of Ceftolozane/Tazobactam and Other Parenteral Antimicrobials Against Escherichia Coli, Klebsiella Pneumoniae, and Pseudomonas Aeruginosa from US Hospitals." *Clinical Therapeutics* 37 (7): 1564–71. doi:10.1016/j.clinthera.2015.05.501.

Sutherland, Christina A., Verastegui, Jamie E. and Nicolau, David P. 2016. "In Vitro Potency of Amikacin and Comparators against E. coli,K. Pneumoniae and P. Aeruginosa Respiratory and Blood Isolates."

Annals of Clinical Microbiology and Antimicrobials. doi:10.1186/s12941-016-0155-z.

Tavio, M. D., Vila, J., Ruiz, J., Martin-Sanchez, A. M. and Anta, De M. T. J. 1999. "Mechanisms Involved in the Development of Resistance to Fluoroquinolones in Escherichia Coli Isolates." *Journal of Antimicrobial Chemotherpy* 44: 735–44.

Tickell, Kirkby D., Brander, Rebecca L., Atlas, Hannah E., Pernica, Jeffrey M., Walson, Judd L. and Pavlinac, Patricia B. 2017. "Identification and Management of Shigella Infection in Children with Diarrhoea: A Systematic Review and Meta-Analysis." *The Lancet Global Health* 5 (12): e1235–48. doi:10.1016/S2214-109X(17)30392-3.

Van heirstraeten, Liesbet, Leten, Gert, Lammens, Christine, Goossens, Herman and Malhotra-kumar, Surbhi. 2012. "Increase in Fluoroquinolone Non-Susceptibility among Clinical Streptococcus Pyogenes in Belgium during 2007-10." *Journal of Antimicrobial Chemotherapy* 67 (11): 2602–5. doi:10.1093/jac/dks281.

Yan, S. Steve, Schreckenberger, Paul C., Zheng, Xiaotian, Nelson, Nancy A., Harrington, Susan M., Tjhio, Joyce and Fedorko, Daniel P. 2008. "An Intrinsic Pattern of Reduced Susceptibility to Fluoroquinolone in Pediatric Isolates of *Streptococcus Pyogenes*." *Diagnostic Microbiology and Infectious Disease* 62 (2): 205–9. doi:10.1016/j.diagmicrobio.2008.04.018.

Yoo, Sunmi, Pai, Hyunjoo, Byeon, Jeong Hum, Kang, Youn Ho, Kim, Shukho and Lee, Bok Kwon. 2004. "Epidemiology of *Salmonella enterica* serotype Typhi Infections in Korea for Recent 9 Years: Trends of Antimicrobial Resistance." *Journal of Korean Medical Science* 19 (1): 15–20. doi:10.3346/jkms.2004.19.1.15.

In: Ciprofloxacin
Editor: Mohamed Said Attia
ISBN: 978-1-53614-534-2

Chapter 5

METHODS OF ANALYSIS, NEW APPLICATIONS AND COMMON ADVERSE EFFECTS OF SOME FLUOROQUINOLONES

Vania Maslarska[1,*], Stanislav Bozhanov[1] and Magdalena Kondeva[2]
[1]Department of Chemistry, Faculty of Pharmacy, Medical University-Sofia, Bulgaria
[2]Department of Pharmacology, Pharmacotherapy and Toxicology, Faculty of Pharmacy, Medical University-Sofia, Bulgaria

ABSTRACT

Fluoroquinolones are broad-spectrum antibiotics used to prevent and treat a wide range of bacterial infections. Bactericidal activity of quinolones is related to a combination of: DNA fragmentation, increased reactive oxygen species (ROS) production and activation of programmed cell death systems.

Over the last few years, the level of resistance to commonly prescribed antibiotics is significant and is recognized as a public health

* Corresponding Author: vmaslarska@mail.bg.

problem of global importance. The data from the literature on the mechanisms of resistance to fluoroquinolones are increasing. Some mechanisms of fluoroquinolone resistance occur principally through chromosomal mutation in genes encoding the quinolone targets (DNA gyrase and topoisomerase IV), and to a lesser extent through decreased permeability (implicating upregulation of the AcrAB-TolC multidrug efflux pump). Additionally, plasmid-mediated quinolone resistance mechanisms (Qnr proteins, which protect the quinolone targets; the acetylation of ciprofloxacin and norfloxacin; and the plasmid-mediated efflux pump), have also been described and are epidemiologically relevant.

The great importance of these drugs requires development of effective analytical methods involving high sensitivity and resolution. The spectroscopy and the liquid chromatography are well established methods in the field of pharmaceutical analysis. Various spectroscopic and high performance liquid chromatographic methods for determination of fluoroquinolones, their related impurities and co-administered drugs in the bulk drug forms and pharmaceutical formulations are reviewed.

Some adverse drug reactions are common during the therapy with fluoroquinolones: triceps ruptures and for ciprofloxacin – negative myoclonus (brief sudden loss of muscle activity).

During the past years, some authors give information about the new application of fluoroquinolones as possible anticancer agents. Ofloxacin, sparafloxacin, ciprofloxacin and moxifloxacin are predicted to be the most potent inhibitors of topoisomerase II (Topo2a and Topo2b). It is known that DNA topoisomerases play a major role in DNA relaxation, which is an important step in DNA replication. Topoisomerase II is considered an important target for the development of anticancer drugs. Literature data about methods of analysis, new applications and common adverse effects of fluoroquinolones (in particular ciprofloxacin) will be summarized in this chapter.

Keywords: ciprofloxacin, fluoroquinolones, spectral methods, HPLC methods, adverse effects, drug interactions

Acronyms

ACN	Acetonitrile
ATPS	Aqueous two-phase systems
BCP	Bromocresol Purple

BH	Bromhexine
BTB	Bromothymol Blue
CIP	Ciprofloxacin
CL	Chloranilic acid
CLS	Classical least squares
CWT	Continuous wavelet transform
DANO	Danofloxacin
Deg Prod	Degradation product
DEX	Dexamethasone
DIC	Dicyclomine
DCF	Diclofenac
DAD	Diode Array Detector
DEA	Diethylamine
DCM	Dichloromethane
EDA	Ethylenediamine
ENRO	Enrofloxacin
EOPO	Thermoseparating copolymers composed of ethylene oxide (EO) and propylene oxide (PO)
FIA	Flow injection analysis
FLD	Fluorescence detector
ILS	Inverse least square
IS	Internal standard
LEVO	Levofloxacin
LIN	Linezolid
LLE	Liquid–liquid extraction
LOME	Lomefloxacin
MEB	Mebeverine hydrochloride
MEPS	Microextraction by packed sorbent
MET	Metronidazole
MIPF-SPME	Molecularly imprinted fiber – solid phase microextraction technique
MeOH	Methanol
MOXI	Moxifloxacin
NDA	Nalidixic acid

NOR	Norfloxacin
OFL	Ofloxacin
ORN	Ornidazole
OXO	Oxolinic acid
PCR	Principal Component Regression
PDA	Photodiode array
PLS	Partial least squares
PP	Protein precipitation
PYR	Pyrimethamine
QN	Quinine
3-HQN	3-Hydroxyquinine
Rel sub	Related substances
SDS	Sodium dodecyl sulphate
SGF	Savitsky–Golay filters
SOS	Sodium octane sulfonate
SPE	Solid phase extraction
SDM	Sulfadimidine
SPAR	Sparfloxacin
TFA	Trifluoroacetic acd
TEA	Triethylamine
TeTA	Triethanolamine
TIN	Tinidazole
TRIM	Trimethoprim
UF	Umbeliferone
UV	Ultraviolet

INTRODUCTION

Ciprofloxacin (CIP) is an antibacterial agent of the fluoroquinolones group. Although it is of the second generation, its broad spectrum of action determines its wide use, despite the presence of new (third and fourth generation) representatives of fluoroquinolone antibiotics with improved properties. Since CIP is important in clinical practice, there is an increased growth of production and development of new (including combined) dosage forms. The increasing use of antibiotics (and in particular CIP) inevitably requires them to be determined in a variety of matrices, for example, in environmental samples [1, 2], water systems [3, 4] and food [5, 6]. Of course, the determination of CIP in substances, in different dosage forms and in biological media plays a key role in the manufacturing process, quality control and therapeutic effect of drugs.

Various analytical techniques for determining CIP have been described in the available literature. The spectral methods (in the visible and ultraviolet range of the spectrum), and the methods based on high-performance liquid chromatography take the leading place, and will be discussed later. Among the other analytical techniques used to determine CIP, mention may be made of titrimetry [7], electroanalytical methods [8-13], fourier transform infrared spectroscopy [14, 15], luminescence and spectrofluorimetric methods [16], radio analytical methods [17], as well as some separation techniques such as thin-layer chromatography [18], micellar liquid chromatography [19] and capillary electrophoresis [20-24].

A titrimetric method for the analysis of CIP in tablets and injectable solutions [7] has been developed. The method is based on the residual titration of cerium (IV) sulphate in acidic medium with standard solution of ammonium iron sulphate and ferrous indicator. The titrimetric method is applicable in the range 2-12 milligrams.

Potentiometric titration has been performed, using ion pair CIP hydrochloride–molybdophosphoric acid and CIP selective electrodes [8]. The concentration range from 4.0×10^{-6} to 1.0×10^{-1} M and detection limit were found to be 1.2×10^{-6} M, respectively. The method has been applied for analysis of CIP in tablets. Another method for analysis of CIP in tablets has been developed based on titration with standard Ag^{+} or Fe^{3+} solutions in electrical micro-titration system with capacitively coupled contactless conductivity detector where the formation of the reaction products leads to a change in the conductivity of the solution [9]. Linear working ranges of 2.0 – 8.0 mmol/L and 1.0 – 5.0 mmol/L have been established for Ag^{+} or Fe^{3+} standard solutions respectively. The results have been in good agreement with those obtained by reference method. Voltammetric techniques have been used to determine CIP in tablets [10-13], eye drops [12], plasma [30], serum [10] and urine [11, 13]. Some of the methods are based on the use of modified glassy carbon electrodes with alizarin red [10] and graphene [11]. $MgFe_2O_4$ nanoparticles as electrochemical sensor [13], as well as an enhancement effect of an anionic surfactant: sodium dodecyl benzene sulfonate [12] have also been used. All methods have been found to be simple and selective, providing good results in the analysis of CIP in pharmaceutical formulations and biological media.

Fourier transform infrared spectroscopy method has been developed for quantification of CIP in tablets [14]. Sample preparation consists of dissolving the powdered tablets in phosphate buffer (pH 6) and methanol. The linear range has been found to be of 2 - 20 μg/ml, with LOD and LOQ of 0.068 μg/ml and 0.450 μg/ml respectively. On the other hand, solvent free method for determination of CIP has been elaborated by application of diffuse reflectance infrared fourier transform spectroscopy [15]. For sample preparation, an appropriate quantity of CIP hydrochloride (working range of 0.3 – 1.5% w/w) has been diluted with dry potassium bromide. The developed method has been applied in analysis of three different brands of CIP tablets. As advantage of both methods relatively simple sample preparation should be mentioned.

Luminescence methods have attracted wide attention due to their high sensitivity, lower limit of detection and wide linear ranges. Flow injection analysis (FIA) coupled with chemiluminescence detection is a powerful analysis tool, which enjoys unique features involving automation, miniaturization, versatility, and inexpensiveness. FIA has been applied in various areas of analytical practice, for example in pharmaceutical, environmental, food and beverages and biomedical analysis [25]. Review papers, devoted to the use of chemiluminescence methods (coupled with FIA) for the determination of pharmaceuticals [26] and in particular of fluoroquinolones [16], can be found in the available literature.

Spectrofluorimetric methods are also used for determination of CIP in pharmaceutical formulations and in biological samples. The majority of the spectrofluorimetric methods include measuring native fluorescence of the drug in various solvents, measuring fluorescence intensity after formation of charge transfer complexes, chemometric methods, lanthanide sensitized fluorescence methods [16].

Radioanalytical methods have been used for investigation of the properties and biodistribution of CIP labelled with $^{99}Tc^{m}$ [17]. It has been found that radiolabelling efficiency of $^{99}Tc^{m}$-CIP was higher than 95%. Biodistribution studies in inflamed mice have shown that $^{99}Tc^{m}$-CIP is rapidly distributed after i.v. administration with a predominant renal clearance. The radioactive preparation is able to localize both bacterial and sterile inflammations but its accumulation may be due only to increased blood flow together with enhanced vascular permeability.

Separating techniques play an important role in the analysis of active substances, their impurities and degradation products. Thin-layer chromatography is a popular technique used in drug analysis. CIP and Ornidazole (ORN) have been determined in human plasma by high performance thin layer chromatography [18]. Tinidazole (TIN) has been used as an internal standard. Extraction of the plasma samples has been performed using methanol: formic acid (5.5:0.5 v/v), and mobile phase, consisting of chloroform: methanol: triethylamine (9.0: 0.8: 0.4 v/v/v). The working concentration range has been determined to be 100-700 ng/ml. The sensitivity of the method was found to be suitable for handling various plasma levels of the drugs.

Another alternative method is micellar liquid chromatography. An advantage of this technique is the use of mobile phases with a small amount of organic solvents, resulting in lower toxicity of these phases and the release of safe waste solutions. A simple micellar liquid chromatographic (MLC) method for the determination of CIP and Enoxacin has been developed [19]. The mobile phase consists of 75 mM sodium dodecyl sulphate: 10 mM phosphate buffer: 18 mM Tetrabutylammonium bromide solution/3% (v/v) 1-propanol at pH 3.0. Tosufloxacin was used as an internal standard. The linear concentration range of application was been 0.10–5.00 μg/ml for both compounds. The method shows good recoveries for the two fluoroquinolones. The proposed method has been applied to human serum samples.

Capillary electrophoresis is an attractive analytical technique characterized by rapidity, low reagent and sample consumption and high separation efficiency. Capillary electrophoresis has been used for determination of CIP in drug substance [20] and in tablets formulations [21, 22]. It is interesting to note the simple procedure for sample preparation - tablets have been dissolved in sodium hydroxide and further diluted with water prior to injection in the capillary electrophoretic system equiped with capacitively-coupled contactless conductivity detector [22]. Quinolones, and in particular CIP, are widely used in veterinary medicine. Their residues may remain in edible tissues. CIP has been determined in milk [22], pork, chicken, swine liver and swine kidney [23] and in pig plasma samples [24]. Simple dillution has been applied for determination of CIP in milk samples by capillary electrophoretic system equiped with capacitively-coupled contactless conductivity detector [22]. However, more complicated procedures have been required for complex biological samples [23, 24]. It has been found that using a field amplified sample stacking–sweeping technique, the sensitivity for ciprofloxacin has been improved around 400-fold compared to conventional capillary electrophoresis method [23].

Despite the diversity and some advantages of the above-mentioned analytical techniques, spectral methods in the ultraviolet and visible spectra, as well as high-performance liquid chromatographic methods continue to be essential tools for the analysis of CIP. Spectroscopic and high-performance liquid chromatography (HPLC) techniques are well established methods, which play a significant role in the field of pharmaceutical analysis, regarding manufacturing process, quality control and drugs determination in biological samples.

Relatively simple procedures, low reagent and sample consumption, speed, precision and accuracy combined with accessibility and comparatively low cost of common apparatus make spectroscopic methods attractive. Direct methods are suitable for determining drug substances. For more complicated samples, when simultaneous determination of drugs with overlapping spectra is necessary, a derivative spectrophotometry can be applied, often in combination with chemometric approaches.

On the other hand, the high performance liquid chromatographic method is characterized by excellent specificity and sufficient precision and accuracy. The wide diversity of chromatographic columns available, and presence of universal and specific detectors, make the analysis of virtually all pharmaceutical compounds possible. This determines HPLC as a unique analytical technique, particularly suited for the analysis of complex samples. However, HPLC requires more complicated and expensive equipment, relatively higher organic solvent consumption and skilled personnel.

The purpose of this paper is to summarize the latest applications of spectral (in ultraviolet and visible spectra) and high-performance liquid chromatographic methods for the determination of CIP in bulk drug, pharmaceutical formulations and in biological samples. Articles published in the period 2012-2017 are covered.

METHODS

Spectral Methods

Ultraviolet Spectrophotometric Methods

Direct UV, derivative and chemometric spectrophotometric methods have been used for the analysis of CIP, alone [27-32] or in combination with other drugs [33-46], in pure and in pharmaceutical dosage forms. Simple UV spectrophotometric methods, based on direct measurements in water solutions, have been developed for the estimation of CIP in ophtalmic solutions [27] and tablets [28, 29]. Direct measurements have also been applied in 0.1 N HCl and in 0.1 N NaOH [30, 31]. Both methods have been used in the quality control of CIP tablets. The working linear range for CIP in the above mentioned methods was determined to be around 2-10 μg/ml. Derivative spectrophotometry, especially in combination with chemometric and signal processing techniques offers solutions for various analytical problems, for example those associated with matrix interferences, resolution of multicomponent systems or overlapping spectra. Derivative techniques can be used for spectrophotometric data treatment, to improve the accuracy of analyses of mixtures. Various applications of derivative spectrophotometry techniques can be found in the available literature [47, 48]. Three UV spectrophotometric methods (zero order, first order, and second order) [32] have been developed and successfully applied to estimate the amount of CIP Hydrochloride in pharmaceutical formulations. The developed methods have been found to be accurate, sensitive and precise. CIP and Dexamethasone (DEX) have been simultaneously determined in ear drops and ophthalmic solutions [33, 34]. Five UV spectrophotometric methods have been developed to determine both drugs in ear drops. The first method has been the well established dual wavelength method. The second and third methods have utilized the isoabsorptive point, absorbance subtraction and absorbance ratio. The other two methods have been the manipulating ratio spectra namely, ratio subtraction and ratio difference [33]. The linear ranges for CIP and DEX have been determined to be 5-30 μg/ml and 5-50 μg/ml respectively. The first derivative ratio has been used for determination of both drugs in ophthalmic solutions [34]. The respective linear ranges have been determined to be 6-18 μg/ml for CIP and 2-6 μg/ml for DEX. The developed methods have been found to be suitable for routine analysis, with minimum manipulation steps and without preliminary separation of the two drugs. Chemometric assisted zero order UV spectrophotometry has been used for determination of CIP and Diclofenac (DCF) [35]. Linear ranges have been determined to be 2-10 μg/ml and 4-32 μg/ml for CIP and DCF respectively. The method has been applied for Chitosan dental films developed for treatment of periodontitis. A spectrophotometric method for determination of CIP and Mebeverin hydrochloride (MEB) has been developed [36]. The first and second derivative spectra permitted individual and simultaneous determination of CIP and MEB in a concentration range of 4-28 μg/ml by measuring the amplitude of peak to base line and the area under the peak at selected spectrum intervals. For resolving the interference of Metronidazole with CIP in pharmaceutical dosage forms a zero order and signal processing spectrophotometric techniques have been applied [37]. The respective linear ranges have been determined to be 1-10 μg/ml for both drugs. The proposed methods do not need any sophisticated apparatus and could be easily applied in quality control laboratories. CIP and ORN have been determined in tablet dosage forms by simultaneous equations [38, 39] and absorption ratio methods [38]. The obtained results were in good agreement with the corresponding labelled amount. CIP and TIN have been determined in tablet dosage forms by simultaneous equation [40-44], first order derivative spectra [41], isoabsorptive point [42] and absorbance ratio [41, 44] methods. On the other hand CIP, TIN and Dicyclomine (DIC) have been also determined by simultaneous equation method in tablet formulations [45]. CIP and Bromhexin (BH) were determined by ultraviolet spectrophotometry in degradation studies in different media. The method has been applied to combined tablet dosage forms [46].

Visible Spectrophotometric Methods

CIP has the ability to form complexes with different metal ions. This ability is used to create many spectrophotometric methods for the analysis of CIP in various matrices [48, 49]. A spectrophotometric method based on a charge transfer complexation of CIP with Chloranilic acid (CL) has been elaborated [50]. The achieved linear range has been determined to be of 5.6 - 120 μg/ml. The proposed method has recovery within the range stated in the official compendium. CIP in infusions [51] and tablets [52] have been determined by ion-pair formation methods. The proposed methods have been based on the ion-pairs formation between CIP hydrochloride and Bromocresol Purple (BCP) or Bromothymol Blue (BTB) [51]. Complexation of CIP with Ni (II) tetrathiocyanate has also been used [52]. The results obtained by this method have been found to be in good agreement with reference methods. A method, based on the oxidation of CIP by a known excess of Ceric Ammonium Sulphate in sulphuric acid medium has been elaborated [53]. Subsequently, unreacted Ce (IV) has been determined using Amaranth dye. The method has been succesfully applied to tablets with linear working range of 2 - 13 μg/ml. Complex formation with Fe (III) has also been used for determination of CIP in ophtalmic solutions [54] and in tablets [55]. The working linear ranges have been determined to be of 50 -100 μg/ml [54] and 0.5 - 50 μg/ml [55] respectively. It is interesting to note the development of flow injection method for the quantitative determination of CIP using iron extracted from soil as green reagent [55].

Table 1 summarizes the reported spectrophotometric methods for analysis of CIP alone and in combination with other drugs. The drugs are tabulated in alphabetical order.

Table 1. Ultraviolet and visible spectrophotometric methods for analysis of CIP, alone and in combination with other drugs

Drugs	Matrix	Methods/Reagents	λ, nm	Ref.
Ultraviolet spectrophotometry				
CIP	ophtalmic solutions	direct method in water solutions	275	[27]
CIP	tablets	direct method in water solutions	275	[28]
CIP	tablets	direct method in water solutions	278	[29]
CIP	tablets	direct method in 0.1M HCl	273	[30]
CIP	tablets	direct method in 0.1 N HCl direct method in 0.1 N NaOH	294	[31]
CIP	tablets	zero order first order second order	272 274 274	[32]
CIP BH	tablets	degradation studies, 1M HCl, 1M NaOH, 6% H_2O_2, distilled water	200-400	[46]
CIP DEX	ear drops	dual wavelength method absorbance subtraction method absorbance ratio method ratio subtraction method ratio difference method	336.5-254.5 254.5-336.5 261.5 331.5 238.5 238.5 240-285	[33]
CIP DEX	ophtalmic solutions	first order derivative ratio spectra	325 254	[34]
CIP DCF	chitosan dental films	zero order spectra; chemometric techniques (CLS, ILS, PLS, PCR)	230-310	[35]
CIP MEB	tablets	first derivative second derivative	342 326	[36]
CIP MET	tablets	area under the curve simultaneous equation signal processing, SGF signal processing, CWT	273–283; 307–317 280; 311 262 257	[37]

Drugs	Matrix	Methods/Reagents	λ, nm	Ref.
CIP ORN	tablets	simultaneous equations, absorbance ratio	272 319 272 292	[38]
CIP ORN	tablets	simultaneous equations	270 319	[39]
CIP TIN	tablets	simultaneous equations	281.7 310.9	[40]
CIP TIN	tablets	simultaneous equations absorbance ratio first order derivative spectra	276 317 298 276 262 307	[41]
CIP TIN	tablets	simultaneous equations isoabsorptive point	280 310 291	[42]
CIP TIN	tablets	simultaneous equations absorbance ratio	271 318 292 271	[43]
CIP TIN	tablets	simultaneous equations absorbance ratio	272 365 299 277	[44]
CIP TIN DIC	tablets	simultaneous equations	274 366 218	[45]
Visible spectrophotometry				
CIP	tablets	charge-transfer complexation, with CL	520	[50]
CIP	infusions	ion-pair complexation, with BCP with BTB	440 450	[51]
CIP	tablets	ion-pair complexation, Ni (II) tetrathiocyanate	623	[52]
CIP	tablets	redox reaction, Ce (IV) sulphate, amaranth dye	523	[53]
CIP	ophtalmic solutions	first derivative complexation with Fe (III)	386	[54]
CIP	tablets	FIA, complexation with Fe (III) extracted from soil	440	[55]

High Performance Liquid Chromatography (HPLC) Methods

In the analysis of ciprofloxacin, many High Performance Liquid Chromatography (HPLC) methods with different detection techniques are applied. The most common is HPLC with ultraviolet (HPLC-UV) or fluorescence detection (HPLC-FLD). Another detector combined with the HPLC system is mass detector (MS) (HPLC-MS). The pharmaceutical formulations are complex matrices. Physiological fluids (blood, bile, saliva, and urine) and tissues homogenates require a more complex technique of separation. This is due to the presence of endogenous substances that may appear on the chromatogram or electropherogram during analysis. The base factor is to optimize the conditions of the analysis (use of the proper solvent or buffer) and the sample preparation. In this case the sample preparation may involve dilution which might be applied for urine, protein precipitation or extraction applied in more complex matrices (blood, serum, tissue homogenates). This part reports information on methods for determining CIP in different matrices. The methods are divided according to the analytical technique used and preconditioning of samples for analysis.

In the Table 2 are presented analytical techniques for quantitative analysis of this drug in pharmaceutical formulation. Most of them are based on reversed phase HPLC. The most common applied detectors are UV [56-60, 62, 63, 65-73, 76, 77, 80-82] and photodiode array detector (PDA) [64, 74-75, 78-79]. The other detector that can be applied is fluorescence detector (FLD) [61]. The mobile phase is a mixture of water or aqueous buffer and organic solvent. Triethylamine (TEA) is used as an addition to mobile phase. TEA is an ion pair reagent added to water that improves the shape of the peak. Its content does not exceed 1%, and the pH of the mobile phase is slightly acidic [56, 65, 67, 68, 72, 80, 82]. The proper pH value is adjusted with orthophosphoric acid or acetic acid [61]. Small changes in pH of the mobile phase have a great influence to the chromatographic behavior of these substances [58]. The addition of ion pair reagent improves the quality of the separation due to the presence of the negatively charged carboxyl group. The other polar constituent might be the phosphate buffer consisting of either sodium or potassium phosphates in the following range of concentrations 10–50 mM [63, 64, 66, 67, 74, 77-79, 81]. The most common organic solvent in HPLC separation is acetonitrile (ACN) [56–63, 66–70, 72–75, 77–82]. Its content is within the range 10 – 75% for isocratic elution [56–63, 66–70, 72–75, 77–82]. The pre-dominant type of chromatographic columns used for RP-HPLC analysis are C18 and C8 (Table 2). In some cases C8 column as stationary phase is preferable [64]. The authors have attained the best chromatographic separations within run time of 10 minutes. The peaks of DEX showed high tailing on C18, Phenyl-2, and Cyano- columns but symmetrical good peaks were achieved on C8. HILIC columns were also applied in CIP and ORN analysis [70]. The main advantage to using HILIC columns is the fact that they can be used for separation of ionized compounds. The HILIC columns are suitable for MS detection due to the high content of organic solvent. HILIC separation is a normal type of separation, but the typical reversed phase eluents are used. It is helpful when the poor retention of the analyte is observed in the column. The methanol is often used in addition to ACN, and it can be used in both isocratic [65, 71, 72, 76, 101] and gradient elution [95, 101]. ACN, water, and methanol (and their mixtures) might be used as the solvents for stock solutions [71, 72, 76]. The other contents of the mobile phase might be diethylamine (DEA) [58], sodium-1-octane sulfonate (SOS) as an ion pairing reagent [62], acetic acid (in FLD detection) [61]. Other authors [62] reported the use of SOS in mobile phase as an ion pairing reagent to the mobile phase and vary the ratio of buffer and acetonitrile can improve resolution and peak parameters. They obtained the optimum separation and good peak shapes of CIP, DEX and Ethylenediamine (EDA) as internal standard (IS).

All aforementioned techniques require proper sample preconditioning. In the Table 3 are summarized reported HPLC methods for CIP determination in various biological samples: blood serum [64, 68, 93], urine [64], human plasma [84, 85, 87, 89, 95, 97-101] blood plasma of broiler chicken [86], rabbit plasma [88], sputum [94], fish tissue [96], milk, egg, shrimp [83], cell culture medium (cell lysate) [90], porcine and bovine meat [91], raw goat milk [92].

Table 2. HPLC methods – pharmaceutical preparations

Drugs	Matrix	Detection	Stationary phase	Chromatographic conditions	Ref.
CIP	tablets, capsules	UV 278 nm	X BridgeC18, (150 x 4.6, 3.5μm)	0.025M H_3PO_4(pH 3.0 ± 0.1, TeTA): ACN (60:40 v/v)	[56]
CIP	tablets	UV 290 nm	LiChrosorb C18, (250 x 4.6, 5μm)	0.3% H_3PO_4: ACN (65:35 v/v)	[57]
CIP	suspensions tablets	UV 278 nm	μ-Bondapak ODS-C18 (250 x 4.6, 10 μm)	ACN: 0.025M H_3PO_4 (pH 3.0 ± 0.1 DEA) (70:30 v/v)	[58]
CIP	tablets	UV 275 nm	C18 X terra (150 x 4.6, 5 μm)	Phosphate buffer 5.3 mM (3.5 ± 0.1, H_3PO_4): ACN (60:40 v/v)	[59]
CIP	tablets	UV 278 nm	Bondapak C18 (250 x 4.6)	0.025M H_3PO_4 (pH 3.0 ± 0.1 TEA): ACN (87:13 v/v)	[60]
CIP	bulk drug	FLD 250/410 nm	Kromasil 100 C18 (250 x 4.6, 5μm)	H_2O: ACN: CH_3COOH (87:12:1 v/v/v)	[61]
CIP DEX	ophthalmic solutions	UV 240 nm	ACE C18, (250 x 4.6, 5μm)	SOS buffer (pH 3.8): ACN (65:35 v/v)	[62]
CIP DEX	eye drops	UV 254 nm	Chromosil C18, (250 x 4.6, 5μm)	phosphate buffer (pH 4): ACN (65:35 v/v)	[63]
CIP DEX	eye drops	PDA 270 nm	Hypersil BDS C8, (250 x 4.6, 5μm)	phosphate buffer (pH 3.0): MeOH (41:59 v/v)	[64]
CIP DEX	eye/ear drops	UV 254 nm	C18 (250 x 4.6, 5μm)	MeOH: H_2O: TEA (55:45:0.6 v/v/v)	[65]
CIP LEVO OFL NOR	tablets	UV 280 nm	Eurosphere C18, (250 x 4.6)	0.01M KH_2PO_4 (pH 3): ACN (82:18 v/v)	[66]
CIP MET	tablets	UV 298 nm	Lichrospher C18 (100 x 4.6, 5μm)	KH_2PO_4 (50mM, pH 3.5): ACN (80:20 v/v)+TEA (7.5 mM)	[67]
CIP MET	tablets	UV 290 nm	LiChrosorb C18 (250 x 4.6, 5μm)	TEA:H_3PO_4:ACN (0.02:80:20 v/v/v).	[68]

Drugs	Matrix	Detection	Stationary phase	Chromatographic conditions	Ref.
CIP ORN	tablets	UV 299 nm	Capcellpak C18, (250 x 4.6, 5µm)	ACN: H_2O (70:30 v/v), (pH 2.8, H_3PO_4)	[69]
CIP ORN	tablets	UV 289 nm	Phenomenex Luna C18 (250 x 4.60, 5µm)	ACN: H_2O (pH 2.5, H_3PO_4) (75:25 v/v)	[70]
CIP PHENA	tablets	UV 295 nm	Enable C18 (250 x 4.6, 5µm)	MeOH: H_2O (80:20 v/v)	[71]
CIP QN	binary mixtures	UV 236 nm	Purospher Star C18e (250 x 4.6, 5µm)	ACN: MeOH: 0.1% TEA (1:6:3 v/v/v), (pH 3.8 H_3PO_4)	[72]
CIP TIN	tablets	UV 316 nm	Agilent XDB C18, (150 x 4.6, 5µm)	ACN: 0.1% H_3PO_4 (20:80 v/v)	[73]
CIP TIN	tablets	PDA 278.5 nm 327.5 nm	Purospher Star C18, (100 x 2.1, 2µm)	phosphate buffer (pH 3 H_3PO_4): ACN (80:20 v/v)	[74]
CIP TIN	tablets	PDA 316 nm	Inertsil C18 (250 x 4.6, 5µm)	0.17% H_3PO_4: ACN (82:18 v/v)	[75]
CIP TIN	tablets	UV 225 nm	Zorbax Rx-C18 (150 x 4.6, 5µm)	H_3PO_4: MeOH (70:30 v/v), (pH 3)	[76]
CIP TIN	tablets	UV 316 nm	Inertsil C18 (250 x 4.6, 5µm)	phosphate buffer (pH 6.8): ACN (82:18 v/v)	[77]
CIP TIN EDA	tablets	PDA 278 nm 317 nm	X-Terra C18 (150 x 4.5, 5µm)	A: KH_2PO_4 buffer (pH 4.5) B: KH_2PO_4 buffer (pH 4.5): ACN (50:50 v/v) gradient mode	[78] [79]
CIP deg prod	bulk drug	UV 278 nm	C18, S5ODS (250 x 4.6, 5µm)	0.025M H_3PO_4 (pH 3.0 TEA): ACN (87:13 v/v)	[80]
CIP deg prod	bulk drug	UV 278 nm	Phenomenex C18 (250 x 4.6, 5µm)	KH_2PO_4 buffer (pH 3): ACN (80:20 v/v)	[81]
CIP rel sub	bulk drug	UV 278 nm	Inertsil C18, (250 x 4.0, 5µm)	0.15% H_3PO_4 (pH 3.0 TEA):ACN gradient mode	[82]

Table 3. HPLC methods – biological samples

Drugs	Matrix	Sample preparation	Detection	Stationary phase	Chromatographic conditions	Ref.
CIP	milk egg shrimp	LLE by ATPS (copolymers EOPO)	UV 274 nm	Eclipse XDB-C18, (250x4.6, 5μm)	$MeOH:H_2O$ (pH 3.0) (27:73 v/v)	[83]
CIP SDM (IS)	plasma	PP (ACN)	UV 277 nm	ACE®5 C18 (250x4.6, 5μm)	Phosphate buffer (pH 2.7) :ACN (77:23 v/v)	[84]
CIP PhAc (IS)	human plasma	LLE (0.1 M phosphate buffer pH 7.4 DCM)	UV 276 nm	Bondapack C18 (250x4.6, 10μm)	ACN: 0.1 M KH_2PO_4 (20:80 v/v) (pH 3)	[85]
CIP	blood plasma of broiler chicken	PP (ACN)	UV 229 nm	-	Phosphate buffer: ACN (50:50 v/v)	[86]
CIP UF (IS)	human plasma	PP (ACN)	UV 280 nm	Hypersil BDS C18 (150x4.6, 5 μm)	0.1% TEA: ACN (80:20 v/v), pH 2.5 H_3PO_4)	[87]
CIP LEVO (IS)	rabbit plasma	LLE (MeOH)	UV 277 nm	PhenomeneC18 (250x4.6, 3.5μm)	KH_2PO_4 buffer (pH 4.5): ACN (3:7 v/v)	[88]
CIP LEVO (IS)	human plasma	PP (ACN)	UV 276.6 nm	Lachrom C18, (250x4.6, 5 μm)	Phosphate buffer 20 mM (pH 3.0±0.1 TeTA):ACN (13:87 v/v)	[89]
CIP	cell culture medium cell lysate	PP ($HClO_4$)	PDA 275 nm	Zorbax SB C18, (150x4.6, 5 μm)	ACN: 0.05 M Na_2HPO_4 (80:20 v/v)	[90]
CIP DANO ENRO OXO	porcine bovine meat	ultrasonication in a micellar solution filtration	FLD 260/366 nm 280/455 nm	Kromasil C18 (150x4.6, 5μm)	0.05 M SDS: 7.5% 1-propanol: 0.5% TEA (pH 3)	[91]

Drugs	Matrix	Sample preparation	Detection	Stationary phase	Chromatographic conditions	Ref.
CIP DEX	human serum urine	dilution and centrifugation	PDA 270 nm	Hypersil BDS C8 (250x4.6, 5μm)	Phosphate buffer (pH 3.0): MeOH (41:59 v/v)	[64]
CIP ENRO	raw goat milk	SPE C18 (H_2O + 2% TFA): ACN: MeOH (77:15:8 v/v/v)	FLD 280/448 nm	Chromolith Performance RP-18e (100x4.6, 5 μm), RP-18 pre-column	H_2O (4% CH_3COOH): ACN:MeOH (84:8:8 v/v/v)	[92]
CIP ENRO TRIM	blood serum of poultry	PP($HClO_4$)	UV 278 nm	Kromasil 100-5 C18 (150x4.6, 5 μm)	50 мM Acetate buffer (pH 3.0): ACN (86 : 14 v/v)	[93]
CIP LEVO ENRO(IS)	human sputum	Dilution, Centrifugation, (MEPS)	PDA 279 nm 295 nm	Discovery C8 (250x4.6, 5μm)	Phosphate buffer (30 mM, pH 2.5 1% TEA): ACN (86:14 v/v)	[94]
CIP LEVO NOR OFL	plasma serum	Deproteination (TFA), MIPF-SPME	UV 280 nm	Eurosphere C18(250x4.65μm)	0.01 M KH_2PO_4 (pH 3): ACN (82:18 v/v)	[68]
CIP LIN	human plasma	MEPS	PDA 277 nm 251 nm	Poroshell 120 SB C18 (50x2.1, 2.6 μm)	A: 10 mM NH_4Ac (pH 3.5 HCl) B: ACN: MeOH (80:20 v/v) gradient mode	[95]
CIP NDA	fish tissue	LLE (MeOH)	UV 282 nm 266 nm	ChromosilC18 (250x4.6, 5μm); C18 (150x4.6, 5μm); C8(150x4.6, 5μm)	CIP: MeOH:0.25M H_3PO_4 (80:20 v/v) NDA: ACN: 0.5 M KH_2PO_4 buffer (30:70 v/v)	[96]
CIP ORN TIN (IS)	human plasma	LLE (MeOH: HCOOH)	UV 300 nm	Eurosphere 100 C18 (250x4.6, 5 μm)	ACN: MeOH: H_2O: TEA (40:20:40: 1% v/v/v/v)	[97]
CIP QN	human plasma	PP (ACN)	PDA 275 nm 254 nm 254 nm	Zorbax-CN (150x4.6, 5 μm)	ACN: 0.02 M KH_2PO_4 (pH 2.8) (42:58 v/v)	[98]

Table 3. (Continued)

Drugs	Matrix	Sample preparation	Detection	Stationary phase	Chromatographic conditions	Ref.
3-HQN PYR (IS)						
CIP, OFL (IS)	human plasma	PP ($CHCl_3$)	LC-MS/MS m/z 332/231.3 m/z 362.2→261.0 for IS	C18, (75x 4.6, 5 µm)	0.2% HCOOH: MeOH (10:90 v/v)	[99]
CIP MOXI SPAR DA-7157, prodrug DA-7218 (DA1)	human plasma	PP (ACN)	DAD 278nm; FLD 292/525 nm	Atlantis dC18(150x4.6, 5 µm)	ACN: 0.1% TFA (v/v) gradient mode	[100]
CIP, OFL (IS)	human plasma	LLE (ether: methylene chloride 7:3 v/v)	LC-MS/MS MS/MS (MRM mode) (M+H)+ ions m/z 332.1→231.1 m/z 362.1→261.1)	Phenomenex Luna phenyl-hexyl (50x2.0, 5 µm)	MeOH: 5 mM NH_4Ac(pH 3.0) (35:65 v/v)	[101]

Sample Preparation

Sample preparation or sample pre-treatment is a fundamental and critical part of any bioanalytical method. It has a high impact on the quality of the data and it is usually the most time-consuming step of drug analysis in biological matrices, accounting for 80% of the total analysis time. Biological matrices (e.g., blood, plasma/serum, tissue, urine, saliva) which contain the drug/analyte under investigation have different degrees of complexity and comprise several components, such as salts, acids, basis, proteins, cells and lipids. Sample preparation aims at selective isolation of the analyte from the matrix by removing the precipitation compounds (Table 3). Three main approaches are applied in the preparation of biological samples. Protein precipitation, liquid-liquid extraction (LLE) and dilution is typically applied prior to analysis. Protein precipitation is mainly performed using solvents such as ACN [84, 86, 87, 89, 98, 100], methanol [88, 64], a mixture of ACN and methanol [24, 96], perchloric acid and methanol [90, 93], formic acid and methanol [97], trichloroacetic acid (TCA) [68], chloroform [99], and without deproteination with H_2O (containing 2% TFA/ACN): ACN: MeOH (77:15:8, v/v/v) as eluent [92]. Chen et al. reported the LLE, utilizing aqueous two-phase systems (ATPS). They used a new ATPS formed by thermoseparating copolymers composed of ethylene oxide (EO) and propylene oxide (PO) EOPO [83]. The extraction method comprises LLE with dichloromethane [85], chloroform [99], ether and methylene chloride (7/3, v/v) [101] and dispersive liquid–liquid microextraction by packed sorbent (MEPS) [94, 95]. Other procedures applied in preconditioning are ultrasonication in a micellar solution and filtration [91], dilution and centrifugation [64], dilution, centrifugation and microextraction by packed sorbent (MEPS) [94], deproteination with trichloroacetic acid followed by molecularly imprinted fiber-solid phase microextraction technique (MIPF-SPME) [68].

The dilution is a commonly used method in sample preconditioning of pharmaceutical formulations. The analysis of the quantity of CIP with separation techniques requires also the use of the internal standard. The addition of the internal standard ensures the repeatability of the results and improves the precision of the assay.

The limit of detection (LOD) and limit of quantification (LOQ) strongly depended on both the used matrix and applied detector. The LOD and LOQ for pharmaceutical formulations were even of the order of 0.02 ng/ml for fluorescent detection and 0.03 μg/ml for UV detection. The detection limit for the biological matrices such as plasma, urine, and serum were higher. The MS/MS detector was more sensitive for the analyte than UV or FLD; however, for routine clinical practice it is not always necessary to detect very low concentrations because peak and trough concentrations are on the order of mg/l [99, 101]. However, if the lower level of quantification is required, mass detection can be applied [99, 101]. The MS/MS ion transitions were monitored as 332.0→231.3 for ciprofloxacin and 362.2→261.0 for IS [101].

MECHANISMS OF RESISTANCE AND NEW APPLICATIONS OF FLUOROQUINOLONES

Mechanisms of Resistance

There are 3 main mechanisms of resistance to fluoroquinolones:

1. chromosomal mutations in genes, encoding the quinolone targets (DNA gyrase (GyrA and GyrB) and topoisomerase IV (ParC and ParE));
2. decreased permeability (overexpression of the AcrAB-TolC multidrug efflux pumps or changes in outer membrane proteins: e.g., OmpF and OmpC);
3. plasmid-mediated quinolone resistance mechanisms (Qnr proteins, that protect the quinolone targets; the acetylation of CIP and norfloxacin by Aac (6')-Ib-cr; and the plasmid-mediated efflux pumps, QepA and OqxAB) [102, 103].

In contrast to fluoroquinolone resistance mechanisms such as chromosomal mutations and efflux pumps, qnr genes are often located on mobile plasmids and can be shared between bacterial cells through the process of horizontal gene transfer.

In their study [104], they screened more than 12 terabases of DNA for novel qnr fluoroquinolone resistance genes and were able to identify 20 putatively novel qnr genes.

Similarly to many other resistance genes, qnr genes are hypothesized to have originated from harmless environmental bacteria and subsequently mobilized into human pathogens. Recent reports suggest that qnr genes are ubiquitously present in microbial communities from many environments, including marine and lake water, soil, river sediment, and the human microbiome [105-109]. Boulund et al. (2017) found that the nine selected for experimental validation qnr genes, six consistently showed an increased MIC to CIP at levels comparable to previously established qnr variants, when expressed in E. coli [104]. The results of this study indicate, however, that no known or novel qnr genes are ubiquitously spread in high abundance across the metagenomes of the individuals included in their study, suggesting that horizontally transferrable qnr fluoroquinolone resistance genes are rare in the human microbiome.

Other literature data confirmed that in the resistance mechanisms to quinolones, may play role of the mitochondrial enzyme succinate dehydrogenase. When the activity of this enzyme was decreased, it was observed higher production of superoxide ions. The authors found that inhibiting succinate dehydrogenase is sufficient to increase sensitivity to CIP in LLQR E. coli (Low-Level Quinolone-resistant Escherichia coli) [102].

ROS, including superoxide radical $\bullet O_2^-$, peroxide O_2^{2-}, and hydroxyl radicals •OH, are present in bacteria at low levels during normal aerobic respiration and are mitigated by antioxidant defenses in bacteria including superoxide dismutase (SOD) and catalase [110]. In bacteria, superoxide disrupts enzyme iron sulfur clusters, resulting in an increased free ferrous iron pool [111]. This free iron further localized at the DNA, proteins and lipids, allowing Fenton chemistry to occur within the diffusion lengths of hydroxyl radical for increased deleterious effects from ROS species [112]. Furthermore, it was recently shown that enhancing the endogenous production of superoxide and peroxide in E. coli by single-gene deletions potentiated antibiotic activity [113]. In their study, Courtney et al. (2017) found that superoxide-generating nanoparticles in combination with CIP increased bactericidal effects of the CIP against a range of MDR Gram-negative clinical isolates [110].

New Applications

Anticancer Activity

DNA topological states depend upon the activity of topoisomerase I and II [114]. Their activity is important for cellular activities like replication, recombination, transcription and DNA repair [115]. Topoisomerase II is present in two isoforms: Top2a and Top2b in mammals [116]. Top2a is actively involved in replicating cells while Top2b is constitutively expressed in specific cellular processes like neural development [117]. Human Topo2 is the target of several anticancer agents [118], which includes doxorubicin, amascrine, mitoxantrone and etoposide [119].

There are literature data that quinolone-induced inactivation of Topo II at high concentrations is proposed to involve direct binding of quinolones to DNA [120]. Moxifloxacin inhibited purified human topoisomerase II and acted synergistically with VP-16 at the purified enzyme level and enhanced its anti-proliferative effects in THP-1 and Jurkat cells [121]. According these information, [122] they investigated in silico molecular interactions of 13 fluoroquinolones (CIP, enoxacin, finafloxacin, flumequine, gatifloxacin, levofloxacin, lomefloxacin, moxifloxacin, norfloxacin, ofloxacin, prulifloxacin, sarafloxacin, sparafloxacin) with human DNA topoisomerase II a and b. Molecular docking studies showed that fluoroquinolones had formation of hydrogen bond and good binding affinity with human Topo2a and Topo2b. Ofloxacin, sparafloxacin, CIP and moxifloxacin are predicted to be the most potent inhibitors among the

13 fluoroqinolones docked. This in silico study suggests that fluoroquinolones could be repositioned as DNA topoisomerase II inhibitors hence can be used as anticancer drugs.

Several key tumor suppressor pathways are inactivated during the development of most, if not all, human cancers. A prime example of such frequently inactivated tumor suppressor is p53, an important regulator of cellular responses to stress stimuli, such as hypoxia, DNA damage, oncogene activation, telomere shortening or metabolic stress [123]. Its function is commonly lost in cancers by mutations in the p53 gene or by overexpression of cellular inhibitory proteins Mdm2 and MdmX (also known as Mdm4 or HdmX) that cooperate to inhibit p53-mediated transcription by binding to its transactivation domain and by targeting p53 for proteasomal degradation [124]. Mdm2 and MdmX are essential for keeping p53 activity low in normal untransformed and unstressed cells, but their overexpression is estimated to contribute to the loss of p53 activity in up to two million cancer cases worldwide every year [125]. MdmX has been identified as a key therapeutic target in malignant melanoma, with MdmX protein levels increased in over 60% of tumors [126]. In their study [127] Valianatos et al. (2017), found that enoxacin and CIP, but not ofloxacin, inhibited the growth and viability of human melanoma cell line A375, by strongly activation of wild type p53-dependent transcription, without causing significant DNA damage. Their results suggest that some clinically approved fluoroqinolones, like CIP and enoxacin, could potentially be repurposed as activators of p53 tumor suppressor in cancers overexpressing Mdm X oncoprotein.

Inhibitors of Urease and Radical Scavenging Potency

Channar et al. (2017) investigated newly synthetized CIP-, sulfadiazine- and amantadine-based sulfonamides as potent inhibitors of urease and free radical scavengers [128]. Ureae-delivering microscopic organisms have harmful effects on human health. Thus, in human beings the ureas of Helicobacter pylori cause afflictions of the gastrointestinal and urinary tract, for example, stomach disease and peptic ulcers [129, 130]. The authors found that one of the CIP-based sulfonamide exhibited a mixed type of inhibition on the urease, but didn't revealed stronger radical scavenging potency in comparison to the reference vitamin C [128].

QUINOLONES – ADVERSE EFFECTS AND DRUG INTERACTIONS

Mechanism of Action

Bactericidal activity of quinolones has been related to a combination of DNA fragmentation (by inhibiting bacterial DNA gyrase and topoisomerase IV), reactive oxygen species (ROS) production and programmed cell death (PCD) systems mediated by toxin-antitoxin (TA) modules such as mazEF [102]. Quinolones produce alterations to the cellular respiration and iron metabolism, which resulting in cellular damage [131, 132].

Adverse Effects

Gastro-Intestinal (GI) Adverse Effects

The most common adverse reactions involve the GI tract, with 3% to 17% of patients reporting mostly mild nausea, vomiting, and/or abdominal discomfort. Diarrhea and antibiotic-associated colitis have been unusual [133].

Adverse Effects on Muscles and Skeleton

Some adverse drug reactions are common during the therapy with fluoroquinolones: triceps ruptures and for CIP – pronounced negative myoclonus (brief sudden loss of muscle activity in agonist muscles followed by a compensatory jerk of the antagonistic muscles, appearing as involuntary jerky movements) [134].

Achilles tendon rupture or tendinitis has occurred rarely. Renal disease, hemodialysis and steroid use may be predisposing factors. All these agents can produce arthropathy in several species of immature animals. Traditionally, the use of quinolones in children has been contraindicated for this reason. However, children with cystic fibrosis given CIP, norfloxacin and nalidixic acid have had few, and reversible, joint symptoms. Therefore, in some cases the benefits may outweigh the risks of quinolone therapy in children [133].

CNS Side Effects

CNS side effects predominantly mild headache and dizziness have been observed. Rarely, hallucinations, delirium and seizures have occurred, predominantly in patients who also were receiving theophylline or a non-steroidal anti-inflammatory drug [133].

Hypersensitivity

Rashes, including photosensitivity reactions, also can occur [133].

Hematological Adverse Effects

Leukopenia, eosinophilia and mild elevations in serum transaminases occur rarely [133].

Cardiac Adverse Effects

QT interval prolongation has been observed with sparfloxacin and to a lesser extent with gatifloxacin and moxifloxacin. Quinolones probably should be used only with caution in patients on class III (amiodarone) and class IA (quinidine, procainamide) antiarrhythmics [133].

Drug Interactions

CIP and pefloxacin inhibit the metabolism of theophylline, and toxicity from elevated concentrations of the methylxanthine may occur. Non-steroidal anti-inflammatory drugs may augment displacement of y′-aminobutyric acid (GABA) from its receptors by the quinolones [133].

REFERENCES

[1] Petrović, Mira; Maria, Dolores Hernando; Silvia Díaz-Cruz, M; Damià, Barceló. "Liquid Chromatography-Tandem Mass Spectrometry for the Analysis of Pharmaceutical Residues in Environmental Samples: A Review." *Journal of Chromatography A*, 1067, no. 1–2, (2005), 1–14. doi:10.1016/j.chroma.2004.10.110.

[2] Gros, Meritxell; Mira, Petrovic; Damià, Barceló. "Multi-Residue Analytical Methods Using LC-Tandem MS for the Determination of Pharmaceuticals in Environmental and Wastewater Samples: A Review." *Analytical and Bioanalytical Chemistry*, 386, no. 4, (2006), 941–52. doi:10.1007/s00216-006-0586-z.

[3] Kümmerer, Klaus. "Antibiotics in the Aquatic Environment - A Review - Part I." *Chemosphere*, 75, no. 4, (2009), 417–34. doi:10.1016/j.chemosphere.2008.11.086.

[4] Matamoros, Víctor; Diana, Calderón-Preciado; Carmen, Domínguez; Josep, M. Bayona. "Analytical Procedures for the Determination of Emerging Organic Contaminants in Plant Material: A Review." *Analytica Chimica Acta*, 722, (2012), 8–20. doi:10.1016/j.aca.2012. 02.004.

[5] Marazuela, MD; Bogialli, S. "A Review of Novel Strategies of Sample Preparation for the Determination of Antibacterial Residues in Foodstuffs Using Liquid Chromatography-Based Analytical Methods." *Analytica Chimica Acta*, 645, no. 1–2, (2009), 5–17. doi:10.1016/j.aca.2009.04.031.

[6] Kotretsou, Stamatia I. "Determination of Aminoglycosides and Quinolones in Food Using Tandem Mass Spectrometry: A Review." *Critical Reviews in Food Science and Nutrition*, 44, no. 3, (2004), 173–84. doi:10.1080/10408690490441488.

[7] Basavaiah, Kanakapura; Paregowda, Nagegowda; Bankavadi, Chikkaswamy Somashekar; Veeraiah, Ramakrishna. "Spectrophotometric and Titrimetric Determination of Ciprofloxacin Based on Reaction with Cerium (IV) Sulphate."

ScienceAsia, 32, no. 4, (2006), 403–9. doi:10.2306/scienceasia 1513-1874.2006.32.403.

[8] Zhang, Xin; Youli, Wei; Yaping, Ding. "Electrocatalytic Oxidation and Voltammetric Determination of Ciprofloxacin Employing Poly(Alizarin Red)/Graphene Composite Film in the Presence of Ascorbic Acid, Uric Acid and Dopamine." *Analytica Chimica Acta*, 835, (2014), 29–36. doi:10.1016/j.aca.2014.05.020.

[9] Zhang, Xu Zhi; Meng, Shi Huang; Qian, Qian Yang; Dong, Sheng Ding; Jun, Zhao; Wen, Rong Yang; Ke Ming, Qu. "Simple and Cost-Effective Determination of Ciprofloxacin Hydrochloride by Electrical Micro-Titration." *Chinese Chemical Letters*, 28, no. 7, (2017), 1406–12. doi:10.1016/j.cclet.2017.03.019.

[10] Shan, Jun; Yong, Liu; Ruizhen, Li; Can, Wu; Lihua, Zhu; Jingdong, Zhang. "Indirect Electrochemical Determination of Ciprofloxacin by Anodic Stripping Voltammetry of Cd(II) on Graphene-Modified Electrode." *Journal of Electroanalytical Chemistry*, 738, (2015), 123–29. doi:10.1016/j.jelechem.2014.11.031.

[11] Abass, Amina M; Ahmed, Ahmed. "Construction and Potentiometric Study of Ciprofloxacin Selective Electrodes." *International Journal of Research in Pharmacy and Chemistry*, 7, no. 4, (2017), 425–32.

[12] Zhang, Shenghui; Shuang, Wei. "Electrochemical Determination of Ciprofloxacin Based on the Enhancement Effect of Sodium Dodecyl Benzene Sulfonate." *Bulletin of the Korean Chemical Society*, 28, no. 4, (2007), 543–46.

[13] Ensafi, Ail A; Ali, R. Allafchain; Mohammadzadeh, R. "Characterization of $MgFe_2O_4$ Nanoparticles as a Novel Electrochemical Sensor: Application for the Voltammetric Determination of Ciprofloxacin." *Analytical Sciences*, 28, no. July, (2012), 705–10. doi:10.1039/c1jm11909e.

[14] Pandey, S; Pandey, P; Tiwari, G; Tiwari, R; Rai, AK. "FTIR Spectroscopy: A Tool for Quantitative Analysis of Ciprofloxacin in Tablets." *Indian Journal of Pharmaceutical Sciences*, 74, no. 1, (2012), 86–90. doi:10.4103/0250-474X.102551.

[15] Bhongade, Bhoomendra; Sirajunisa, Talath; Sunil, Dhaneshwar. "A Validated Method for the Quantitation of Ciprofloxacin Hydrochloride Using Diffuse Reflectance Infrared Fourier Transform Spectroscopy." *International Journal of Spectroscopy*, 2014, (2014). http://dx.doi.org/10.1155/2014/294612%0AResearch.

[16] Kaur, Kuldeep; Baldev, Singh; Ashok, Kumar Malik. "Chemiluminescence and Spectrofluorimetric Methods for Determination of Fluoroquinolones: A Review." *Analytical Letters*, 44, no. 9 (2011), 1602–39. doi:10.1080/00032719.2010.520392.

[17] Gano, L; Patrick, L; Cantinho, G; Pena, H; Martins, T; Marques, E. "Ciprofloxacin in Imaging of Infective Versus Sterile Inflammation." In International Symposium on *Modern Trends in Radiopharmaceuticals for Diagnosis and Therapy*, 30 March - 3 April, 213–20. Lisbon (Portugal): International Atomic Energy Agency, Vienna (Austria), 1998.

[18] Rote, Ambadas Ranganath; Ravindranath, Bhanudas Saudagar. "New Analytical Method Development and Validation of Ciprofloxacin and Ornidazole in Human Plasma by High Performance Thin Layer Chromatography." *Pharmaceutical Methods*, 7, no. 2, (2016), 89–93. doi:10.5530/phm.2016.7.13.

[19] Vílchez, José Luis; Lilia, Araujo; Avismelsi, Prieto; Alberto, Navalón. "Determination of Ciprofloxacin and Enoxacin in Human Serum Samples by Micellar Liquid Chromatography." *Analytica Chimica Acta*, 516, (2004), 135–40. doi:10.1016/j.aca.2004.04.025.

[20] Michalska, Katarzyna; Genowefa, Pajchel; Stefan, Tyski. "Determination of Ciprofloxacin and Its Impurities by Capillary Zone Electrophoresis." *Journal of Chromatography A*, 1051, (2004), 267–72.

[21] Faria, Adriana F; Marcus, VN. de Souza; Marcone, AL. de Oliveira. "Validation of a Capillary Zone Electrophoresis Method for the Determination of Ciprofloxacin, Gatifloxacin, Moxifloxacin and Ofloxacin in Pharmaceutical Formulations." *Journal of the Brazilian Chemical Society*, 19, no. 3, (2008), 389–96. doi:10.1002/jssc.200 700272.

[22] Montes, Rodrigo HO; Mariana, C. Marra; Monike, M. Rodrigues; Eduardo, M. Richter; Rodrigo, AA. Muñoz. "Fast Determination of Ciprofloxacin by Batch Injection Analysis with Amperometric Detection and Capillary Electrophoresis with Capacitively Coupled Contactless Conductivity Detection." *Electroanalysis*, 26, no. 2, (2014), 432–38. doi:10.1002/elan.201300474.

[23] Xu, Xiaoying; Lihong, Liu; Zhimin, Jia; Yang, Shu. "Determination of Enrofloxacin and Ciprofloxacin in Foods of Animal Origin by Capillary Electrophoresis with Field Amplified Sample Stacking-Sweeping Technique." *Food Chemistry*, 176, (2015), 219–25. doi:10. 1016/j.foodchem.2014.12.054.

[24] Hernández, Margarita; Carme, Aguilar; Francesc, Borrull; Marta, Calull. "Determination of Ciprofloxacin, Enrofloxacin and Flumequine in Pig Plasma Samples by Capillary Isotachophoresis-Capillary Zone Electrophoresis." *Journal of Chromatography B: Analytical Technologies in the Biomedical and Life Sciences*, 772, no. 1, (2002), 163–72. doi:10.1016/S1570-0232(02)00071-5.

[25] Fletcher, P; Andrew, KN; Calokerinos, aC; Forbes, S; Worsfold, PJ. "Analytical Applications of Flow Injection with Chemiluminescence Detection--a Review." *Luminescence: The Journal of Biological and Chemical Luminescence*, 16, (2001), 1–23. doi:10.1002/bio.607.

[26] Waseem, Amir; Mohammad, Yaqoob; Abdul, Nabi. "Analytical Applications of Flow Injection Chemiluminescence for the Determination of Pharmaceuticals– A Review." *Current Pharmaceutical Analysis*, 9, no. 4, (2013), 363–95. doi:10.2174/ 1573412911309990002.

[27] Cazedey, Edith Cristina Laignier; Hérida, Regina Nunes Salgado. "Spectrophotometric Determination of Ciprofloxacin Hydrochloride in Ophthalmic Solution." *Advances in Analytical Chemistry*, 2, no. 6, (2012), 74–79. doi:10.5923/j.aac.20120206.01.

[28] Fereja, Tadesse Haile; Muluneh, Fromsa Seifu; Tizita, Yirga Mola. "UV-Visible Spectrophotometric Method Development and Quantification of Ciprofloxaciline in Tablets Dosage Form."

American Journal Pharmacy and Pharmacology, 2, no. 1, (2015), 1–8.

[29] Naveed, Safila; Nimra, Waheed. "Simple UV Spectrophotometric Assay of Ciprofloxacin." *Mintage Journal of Pharmaceutical and Medical Sciences*, 3, no. 4, (2014), 10–13. doi:10.4236/oalib. 1100615.

[30] Navarro, Maikel Pérez; Yaslenis, Rodríguez Hernández; Yania, Suárez Pérez. "Validación Del Método Por EspectrofotometríaUltravioleta Para Control de Calidad de Clorhidrato de CiprofloxacinaEnTabletasCiprecu." *RevistaCubana de Farmacia*, 48, no. 2, (2014), 199–212. [Validation of the Ultraviolet Spectrophotometry Method for the Quality Control of Ciprofloxacin Chlorhydrate in Ciprecu Tablets. *Cuban Journal of Pharmacy*, 48, no. 2, (2014), 199-212]. http://scielo.sld.cu/pdf/far/v48n2/far05214.pdf%5Cnhttp://ovidsp.ovid.com/ovidweb.cgi?T=JS&PAGE=reference&D=emed12&NEWS=N&AN=2015687948.

[31] Naveed, Safila; Huda, Kafeel; Ramsha, Rukh. "Spectrophotometric Method for the Estimation of Ciprofloxacin in Different Medium." *International Journal of Pharmaceutical Research and Drug Development*, 1, no. 1, (2014), 27–30.

[32] Rekha, Kharat; Jadhav, Santosh; Tamboli, Dilshadbee; Tamboli, Ashpak. "Estimation of Ciprofloxacin Hydrochloride in Bulk and Formulation by Derivative UV-Spectrophotometric Methods." *International Journal of Advances in Scientific Research*, 1, no. 03, (2015), 137–44. doi:10.7439/ijasr.

[33] Fouad, Manal Mohamed. "Novel Spectrophotometric Methods for Simultaneous Determination of Ciprofloxacin Hydrochloride and Dexamethasone Sodium Phosphate in Their Binary Mixture." *Indo American Journal of Pharmaceutical Research*, 5, no. 07, (2015), 2470–80.

[34] Bantarapiwat, K; Rojsanga, P; Ruangwises, N; Buranaphalin, S. "Simultaneous Determination of Ciprofloxacin Hydrochloride and Dexamethasone in Ophthalmic Solution by High Performance Liquid Chromatography and Derivative Spectrophotometry

Chromatography." *Mahidol University Journal of Pharmaceutical Sciences*, 43, no. 4, (2016); 183–92.

[35] Charyulu, R Narayana; Mohammed, Gulzar Ahmed; Prashant, Nayak; Mudit, Dixit. "Simultaneous Analysis and Validation of Ciprofloxacin-Diclofenac and Tetracycline- Diclofenac by Using UV Spectrophotometer." *International Journal of Pharmaceutical Sciences Review and Research*, 28, no. 39, (2014), 207–13.

[36] Mohammmed, Maha A; Muna, A. Kadhum. "Simultaneous Determination of Ciprofloxacin Hydrochloride and Mebeverin Hydrochloride by Derivative Spectrophotometry." *Ibn Al-Haitham Journal for Pure and Applied Science*, 27, no. 3, (2014), 448–61.

[37] Attia, Khalid AM; Mohammed, W. I. Nassar; Mohamed, B. El-Zeiny; Ahmed, Serag. "Zero Order and Signal Processing Spectrophotometric Techniques Applied for Resolving Interference of Metronidazole with Ciprofloxacin in Their Pharmaceutical Dosage Form." *Spectrochimica Acta - Part A: Molecular and Biomolecular Spectroscopy*, 154, (2016), 232–36. doi:10.1016/j.saa.2015.10.040.

[38] Grewal, AS; Patro, SK; Kanungo, SK; Bhardwaj, SK. "Simultaneous Spectrophotometric Estimation of Ciprofloxacin and Ornidazole It Tablet Dosage Form." *International Journal of Pharmaceutical Science and Research*, 3, no. 08, (2012), 2716–20.

[39] Krishna, J; Ramya, B; Sandhya, Naga; Sanayaima, Huidrom; Prasad, VVLN. "Development and Validation of UV Spectrophotometric Method for the Simultaneous Estimation of Ciprofloxacin Hydrochloride and Ornidazole in Combined Pharmaceutical Dosage Form." *Journal of Advanced Pharmacy Education and Research*, 4, no. 4, (2014), 405–8.

[40] Pavanipadmapriya, B. "New Spectrophotometric Multicomponent Estimation of Ciprofloxacin and Tinidazole Tablets." *International Journal of ChemTech Research*, 5, no. 1, (2013), 42–46.

[41] Patil, Manaswi; Vrushali, Tambe; Vijaya, Vichare; Reshma, Kolte. "Validated Simultaneous UV Spectrophotometric Methods for Estimation of Ciprofloxacin and Tinidazole in Tablet Dosage

Form." *International Journal of Pharmacy and Pharmaceutical Sciences*, 4, no. 3, (2012), 182–85. doi:ISSN- 0975-1491.

[42] Bhalerao, Swapnil R; Ambadas, R. Rote. "Application of UV Spectrophotometric Methods for Estimation of Ciprofloxacin and Tinidazole in Combined Tablet Dosage Form." *International Journal of Pharmacy and Pharmaceutical Sciences*, 4, no. 3, (2012), 464–67.

[43] Gummadi, Sowjanya; Devi, Thota; Sri, Valli Varri; Pratyusha, Vaddi; Venkata, Lakshmi Narasimha Seshagiri Rao Jillella. "Development and Validation of UV Spectroscopic Methods for Simultaneous Estimation of Ciprofloxacin and Tinidazole in Tablet Formulation." *International Current Pharmaceutical Journal*, 1, no. 10, (2012), 317–21.

[44] Prathyusha, V; Abdul Rahaman, SK; Revathi, S; Renuka, G. "Development and Validation of UV Spectrophotometric Methods for Simultaneous Estimation of Ciprofloxacin and Tinidazole in Tablet Dosage Form." *International Journal of Pharmacy and Industrial Research*, 3, no. 3, (2013), 259–300.

[45] Raghunath, Malathi; Amol, Dhamne; Vaishali, Mistry; Vaidhun, Bhaskar. "Validated UV Spectrophotometric Method for Estimation of Fixed Dose Combination of Ciprofloxacin, Tinidazole and Dicyclomine in Bulk and Tablet Formulation." *World Journal of Pharmacy and Pharmaceutical Sciences*, 4, no. 3, (2015), 1117–27. http://www.wjpps.com/download/article/1425133012.pdf.

[46] Nagapara, Avinash M; Hasmukh, C Nagapara; Darshan, Madiya; Shital, Faldu. "Degradation Study of Ciprofloxacin Hydrochloride, Bromhexine Hydrochloride and Their Combined Pharmaceutical Dosage Form by Spectrophotometry." *Pharma Tutor*, 2, no. 7, (2014), 102–9.

[47] Bosch Ojeda, C; Sanchez Rojas, F. "Recent Applications in Derivative Ultraviolet/Visible Absorption Spectrophotometry: 2009-2011. A Review." *Microchemical Journal*, 106, (2013), 1–16. doi:10.1016/j.microc.2012.05.012.

[48] Kaur, Kuldeep; Ashwini, Kumar; Ashok, Kumar Malik; Baldev, Singh; Rao, ALJ. "Spectrophotometric Methods for the Determination of Fluoroquinolones: A Review." *Critical Reviews in Analytical Chemistry*, 38, no. 1, (2008), 2–18. doi:10.1080/10408340701804400.

[49] Uivarosi, Valentina. "Metal Complexes of Quinolone Antibiotics and Their Applications: An Update." *Molecules*, 18, no. 9, (2013), 11153–97. doi:10.3390/molecules180911153.

[50] Igboasoiyi, AC; Attih, EE; Ofoefule, SI; Umoh, ED; Udoh, OC "Spectrophotometric Determination of Ciprofloxacin Using Charge-Transfer Complexation Technique." *International Journal of Innovative Research and Development*, 3, no. 11, (2014), 177–82.

[51] Qassim, Ameen W. "Spectrophotometric Determination of Ciprofloxacin Hydrochloride In Pharmaceutical Formulation Ciproxin." *International Journal of Advanced Scientific and Technical Research*, 3, no. 5, (2015), 135–46.

[52] Patel, MN; Bhatt, BS; Gandhi, DS; Dosi, PA; Parmar, PA. "Spectrophotometric Determination of Ciprofloxacin by Ion Pair Formation." *Journal of Analytical Chemistry*, 67, no. 7, (2012), 655–60. doi:10.1134/S1061934812050103.

[53] Rajitha, B; Sayaji, Rao; Vinod Kumar, T. "Spectrophotometric Determination of Drugs & Pharmaceuticals Using Cerium(IV) as Oxidant and Amaranth Dye as Analytical Reagent." *IOSR Journal of Applied Chemistry*, 8, no. 5, (2015), 15–23. doi:10.9790/5736-08511523.

[54] Cazedey, CL; Edith, Rudy Bonfilio; Magali, B. Araújo; Hérida, RN. Salgado. "A First-Derivative Spectrophotometric Method for the Determination of Ciprofloxacin Hydrochloride in Ophthalmic Solution." *Physical Chemistry*, 2, no. 6, (2013), 116–22. doi:10.5923/j.pc.20120206.06.

[55] Palamy, Sysay; Wirat, Ruengsitagoon. "Reverse Flow Injection Spectrophotometric Determination of Ciprofloxacin in Pharmaceuticals Using Iron from Soil as a Green Reagent."

Spectrochimica Acta - Part A: Molecular and Biomolecular Spectroscopy, 190, (2018), 129–34. doi:10.1016/j.saa.2017.09.032.

[56] Scherer, R; Jessica, Pereira; Juliete, Firme; Mariana, Lemos; Mayara, Lemos. "Determination of Ciprofloxacin in Pharmaceutical Formulations Using HPLC Method with UV Detection." *Indian Journal of Pharmaceutical Sciences*, 76, no. 6, (2014), 467–578.

[57] Maslarska, Vania; Bozhanov, S; Tsvetkova, B; Peikova, L; Zareva, N. "RP-HPLC Method for Determination of Ciprofloxacin in Pharmaceutical Dosage Forms." *Pharmacia*, 63, no. 1, (2016), 3–8.

[58] Hasan, Najmul; Farhan, Ahmed Siddiqui; Nawab, Sher; Nighat, Shafi; Arif, Zubair; Muhammad, Afzal. "Development and Validation of a Reverse Phase HPLC Method for the Analysis of Ciprofloxacin and Its Application in Bulk and Different Dosage Formulations." *World Applied Sciences Journal*, 31, no. 5, (2014), 730–40. doi:10.5829/idosi.wasj.2014.31.05.8393.

[59] Bera, AK; Kumar De, A; Pal, B "RP-HPLC Method Development and Validation for the Determination of Ciprofloxacin from Marketed Tablet Dosage Forms." *Journal of Chemical and Pharmaceutical Research*, 6, no. 5, (2014), 1214–18. https://www.scopus.com/inward/record.uri?eid=2-s2.0 8490710 4403&partnerID=40&md5=f2ad0295f9514c05b5bd9d02ecf10419.

[60] Ali, Karima F. "Estimation and Evaluation of the Effect of PH on Ciprofloxacin in Drug Formulations." *Journal of Chemical and Pharmaceutical Research*, 6, no. 4, (2014), 910–16.

[61] Torres, Nádia Hortense; Juliana, Heloisa; PinêAmérico, Carina Nazato; Franz, ZirenaVilca; Luiz, Fernando; Romanholo, Ferreira; et al. "Optimization Methodology for Detection of Antimicrobial Ciprofloxacin by HPLC-FLD." *International Journal of Engineering Research and Development*, 4, no. 2, (2012), 59–62.

[62] Bantarapiwat, K; Rojsanga, P; Ruangwises, N; Buranaphalin, S. "Simultaneous Determination of Ciprofloxacin Hydrochloride and Dexamethasone in Ophthalmic Solution by Reversed Phase High Performance Liquid Chromatography." *Mahidol University Journal of Pharmaceutical Sciences*, 43, no. 4, (2010), 183–92.

[63] Prakash, Katakam; Karanam, R. Sireesha. "Simultaneous Determination of Ciprofloxacin Hydrochloride and Dexamethasone Sodium Phosphate in Eye Drops by HPLC." *E-Journal of Chemistry*, 9, no. 3, (2012), 1077–84. doi:10.1155/2012/187824.

[64] Razzaq, S; Ashfaq, M; Mariam, I; Khan, IU; Razzaq, M; Ghulam, S. "Stability Indicating RP-HPLC Method for Simultaneous Determination of Ciprofloxacin and Dexamethasone in Binary Combination." *Journal of the Chilean Chemical Society*, 62, no. 3, (2017), 3572–77.

[65] Desai, Urvish H; Arpit, H Patwari; Jaydeepkumar, K Maradiya; Mehul, K Sathawara; Bhanubhai, N Suhagia; Ishwarsinh, S Rathod. "RP-HPLC Method for Simultaneous Estimation of Ciprofloxacin and Dexamethasone in Eye/Ear Drops." *International Journal of Pharmaceutical Sciences and Drug Research*, 5, no. 2, (2013), 62–66.

[66] Mirzajani, Roya; Fatemeh, Kardani. "Fabrication of Ciprofloxacin Molecular Imprinted Polymer Coating on a Stainless Steel Wire as a Selective Solid-Phase Microextraction Fiber for Sensitive Determination of Fluoroquinolones in Biological Fluids and Tablet Formulation Using HPLC-UV Detection." *Journal of Pharmaceutical and Biomedical Analysis*, 122, (2016), 98–109. doi:10.1016/j.jpba.2016.01.046.

[67] Budiarti, Agnes; IbnuGholib, Gandjar; Abdul, Rohman. "Liquid Chromatography With UV Detection For Simultaneous Determination Of Ciprofloxacin And Metronidazole." *Jurnal Teknologi*, 72, no. 1, (2015), 45–47. doi:10.11113/jt.v72.3071.

[68] Maslarska, Vania; Tsvetkova, B; Peikova, L; Kostova, B; Rachev, D; Bozhanov, S; Zareva, N. "HPLC assay of model tablet formulations containing metronidazole and ciprofloxacin." *International Journal of Pharmacy and Pharmaceutical Sciences*, 8, (2016), 306-310.

[69] Damerakonda, Kumara Swamy; Hima Bindu, M. "A Novel Validated Stability Indicating Simultaneous Estimation of Ciprofloxacin and Ornidazole by Reverse Phase High Pressure

Liquid Chromatography." *International Journal of Pharmacy and Biological Sciences*, 5, no. 3, (2015), 94–101.

[70] Krishna, JR; Sandhya, BN; Sanayaima, H; Prasad, VVLN. "Development and Validation of UV Spectrophotometric Method for the Simultaneous Estimation of Ciprofloxacin Hydrochloride and Ornidazole in Combined Pharmaceutical Dosage Form." *Journal of Advanced Pharmacy Education and Research.*, 4, no. 4, (2014), 440–43.

[71] Satishkumar, SA; Mohammed, B; Manzoor, A; Anil Kumar, SM; Vijaya Krishna, C. Aradhya; Siddalinga Swamy, MS. "RP-HPLC Method Development and Validation for Simultaneous Estimation of Ciprofloxacin and Phenazopyridine Hydrochloride in Combined Tablet Dosage Form." *World Journal of Pharmacy and Pharmaceutical Sciences*, 4, no. 2, (2014), 775–84.

[72] Sawant, RL; Jadhav, KA; Tanpure, KD; Bharat, AV. "RP-HPLC Methods Development for the Simultaneous Estimation of Quinine and Ciprofloxacin Sawant." *International Journal for Pharmaceutical Research Scholars*, 4, no. 2, (2015), 130–35. doi:10.4172/2155-9872.1000233.

[73] Sirisha, T; Gurupadayya, BM; Sridhar, S. "Simultaneous Determination of Ciprofloxacin and Tinidazole in Tablet Dosage Form by Reverse Phase High." *Tropical Journal of Pharmaceutical Research*, 13, no. 6 (2014): 981–87. doi:10.4314/tjpr.v13i6.23.

[74] Jansari, K; Nirav Patel, B; Parag Patel, R; Nikita Patel, N; Hemant Desai, T. "Development and Validation of Stability Indicating Method for Simultaneous Estimation of Ciprofloxacin Hcl and Tinidazole Using RP-UPLC Method." *IOSR Journal of Pharmacy*, 2, no. 5, (2012), 12–19. doi:10.9790/3013-25401219.

[75] Choudhary, S; Goyal, A; Deep Singh, G. "Dissolution Development of Ciprofloxacin and Tinidazole in Combined Tablet Dosage Form." *International Journal of Pharmacy and Therapeutics*, 6, no. 1, (2015), 33–36.

[76] Kulsum, Syeda; Rahul, Reddy; Kanaka Durga, CM; Padmalatha, M. "A Simple and Validated RP-HPLC Method for the Simultaneous

Estimation of Tinidazole and Ciprofloxacin in Bulk and Pharmaceutical Dosage Forms." *International Journal of Research and Development in Pharmacy and Life Sciences*, 2, no. 1, (2012), 238–43.

[77] Goyal, Anju; Choudhary, Sweety; Gaurav, Deep Singh. "A Validated RP-HPLC Method for Estimation of Ciprofloxacin and Tinidazole in Tablet Dosage Form." *International Journal of Pharmaceutical Chemistry and Analysis*, 2, no. 1, (2015), 22–27.

[78] Balasekhara, Reddy; Sarbudeen, CHM; Balarami Reddy, Y; Durga, D. Rao. "New RP-HPLC Method Development and Validation for Simultaneous Estimation of Tinidazole and Ciprofloxacin and Ethylenediamine Impurities in Tablet Dosage Form." *Medicinal Chemistry and Analysis*, 5, no. 1, (2015), 16–24.

[79] Alapati, VR; DivyaTeja, G; Sunitha, G; Rajesh, CH; Vamsikrishna, L; Panikumar, D Anumolu. "Validated Stability Indicating Liquid Chromatographic Method for Quantification of Ciprofloxacin HCl, Its Related Substance and Tinidazole in Tablet Dosage Form." *International Journal of Pharmacy and Pharmaceutical Sciences*. 6, no. 5, (2014), 611–15. http://www.ijppsjournal.com/Vol6Issue5/9534.pdf.

[80] Adam, Elsadig HK; Mukhtar, El; Mohammed, Abd; Ahmed, EM Saeed. "Stability Study of Ciprofloxacin Hydrochloride under Stress Conditions Using Reverse Phase -High Performance Liquid Chromatography Method." *Der Pharmacia Sinica*, 3, no. 2, (2012), 217–23.

[81] Bushra, Umme; Nazmul, Huda; Mehedi, Mostafa; Zakir, Sultan; Asma, Rahman. "Study of Forced Degradation of Ciprofloxacin Hcl Indicating Stability Using RP-HPLC Method." *Der Pharma Chemica*, 5, no. 6, (2013), 132–37.

[82] Shrinivas, S; Revanasiddappa, M. "Analytical Stability Indicative Method Development and Validation by High Pressure Liquid Chromatography for Assay in Ciprofloxacin Hydrochloride Drug Substances." *American Journal of Analytical Chemistry*, 6, no. August, (2015), 719–30. doi:10.4236/ajac.2015.69069.

[83] Chen, Bo; Juan, Han; Yun, Wang; Chengzhuo, Sheng; Yu, Liu; Guocai, Zhang; Yongsheng, Yan. "Separation, Enrichment and Determination of Ciprofloxacin Using Thermo separating Polymer Aqueous Two-Phase System Combined with High Performance Liquid Chromatography in Milk, Egg, and Shrimp Samples." *Food Chemistry*, 148, (2014), 105–11. doi:10.1016/j.foodchem.2013.10.011.

[84] Vella, Janis; Francesca, Busuttil; Nicolette, Sammut Bartolo; Carmel, Sammut; Victor, Ferrito; Anthony, Serracino-Inglott; Lilian, M. Azzopardi; Godfrey, LaFerla. "A Simple HPLC-UV Method for the Determination of Ciprofloxacin in Human Plasma." *Journal of Chromatography B: Analytical Technologies in the Biomedical and Life Sciences*, 989, (2015), 80–85. doi:10.1016/j.jchromb.2015. 01.006.

[85] Emami, Jaber; Mahboubeh, Rezazadeh. "A Simple and Sensitive High-Performance Liquid Chromatography Method for Determination of Ciprofloxacin in Bioavailability Studies of Conventional and Gastroretentive Prolonged-Release Formulations." *Advanced Biomedical Research*, 5, (2016), 163. doi:10.4103/2277-9175.190995.

[86] Billah, Md Mustahsan; Masud Rana, SM; Mohammad, Salim; Hossain, AKM; Saifuddin, SKM; Azizul, Islam; Zannatul, Naim; Santanu, Barua. "Determination of the Presence and Pharmacokinetic Profile of Ciprofloxacin by TLC and HPLC Method Respectively in Broiler Chicken after Single Oral Administration." *The Journal Of Antibiotics*, 67, no. 7, (2014), 745. http://dx.doi.org/10.1038/ ja.2014.56.

[87] Mallah, E, Arafat, B; Al Khawaja, B; Abu Dayyih, W; Abu, Awad A; Hroub, HA; Hamad, M; Arafat, T. "Relative Bioavailability of Ciprofloxacin Doses (750 and 1000) mg in Healthy Male Volunteers by Using HPLC Method." *Journal of Bioequivalence Studies*, 1, no. 1, (2015), 1–6.

[88] Mallikarjuna Gouda, M; Ramakrishna, Shabaraya A. "Bioanalytical Method Development and Validation for the Quantification of

Ciprofloxacilin HCl in Plasma By HPLC." *European Journal of Pharmaceutical and Medical Research*, 3, no. 3, (2016), 525–28.

[89] Mukti, AnggunAji; Fathul, Jannah; Arief, Nurrochmad; Endang, Lukitaningsih. "Development and Validation Method for Quantitative Determination of Ciprofloxacin in Human Plasma and Its Application in Bioequivalence Test." *Asian Journal of Pharmaceutical and Clinical Research*, 9, no. 3, (2016), 89–95.

[90] Sisto, Francesca; Arianna, Bonomi; Loredana, Cavicchini; Valentina, Coccè; Maria, Maddalena Scaltrito; Gianpietro, Bondiolotti; Giulio, Alessandri; Eugenio, Parati; Augusto, Pessina. "Human Mesenchymal Stromal Cells Can Uptake and Release Ciprofloxacin, Acquiring *in Vitro* Anti-Bacterial Activity." *Cytotherapy*, 16, no. 2, (2014), 181–90. doi:10.1016/j.jcyt.2013.11.009.

[91] Terrado-Campos, David; Khaled, Tayeb-Cherif; Juan, Peris-Vicente; Samuel, Carda-Broch; Josep, Esteve-Romero. "Determination of Oxolinic Acid, Danofloxacin, Ciprofloxacin, and Enrofloxacin in Porcine and Bovine Meat by Micellar Liquid Chromatography with Fluorescence Detection." *Food Chemistry*, 221, (2017), 1277–84. doi:10.1016/j.foodchem.2016.11.029.

[92] Piñero, María Ysabel; MairyFuenmayor, Lourdes Arce; Roberto, Bauza; Miguel, Valcárcel. "A Simple Sample Treatment for the Determination of Enrofloxacin and Ciprofloxacin in Raw Goat Milk." *Microchemical Journal*, 110, (2013), 533–37. doi:10.1016/j.microc.2013.06.008.

[93] Kubasov, AS; Kochetkov, PP; Balyshev, AV; Lobova, PS; Abramov, SV; Abramov, VE. "Simultaneous Determination of Trimethoprim, Enrofloxacin, and Ciprofloxacin in Blood Serum of Poultry." *Journal of Analytical Chemistry*, 71, no. 6, (2016), 637–40. doi:10.1134/S1061934816060071.

[94] Locatelli, Marcello; Maria, Teresa Ciavarella; Donatella, Paolino; Christian Celia, ErsiliaFiscarelli; Gabriella, Ricciotti; Arianna, Pompilio; et al. "Determination of Ciprofloxacin and Levofloxacin in Human Sputum Collected from Cystic Fibrosis Patients Using

Microextraction by Packed Sorbent-High Performance Liquid Chromatography Photodiode Array Detector." *Journal of Chromatography A*, 1419, (2015), 58–66. doi:10.1016/j.chroma. 2015.09.075.

[95] Ferrone, Vincenzo; Maura, Carlucci; Roberto, Cotellese; Paolo, Raimondi; Annadomenica, Cichella; Lorenzo, Di Marco; Giuseppe, Carlucci. "Development and Validation of a Fast Micro-Extraction by Packed Sorbent UHPLC-PDA Method for the Simultaneous Determination of Linezolid and Ciprofloxacin in Human Plasma from Patients with Hospital-Acquired Pneumonia." *Talanta*, 164, no. July 2016, (2017), 64–68. doi:10.1016/j.talanta.2016.11.014.

[96] Rao, Ramamohana; Cyril, Arun Kumar. "Development of New HPLC Method and Identification and Quantification of Nalidixic Acid, Ciprofloxacin in Fish Tissue." *The Experiment*, 4, no. 3, (2012), 243–52.

[97] Rote, AR; Saudagar, RB. "High Performance Liquid Chromatographic Determination of Ciprofloxacin Hydrochloride and Ornidazole in Human Plasma." *Pharmaceutical Analytical Chemistry: Open Access*, 1, no. 1 (2015), 1–4. doi:10.4172/ paco.1000103.

[98] Adegbola, Adebanjo J; Julius, O. Soyinka; Babatunde, A. Adeagbo. "Simultaneous Quantification of Ciprofloxacin, Quinine and 3-Hyrdoxyquinine in Human Plasma Using a HPLC Method." *Asian Journal of Pharmaceutical Research and Health Care*, 8, no. 1, (2016), 11–18. doi:10.18311/ajprhc/2016/673.

[99] Choudhury, Hira; BapiGorain, Anwesha Paul; Pradipta, Sarkar; Shubhasis, Dan; Pragnya, Chakraborty; Tapan, K. Pal. "Development and Validation of an LC-MS/MS-ESI Method for Comparative Pharmacokinetic Study of Ciprofloxacin in Healthy Male Subjects." *Drug Research*, 67, no. 2, (2017), 94–102. doi:10.1055/s-0042-116593.

[100] Cavazos-Rocha, Norma; Idalia, Carmona-Alvarado; Lucio, Vera-Cabrera; Noemí, Waksman-De-torres; María, De La Luz Salazar-Cavazos. "HPLC Method for the Simultaneous Analysis of

Fluoroquinolones and Oxazolidinones in Plasma." *Journal of Chromatographic Science*, 52, no. 10, (2014), 1281–87. doi:10.1093/ chromsci/bmu002.

[101] Sang-Yeon, Kim; Il-Dong, Song; Hyun-Jin, Kim; Yoo-Sin, Park; Shin-Hee, Kim; Min, -A Kang; Do-Wan, Kim; Ju-Seop, Kang. "Quantification of Ciprofloxacin in Human Plasma by Validated LC-MS/MS Using Ofloxacin as an Internal Standard and its Clinical Application". *Current Pharmaceutical Analysis*, 11, no. 4, (2015), 239-47.

[102] Machuca, Jesús; Esther, Recacha; Alejandra, Briales; Paula, Díaz-de-Alba; Jesús, Blazquez; Álvaro, Pascual; José, Manuel Rodríguez-Martínez. "Cellular Response to Ciprofloxacin in Low-Level Quinolone-Resistant Escherichia Coli." *Frontiers in Microbiology*, 8, no. JUL (2017), 1–11. doi:10.3389/fmicb. 2017.01370.

[103] Zhang, Chuan Zhen; Si, Qi Ren; Man, Xia Chang; Pin, Xian Chen; Huan, Zhong Ding; Hong, Xia Jiang. "Resistance Mechanisms and Fitness of Salmonella Typhimurium and Salmonella Enteritidis Mutants Evolved under Selection with Ciprofloxacin *in Vitro*." *Scientific Reports*, 7, no. 1, (2017), 1–9. doi:10.1038/s41598-017-09151-y.

[104] Boulund, Fredrik; Fanny, Berglund; Carl-Fredrik, Flach; Johan, Bengtsson-Palme; Nachiket, P. Marathe; Joakim Larsson, DG; Erik, Kristiansson. "Computational Discovery and Functional Validation of Novel Fluoroquinolone Resistance Genes in Public Metagenomic Data Sets." *BMC Genomics*, 18, no. 1 (2017), 682. doi:10.1186/ s12864-017-4064-0.

[105] Poirel, Laurent; Alain, Liard; Jose, Manuel Rodriguez-Martinez; Patrice, Nordmann. "Vibrionaceae as a Possible Source of Qnr-like Quinolone Resistance Determinants." *Journal of Antimicrobial Chemotherapy*, 56, no. 6, (2005), 1118–21. doi:10.1093/jac/dki371.

[106] Sánchez, María B; Alvaro, Hernández; José, M. Rodríguez-Martínez; Luis, Martínez-Martínez; José, L. Martínez. "Predictive Analysis of Transmissible Quinolone Resistance Indicates

Stenotrophomonas Maltophilia as a Potential Source of a Novel Family of Qnr Determinants." *BMC Microbiology*, *8* (2008), 1–14. doi:10.1186/ 1471-2180-8-148.

[107] Kristiansson, Erik; Jerker, Fick; Anders, Janzon; Roman, Grabic; Carolin, Rutgersson; Birgitta, Weijdegård; Hanna, Söderström; Joakim Larsson, DG. "Pyrosequencing of Antibiotic-Contaminated River Sediments Reveals High Levels of Resistance and Gene Transfer Elements." *PLoS ONE*, 6, no. 2, (2011). doi:10.1371/ journal.pone.0017038.

[108] Flach, Carl Fredrik; Anna, Johnning; Ida, Nilsson; KorneliaSmalla, Erik Kristiansson; Joakim Larsson, DG. "Isolation of Novel IncA/C and IncN Fluoroquinolone Resistance Plasmids from an Antibiotic-Polluted Lake." *Journal of Antimicrobial Chemotherapy*, 70, no. 10, (2015), 2709–17. doi:10.1093/jac/dkv167.

[109] Bengtsson-Palme, Johan; Martin, Angelin; Mikael, Huss; SanelaKjellqvist, Erik Kristiansson; Helena, Palmgren; Joakim Larsson, DG; Anders, Johansson. "The Human Gut Microbiome as a Transporter of Antibiotic Resistance Genes between Continents." *Antimicrobial Agents and Chemotherapy*, 59, no. 10, (2015), 6551–60. doi:10.1128/AAC.00933-15.

[110] Courtney, Colleen M; Samuel, M. Goodman; Toni, A. Nagy; Max, Levy; Pallavi, Bhusal; Nancy, E. Madinger; Corrella, S. Detweiler; Prashant, Nagpal; Anushree, Chatterjee. "Potentiating Antibiotics in Drug-Resistant Clinical Isolates via Stimuli-Activated Superoxide Generation." *Science Advances*, 3, no. 10, (2017), 1–11. doi:10.1126/sciadv.1701776.

[111] Keyer, Kay; James, A. Imlay. "Superoxide Accelerates DNA Damage by Elevating Free-Iron Levels." *Proceedings of the National Academy of Sciences of the United States of America*, 93, no. 24, (1996), 13635–40. doi:10.1073/pnas.93.24.13635.

[112] Keyer, Kay; Amy, Strohmeier Gort; James, A. Imlay. "Superoxide and the Production of Oxidative DNA Damage." *J Bacteriol*, 177, no. 23, (1995), 6782–90.

[113] Brynildsen, Mark P; Jonathan, A. Winkler; Catherine, S. Spina; Cody MacDonald, I; James, J. Collins. "Potentiating Antibacterial Activity by Predictably Enhancing Endogenous Microbial ROS Production." *Nature Biotechnology*, 31, no. 2, (2013), 160–65.

[114] Wang, Shouming; Warren, Miller; John, Milton; Nigel, Vicker; Alistair, Stewart; Peter, Charlton; Prakash, Mistry; David, Hardick; William, A. Denny. "Structure-Activity Relationships for Analogues of the Phenazine-Based Dual Topoisomerase I/II Inhibitor XR11576." *Bioorganic and Medicinal Chemistry Letters*, 12, no. 3, (2002), 415–18. doi:10.1016/S0960-894X(01)00770-3.

[115] Bertozzi, Davide; Raffaella, Iurlaro; Olivier, Sordet; Jessica, Marinello; Nadia, Zaffaroni; Giovanni, Capranico. "Characterization of Novel Antisense HIF-1α Transcripts in Human Cancers." *Cell Cycle*, 10, no. 18, (2011), 3189–97. doi:10.4161/cc.10.18.17183.

[116] Chung, TD; Drake, FH; Tan, KB; Per, SR; Crooke, ST; Mirabelli, CK. "Characterization and Immunological Identification of CDNA Clones Encoding Two Human DNA Topoisomerase II Isozymes." *Proceedings of the National Academy of Sciences of the United States of America*, 86, no. 23, (1989), 9431–35. doi:10.1073/pnas.86.23.9431.

[117] Yang, Xia; Wei, Li; Elizabeth, D. Prescott; Steven, J. Burden; James, C. Wang. "DNA topoisomerase Iiβ and neural development." *Science*, 287, no. 5450, (2000), 131–4.

[118] Nitiss, John L. "Targeting DNA Topoisomerase II in Cancer Chemotherapy." *Nature Reviews Cancer*, 9, no. 5, (2009), 338–50. doi:10.1038/nrc2607.

[119] Shen, Linus L; John, Baranowski; Andre, G. Pernet. "Mechanism of inhibition of DNA gyrase by quinolone antibacterials: specificity and cooperativity of drug binding to DNA." *Biochemistry*, 28, (1989), 3879-85.

[120] Bromberg, Kenneth D; Alex, B. Burgin; Neil, Osheroff. "Quinolone action against human topoisomerase II alfa: stimulation of enzyme

mediated double-stranded DNA cleavage." *Biochemistry*, 42, (2003), 3393–8.

[121] Fabian, I; Reuveni, D; Levitov, A; Halperin, D; Priel, E; Shalit, I. "Moxifloxacin Enhances Antiproliferative and Apoptotic Effects of Etoposide but Inhibits Its Proinflammatory Effects in THP-1 and Jurkat Cells." *British Journal of Cancer*, 95, no. 8 (2006), 1038–46. doi:10.1038/sj.bjc.6603355.

[122] Jadhav, Ashwini Khanderao; Sankunny, Mohan Karuppayil. "Molecular Docking Studies on Thirteen Fluoroquinolines with Human Topoisomerase II a and B." *In Silico Pharmacology*, 5, no. 4, (2017), 1–12. doi:10.1007/s40203-017-0024-2.

[123] Vousden, Karen H; David, P. Lane. p53 in Health and Disease. *Nature Reviews Molecular Cell Biology*, 8, (2007), 275–83.

[124] Wade, Mark; Yao-Cheng, Li; Geoffrey, M. Wahl. "MDM2, MDMX and P53 in Oncogenesis and Cancer Therapy." *Nature Reviews Cancer*, 13, no. 2, (2013), 83–96. doi:10.1038/nrc3430.

[125] Toledo, Franck; Geoffrey, M. Wahl. "Regulating the P53 Pathway: *In Vitro* Hypotheses, *in Vivo* Veritas." *Nature Reviews Cancer*, 6, no. 12, (2006), 909–23. doi:10.1038/nrc2012.

[126] Gembarska, Agnieszka; FlavieLuciani, Clare Fedele; Elisabeth, A Russell; Michael Dewaele, StéphanieVillar; Aleksandra, Zwolinska; et al. "MDM4 Is a Key Therapeutic Target in Cutaneous Melanoma." *Nature Medicine*, 18, no. 8, (2012), 1239–1247. doi:10.1038/ nm.2863.MDM4.

[127] Valianatos, Georgios; BarboraValcikova, Katerina Growkova; Amandine, Verlande; JitkaMlcochova, LenkaRadova; Monika, Stetkova; Michaela Vyhnakova, OndrejSlaby; Stjepan, Uldrijan. "A Small Molecule Drug Promoting MiRNA Processing Induces Alternative Splicing of MdmX Transcript and Rescues P53 Activity in Human Cancer Cells Overexpressing MdmX Protein." *PLoS ONE*, 12, no. 10, (2017), 1–18. doi:10.1371/journal.pone.0185801.

[128] Channar, Pervaiz Ali; Aamer, Saeed; Fernando, Albericio; Fayaz, Ali Larik; Qamar, Abbas; Mubashir, Hassan; Hussain, Raza; Sung, Yum Seo. "Sulfonamide-Linked Ciprofloxacin, Sulfadiazine and

Amantadine Derivatives as a Novel Class of Inhibitors of Jack Bean Urease; Synthesis, Kinetic Mechanism and Molecular Docking." *Molecules*, 22, no. 8, (2017), 1–20. doi:10.3390/molecules 22081352.

[129] Khan, Khalid Mohammed; Zia, Ullah; Muhammad, Arif Lodhi; Muhammad, Ali; Muhammad, Iqbal Choudhary; Atta, Ur Rahman; Zaheer, Ul Haq. "Successful Computer Guided Planned Synthesis of (4R)-Thiazolidine Carboxylic Acid and Its 2-Substituted Analogues as Urease Inhibitors." *Molecular Diversity*, 10, no. 2, (2006), 223–31. doi:10.1007/s11030-005-9000-6.

[130] Amtul, Z; Atta-ur-Rahman, RA Siddiqui; Choudhary, MI. "Chemistry and mechanism of urease inhibition. "*Current Medicinal Chemistry*, 9, (2002), 1323–48.

[131] Dwyer, DJ; Belenky, PA; Yang, JH; MacDonald, IC; Martell, JD; Takahashi, N; Chan, CTY; et al. "Antibiotics Induce Redox-Related Physiological Alterations as Part of Their Lethality." *Proceedings of the National Academy of Sciences of the United States of America*, 111, no. 20, (2014), E2100–2109. doi:10.1073/pnas. 1401876111.

[132] Lobritz, Michael A; Peter, Belenky; Caroline, BM; Porter, Arnaud Gutierrez; Jason, H. Yang; Eric, G. Schwarz; Daniel, J. Dwyer; Ahmad, S. Khalil; James, J. Collins. "Antibiotic Efficacy Is Linked to Bacterial Cellular Respiration." *Proceedings of the National Academy of Sciences of the United States of America*, 112, no. 27, (2015), 8173–80. doi:10.1073/pnas.1509743112.

[133] Simeonova, R. "Adverse Drug Reactions of Sulfonamides, Tuberculostatics and Quinolones." In *Toxicology (for Pharmacy Students/English Language Training)*, edited by M. Mitcheva, 248, n.d.

[134] Samkar, A; Van, FGCM; De Kleermaeker, MGE TeRiele; Verrips, A. "Negative Myoclonus Induced by Ciprofloxacin." *Tremor and Other Hyperkinetic Movements*, 7, (2017), 1–2. doi:10.7916/ D8QC0FXT.

In: Ciprofloxacin
Editor: Mohamed Said Attia
ISBN: 978-1-53614-534-2

Chapter 6

CIPROFLOXACIN: ANALYTICAL METHODS OF ANALYSIS FOR MONITORING IT IN THE ENVIRONMENT

Lucas Moreira Silva, Marcos Vinicius Foguel and Maria Del Pilar Taboada Sotomayor*
Instituto de Química, Universidade Estadual Paulista "Júlio Mesquita Filho", Araraquara, Brazil

ABSTRACT

An antibiotic is a chemical substance that is produced by a certain microorganism, which, in small amounts, inhibits the growth of another microorganism. Among the various classes of antibiotics, fluoroquinolones are widely used in the treatment of different human and animal infections, especially ciprofloxacin, because they have a broad spectrum of action in several species of gram-negative and gram-positive bacteria. However, the inappropriate use of these compounds can cause several side effects. Because of this, scientists have developed techniques and methodologies with high sensitivity, precision and wide selectivity.

* Corresponding Author Email: mpilarts@hotmail.com.

Ciprofloxacin was determined in various biological and environmental matrices using spectroscopic methods, such as ultraviolet-visible spectrophotometry; chromatographic methods coupled to diode arrangement, fluorescence and mass spectrometry detectors; or using electroanalytical techniques, in which several transducer platforms are used, such as metallic or carbonaceous electrodes without modifications on their surface, as well as electrodes modified in different materials with enzymes, peptides, DNA and/or RNA sequences and molecularly imprinted polymers. Thus, this chapter will present a review of efforts reported in the literature for the sensitive and selective detection of this drug.

Keywords: ciprofloxacin, analytical methods, monitoring in the environment

List of Acronyms

AAS	Atomic absorption spectrometry
ac	Alternating current
AMIS	Amperometric magneto-immunosensor
Arg	Arginine
ATP	Adenosine triphosphate
BC	Before Christ
BSA	Bovine serum albumin
CE	Capillary electrophoresis
CTAB	Cetyltrimethylammonium bromide
CZE–ESI-MS–MS	Capillary zone electrophoresis-electrospray ionisation tandem mass spectrometric
D-Ala-D-Ala	D-alanine:D-alanine
DHPS	Deoxyhypusine synthase
DNA	Deoxyribonucleic acid
EIA	Enzyme-linked antibodies
ELISA	Enzyme-linked immunosorbent assay
et al.	*et alibi* (translation: and elsewhere)
FTIR	Fourier-transform infrared

Glu	Gluctamic acid
HPLC	High-performance liquid chromatography
HRP	Horseradish peroxidase
HSA	Human serum albumin
IUPAC	International Union of Pure and Applied Chemistry
LC/MS/MS	Liquid chromatography coupled with electrospray ionization tandem mass spectrometry
MIP	Molecularly imprinted polymer
MLR	Maximum acceptable limits
MWCNT/GCE	Multi-wall carbon nanotubes film modified on the glassy carbon electrode
PAR/EGR	Poly(alizarin red)/electrodeposited graphene
pKa	Acid dissociation constant
R_{ct}	Charge transfer resistance
RNA	Ribonucleic acid
Ser	Serine
SERS	Surface-enhanced Raman spectroscopy
SP	Solid phase
SPE	Solid-phase extraction
TLC	Thin-layer chromatography
TLC–B	Thin-layer chromatography–bioautography
tRNA	Transfer RNA
UV-Vis	Ultraviolet–visible.

INTRODUCTION

Infections Throughout History

Since the emergence of humanity, there have been historical accounts about the infectious diseases that decimated much of the human population around the world. The first recorded account was approximately in 430 BC, by the historian Thucydides, in his book the *History of the*

Peloponnesian War. He described the Plague of Athens, which killed approximately two thirds of the population of the polis, thus favoring the victory of Sparta over Athens in the Peloponnesian War [1].

Thucydides reported the symptoms of the disease and pathologists initially suspected it might have been typhus, smallpox, bubonic plague, or influenza. However, there was no conclusion until 2006, when researchers at the University of Athens analyzed some teeth recovered from a tomb located below Athens city, and the presence of *Salmonella enterica serovar Typhi* was found, thus confirming that typhoid fever was the infection that caused one of the earliest bacterial epidemics of antiquity [2].

During the Middle Ages, a pandemic originating in China, plagued Europe and parts of Asia. The cause of this devastation was the bacterium *Yersinia pestis*, which was transmitted to man through the fleas *Xenopsylla cheopis* of the black rats *Rattus rattus* [3, 4].

This plague was referred to as the Black Death, due to its main symptom, bloody wart-like wounds throughout the body, characterized with secretions of dark color. Other characteristic symptoms were the presence of intense fever, headache, frailty and seizures by the infected individual. As soon as the first symptoms appeared, the individual died between three and five days, due to lack of knowledge of a known medication for the infection [3, 5].

Amid the chaos, some doctors were prepared to take care of the pestilents, thus risking their own life. As a precaution, doctors wore special clothing and masks and avoided approaching contaminated patients, as the disease was extremely contagious. Doctors would slice off the wounds of infected patients with knives that were up to 1.80 m long and advised others to wash their houses with vinegar to prevent the appearance of fleas [4].

The Black Death killed around 100 million people, causing the world's population to fall from 450 million to about 350 million, equivalent to one-third of the world's population at the time. It wouldn't be until the 19th century, that the world's population would recover and reach 450 million [3, 6, 7].

The next epidemic that struck the world was syphilis. Syphilis is a sexually transmitted disease that is caused by the bacterium *Treponema pallidum*. There are records that the first cases of Syphilis on the European continent was in the year 1494. The origin of Syphilis is not known, but there are two theories concerning its origin [8].

The first variant is called the Colombian Theory, in which historians and infectologists claim that syphilis was a disease brought by Christopher Columbus and Martín Alonso Pinzón, from the New World (America) to the Old World (Europe) as an unintentional part of Colombian trade. This theory stems from the timing of the syphilis outbreak and Christopher Columbus' arrival from America. The syphilis epidemic occurred in 1495 in Naples, Italy, approximately three years after Columbus' return from America [8].

The most recent theory seeks to modify the Colombian theory by claiming that the New World was not the origin of syphilis. This version suggests that there was a certain type of non-venomous treponemic bacterium found in skeletons in Guyana, which on the European continent suffered selective evolutionary pressures and thus caused the occasional occurrence of the subspecies of sexually transmitted syphilis [9].

The second variant of this story is called the Pre-Columbian Theory. This version states that syphilis was already present on the European continent before Columbus' journey to the Americas. During the 18th and 19th centuries, a few paleontologists believed that the symptoms presented by syphilis had already been described in ancient Greece by Hippocrates. Skeletons were found in the region of Pompeii and Metaponto in Italy with damage similar to that caused by congenital syphilis, indicating that this bacterium already existed in Europe. Both theories are still accepted, however, the true origin of syphilis is not yet known [10, 11].

At the beginning of the onset of the disease, the term syphilis was not known, the disease had characteristic names depending on the political and religious problems among the countries of Europe, for example, in Italy it was known as French disease; in France, Poland and Germany it was called the Italian disease; in Russia it was known as Polish disease; the Netherlands named it as Spanish disease and the Turks called it Christian disease. In 1530, the word "syphilis" was written by the Italian physician and poet Girolamo Fracastoro in his Latin poem, *Syphilis sive morbus gallicus* ("Syphilis or French disease"). In this poem, the protagonist is a shepherd named Syphilus, who is exhibited as the first man to contract the disease, as a punishment sent by Apollo because he and his followers had defied the gods [12, 13].

The characteristic symptoms that infected people presented were rashes on their hands and feet, muscle aches, headache, malaise, fever, loss of appetite and the appearance of warts in the genital region. The treatments used at the time were not very effective in curing syphilis, but were intended to "expel the foreign substance" from the patients' bodies. There were some very dangerous treatments, for example, the use of bats in wine and olive oil with some herbs, use of laxatives, until blood transfusions and the application of mercury on the warts [3, 14].

Discovery of Microorganisms

From the earliest historical records of mankind to the 17th century, diseases were associated with some kind of imbalance between man and nature or related to religion as a form of punishment from the gods for the disobedience of people. These beliefs began to change as more scientific discoveries emerged. In 1665, the scientist Robert Hooke developed the first optical microscope, in which it was possible to observe in a piece of cork small units in the form of "boxes" or "cells." As Hooke improved his invention and was able to visualize each cell separately, Hooke's discovery pointed to the origin of the cellular theory, where he states that "*all living things are made up of cells*" [15].

In 1673, Antonie van Leeuwenhoek, Dutch merchant and amateur scientist, designed a new microscope where it was possible to observe for the first time a microorganism. Between 1673 and 1723, he wrote a series of letters to the Royal Society of London detailing his observations of what he named as "animalcules." Leeuwenhoek made minute drawings of "animalcules" out of scrapped material from his teeth, his own feces, and rainwater. These drawings were represented as representations of bacteria and protozoa [16].

It wasn't until 1828, that the term *Bacterium* was introduced by the German microbiologist Christian Gottfried Ehrenberg. The genus *Bacterium* was observed to be a non-spore forming, rod-shaped bacteri [17, 18].

Because of Leeuwenhoek's discovery of this "invisible world of microorganisms," the scientific community was extremely enthusiastic about the origin of microorganisms [15].

In the period between the years 1665, even before the discovery of the existence of the cell in 1861, there were several scientists who were against the the theory of spontaneous generation. One of these scientists was the Italian physicist Francesco Redi, who in 1668 demonstrated that insect larvae did not arise spontaneously from rotting flesh [15, 19, 20].

For this experiment, Redi filled two jars with decaying flesh. The first was left open; the flies lay their eggs on the flesh, and the eggs developed into larvae. The second jar was sealed, and as the flies could not lay the eggs on the meat, the larvae did not appear [15, 19, 20].

However, proponents of the theory of spontaneous generation were not satisfied with the result of the experiment; they claimed that spontaneous generation occurred by contact with air. Thus, Redi performed a second experiment in which a jar was covered with a thin net instead of being completely sealed, exposing the decomposing flesh. Since there was no appearance of any larvae, and only air could enter the jar, Redi concluded that because the net prevented flies from entering the jar, it also prevented the flies from beinf able to lay their eggs. Redi's results strongly discredited the old concept that great forms of life could arise in non-living forms [15, 19].

However, in 1745, the concept of spontaneous generation of microorganisms was strengthened by the Englishman John Needham. He discovered that even after heating nutrient broths and placing them in sealed vials, the cooled solutions were soon inhabited by microorganisms. Needham theorized that microbes develop spontaneously from broths [15, 21].

Twenty years later, and Italian scientist, named Lazzaro Spallanzani, proposed that airborne microorganisms would have penetrated Needham's solutions after they had been boiled. Spallanzani elucidated that the nutrient broth, heated after being sealed in a vial had no microbial development. Needham's claim was that the "vital force" needed for spontaneous generation had been extinguished by the heat and was kept out of the jars by the seals [15, 21].

Another scientist at the time was Antoine Laurent Lavoisier, who proved through experimentation the importance of oxygen to life. Because of Lavoisier's findings, Spallanzani's observations were rejected, the argument being that there was not enough oxygen inside the sealed jars for the development of microbial life [15, 21].

This question was still investigated and in 1858, the German scientist Rudolf Virchow challenged the concept of spontaneous generation with a new concept, that he called biogenesis. This concept inferred that living cells could only arise from preexisting living cells. The arguments about spontaneous generation continued until 1861, when the question was finally solved by the French scientist Louis Pasteur [15, 19, 22].

Pasteur developed a series of experiments in order to prove the existence of the microorganisms in the air and that they could contaminate sterile solutions, thus showing that air alone could not create microbes [15, 19].

In his experiment, he filled several bottles with beef broth, which had a short neck opening, and then boiled the contents. Some of the jars he allowed to cool while open, but others he sealed and allowed them to cool.

Within a few days, the open flaks were contaminated with microbes and the sealed flasks were free of microorganisms. Thus, Pasteur concluded through these results that the microbes present in the air were the agents responsible for the contamination of non-living matter, as in the vials of Needham flasks [15, 19].

Pasteur performed another experiment, using the same procedure described previously, but did not use the bottles with a short neck opening. Instead, Pasteur designed a bottle that had a long s-shaped neck [15, 19]. This unique model created by Pasteur allowed the air to enter the flask, however, the curved neck design was able to capture all the microorganisms in the air, avoiding contamination of the culture media [15].

Pasteur's work was decisive and showed that microorganisms could not originate from mystical forces existing in non-living materials. He showed that microorganisms may be present in non-living matter, solids, liquids, and in the air. It also proved that heat extinguished microbial life, and this technique is still routinely used in medical-laboratory procedures to this day [15, 19].

Thus, the appearance of "spontaneous" life in non-living solutions can be attributed to the microorganisms that were already present in the fluids themselves and in the air. Scientists now believe that a form of spontaneous generation probably occurred at the onset of the first form of life on Earth, but they agree that this did not happen under current environmental conditions [15, 19].

Because scientists' discoveries were known to the people of the time, a group of merchants asked Pasteur to find a way to prevent beer and wine from souring. At that time it was believed that air was responsible for the conversion of sugars present in beer and wine. Pasteur discovered the inverse of what was asked, that a group of microorganisms called yeast were responsible for the conversion of sugar into alcohol in the absence of air. The souring of beer and wine was caused by bacteria already present in the medium, which in the presence of oxygen, turns the sugar into vinegar [15, 23].

Table 1. Koch's Postulates [15, 23, 26]

Postulates	
1.	The same pathogen must be present in all cases of the disease and should not be present in healthy individuals.
2.	The pathogen must be isolated from the diseased host and cultured in pure culture.
3.	The pathogen obtained from the pure culture must cause the same disease when inoculated into a susceptible and healthy laboratory animal.
4.	The pathogen must be isolated from the inoculated animal and must be the original organism.

With this discovery, Pasteur created a method in which the beverage is heated, killing the bacteria responsible for deterioration, but without destroying the product. This process is now known as pasteurization and is still used in the food industry today.

However, in the year 1876, a young German physician known as Robert Koch, who was a rival of Pasteur in the race for the discovery of the cause of anthrax disease, discovered a rod-shaped bacterium, now known as *Bacillus anthracis*, in the blood of cattle that had died of anthrax. Koch isolated this bacterium, injected it into healthy animals, and observed that within a few days the animals became ill and died. Koch then removed the blood of the infected animals and was able to isolate the bacteria again [15, 24].

Due to his experimental results, Koch established an order of experimental steps to directly correlate a specific microbe to a specific disease. These steps are now known as Koch's postulates, shown in Table 1. Since their inception to present day, these same criteria have been instrumental in proving which specific microorganism is responsible for the cause of a specific disease [15, 25].

Development of Antibiotics

Even though it was known by the second half of the 19th century that bacteria was the cause of numerous diseases, an effective method to combat these diseases was still unknown. However, in the year 1880, the German bacteriologist Paul Ehrlich observed that bacteria had an affinity for certain dyes. With this observation, he wondered if it would be possible to create chemical substances that would be capable of selectively acting on bacteria without affecting the host. Ehrlich called this idea the "magic bullet" [15, 27–29].

This idea began a systemic and large-scale screening of various chemical compounds capapble of fighting syphilis, a disease virtually incurable at the time. Together with the bacteriologist Sahachiro Hata and the chemist Alfred Bertheim, they performed the synthesis of hundreds of organoarsenic derivatives, starting as a mold molecule the drug Atoxil, which is highly toxic and was used on rabbits infected with syphilis. In 1909, after testing more than 600 compounds, they were able to find the sixth compound in this series of experiments, called "606," which showed the ability to cure rabbits infected with syphilis and proved to be a significant promise for treatment of infected patients with syphilis [15, 27–30].

The drug synthesized by Ehrlich and his collaborators is known as arsphenamine, and the company Hoechst carried out its commercialization until the end of 1910 under the name of Salvarsan. Despite its high toxicity, the creation of this drug was a huge success in the fight against syphilis. It was later synthesized into a more soluble and less toxic variable under the name Neosalvarsan. Neosalvarsan was prescribed until the 1940s, when it was replaced by penicillin. Incredibly, 100 years after the creation of this drug, its mode of action is still unknown [15, 27–30].

Ehrlich's magic bullet idea was the origin of a search of different strategies in the pharmaceutical industry for the development of new antimicrobial drugs. In 1933, in Bayer AG® laboratories, Josef Klarer and Fritz Mietzsch synthesized a new drug based on the sulphamides group, sulfamidocrisoidin, also called KI-730, and commercially branded Prontosil, which was tested by Gerhard Domagk and presented antibacterial activity in various diseases [15, 27–29].

Table 2. Family of antibiotics [15, 27, 34]

Antibiotic Class	Antibiotic Name	Primary Target
Protein Synthesis Inhibitors		
Aminoglycosides	Streptomycin, spectinomycin, tobramycin, gentamicin, amikacin	30S ribosome (mistranslation by tRNA mismatching) 50S
Macrolides	Roxithromycin, spiramycin, clarithromycin, erythromycin, midecamycin, azithromycin.	50S ribosome (stimulating dissociation of the peptidyl- tRNA molecule from the ribosomes during elongation
Tetracyclines	Tetracycline, demeclocycline, oxytetracycline.	30S ribosome (inhibit aminoacyl tRNA binding to ribosome) 30S
Amphenicols	Thiamphenicol, chloramphenicol, florfenicol.	50S ribosome (inhibit elongation step)
Lincosamides	Lincomycin, clindamycin.	50S ribosome (stimulate dissociation of the peptidyl- tRNA molecule from the ribosomes during elongation
Resistomycins	Resistoflavin, resistomycin.	RNA polymerase
Rifamycins	Rifabutin, rifaximin, rifampicin.	DNA-dependent RNA polymerase RNA
Cell Wall Synthesis Inhibitors		
Lipopeptides	Polymixin B	Lipopolysaccharide in the outer membrane
Glycopeptides	Vancomycin	Peptidoglycan units terminal D-Ala-D-Ala dipeptide
β-lactams	Cephalosporin: cefaclor cefadroxil, ceftazidime. Penicillins: penicillin G, cloxacillin, piperacillin, carbenicillin, ampicillin.	Penicillin-binding proteins
DNA Synthesis Inhibitors		
Sulfonamides	Sulfamethoxazole, sulfadiazine, sulfamethazine, sulfapyridine, sulfamerazine.	Competitive inhibitor for DHPS involved in folate synthesis
DNA Synthesis Inhibitors		
Fluoroquinolones	Nalidixic acid, norfloxacin, sparfloxacin, levofloxacin, ciprofloxacin.	Topoisomerase II (DNA gyrase), topoisomerase IV

However, Prontosil was a strong precursor of the active drug, but the active part, sulfanilamide, was not patentable since it was already being used in the paint industry. Since sulfanilamide was not patented and had low production costs, several pharmaceutical companies began mass production of sulfonamide derivatives [15, 27–29].

Another doctor, physician, and researcher who had studies of extreme importance was Alexander Fleming, who in 1928 observed the appearance of a blue mold in specific areas of the Petri plate in which he cultivated *Staphylococcus aureus*. This mold had the capacity to inhibit the growth of bacterial colonies in the area that surrounded it. This mechanism of inhibition observed between colonies in solid culture media is called antibiosis, from which the term antibiotic came to be, is nothing more than a substance produced by a certain type of microorganism, that in low quantities has the capacity to inhibit the action of other microorganisms. The mold observed by Fleming was quickly identified as the fungus *Penicillium notatum*, and its active compound was isolated and called penicillin [15, 27, 28, 31–33].

In 1940, the first clinical trial of penicillin was conducted by a research group led by Howard Florey and Ernst Chain at Oxford University. Due to the war in the United Kingdom, research aimed at the production of large-scale production of penicillin was not possible, causing them to transfer their work to the United States. Since the original culture of *P. notatum* (later renamed *Penicillium chrysogenum*) did not show greater efficiency in the production of the antibiotic, it was replaced by a more prolific strain. This precious organism was first isolated from a moldy melon, purchased at a market in Peoria, Illinois, United States [15, 27, 28, 33].

The works of Paul Ehrlich and Alexander Fleming were of extreme importance and opened new perspectives in the development of antibiotics in the fight against infectious diseases. Currently there are several classes of antibiotics, shown in Table 2, and what differs one class from the other is the chemical structure and its mechanism of action against the bacterium [15, 27, 28, 33].

CIPROFLOXACIN

A class of synthetic antibiotics that is extremely prominent in its broad spectrum of action are the quinolones. The molecule that gave rise to this class was nalidixic acid, thus forming the first generation of compounds of the class, which is a naphthyridine that was isolated in 1962 by George Lesher as a bioproduct of chloroquine synthesis [35].

To obtain the nalidixic acid molecule, the synthesis starts from the condensation between 6-methylpyridin-2-amine and diethyl- (ethoxy-methylidene) -propanedioate, resulting in diethyl -{[(6-methylpyridin-2-yl) amino] methylidene} propanedioate. Subsequently Dowtherm A is refluxed with diethyl phthalate to obtain ethyl 4-hydroxy-1,8-naphthyridine-3-carboxylate. Afterwards, an alkaline hydrolysis of this ester is carried out with potassium hydroxide, which forms the corresponding carboxylic acid, which is 1-alkyl-1,8-naphthyridin-4-one-3-carboxylic acid, also called nalidixic acid. The synthetic route is shown in Figure 1 [36].

The introduction of nalidixic acid during 1962 for the treatment of infectious diseases of the urinary tract was not very successful due to its high toxicity, low action spectrum, and low treatment efficiency [36–38].

This began the search for new compounds that would be able to act with greater efficiency, a broad spectrum of action, and low toxicity, in the fight against urinary tract infections. This search led to the insertion of the piperidic ring at the C7 position, forming pipemidic acid, thus favoring the action in gram-negative bacteria, and including *Pseudomonas spp*, as well as obtaining activity on gram-positive bacteria, due to the fact that the pauperized ring favored entry into the bacterial cell wall [37, 39].

The major breakthrough in the development of new drugs from nalidixic acid was carried out by Hiroshi Koga et al. in 1977 at the Kyorin Company in Japan. They introduced a fluorine molecule in C6, thus forming norfloxacin, and creating the class of fluoroquinolones, giving rise to the second generation of this class of compounds. Norfloxacin was patented in 1978 and favored a significant increase in the action spectrum in both gram-negative and gram-positive bacteria [39–42].

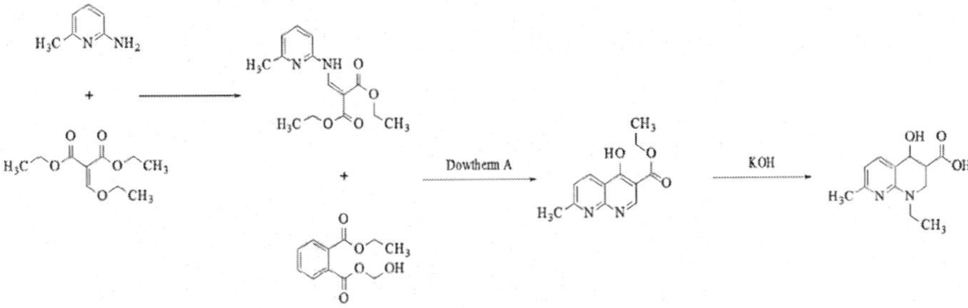

Figure 1. Synthetic route of nalidixic acid [36].

However, in pharmaceutical research, great discoveries are soon suppressed by new ones that present superior power of performance and greater effectiveness. In 1981, three years after the patenting of norfloxacin, a second-generation compound of fluoroquinolones, ciprofloxacin, under the trade name CIPRO® and Bay 09867, was patented and has the patent number EP-B-0 049 355 [38, 41–44].

The synthetic route of ciprofloxacin used by Bayer is shown in Figure 2, and it shows a total yield of 84%. Using as a template the molecule 1- (2,4-dichloro-5-fluorophenyl) -ethanone with the addition of dimethyl carbonate in the presence of sodium hydride, there is the formation of the first intermediate ethyl 3- (2,4-dichloro-5- -fluorophenyl) -3-oxopropanoate. Then ethyl 3- (2,4-dichloro-5-fluorophenyl) -3-oxopropanoate is reacted with (diethoxymethoxy) ethane in acetic anhydride medium, thereby forming ethyl (2Z) -2- (2,4- dichloro-5-fluorobenzoyl) -3-ethoxyprop-2-enoate. Next is the addition of cyclopropanamine, yielding a second intermediate, ethyl (2Z) -3-(cyclopropylamino) -2- (2,4-dichloro-5-fluorobenzoyl) prop-2-enoate, after its formation is carried out the addition of sodium hydride in dimethylformamide medium is performed, thereby bringing about the cyclization of the molecule, causing the formation of two conjugated aromatic rings, yielding a third synthetic intermediate ethyl 7-chloro-1-cyclopropyl-6-fluoro- 4-oxo-1,4-dihydroquinoline-3-carboxylate, and then acid hydrolysis is carried out using 3N hydrochloric acid, thereby obtaining 7-chloro-1-cyclopropyl-6-fluoro-4-oxo-1,4-dihydroquinoline -3-carboxylic acid. The nucleophilic substitution at the C-7 position occurs by the addition of piperazine and N-methylpyrrolidinone, thus forming 1-cyclopropyl-6-fluoro-4-oxo-7- (piperazin-1-yl) -1,4-dihydroquinoline- 3-carboxylic acid, commonly known as ciprofloxacin [45].

Ciprofloxacin IUPAC name is 1-cyclopropyl-6-fluoro-4-oxo-7-piperazinyl-1-quinoline-3-carboxylic acid. It also has a hydrochloride structure, $C_{17}H_{18}FN_3O_3$ HCl with 385.82 g mol^{-1} molar mass, a white powder soluble in water and having a value of 30.00 mg L^{-1} at 20°C, and exhibiting two values of pKa, the first value relating to deprotonation of the carboxylic group, pKa_1 having a value of 6.3; and the second, pKa_2 in the amount of 8.9; concerning deprotonation of the nitrogen of the piperizide ring [46].

In regards to its action spectrum, ciprofloxacin is strongly active against most gram-positive cocci. It is also active against gram-negative aerobic bacilli, presented in Table 3, and has moderate action against mycoplasma, chlamydia, ureplasma and some mycobacteria [37–39, 43].

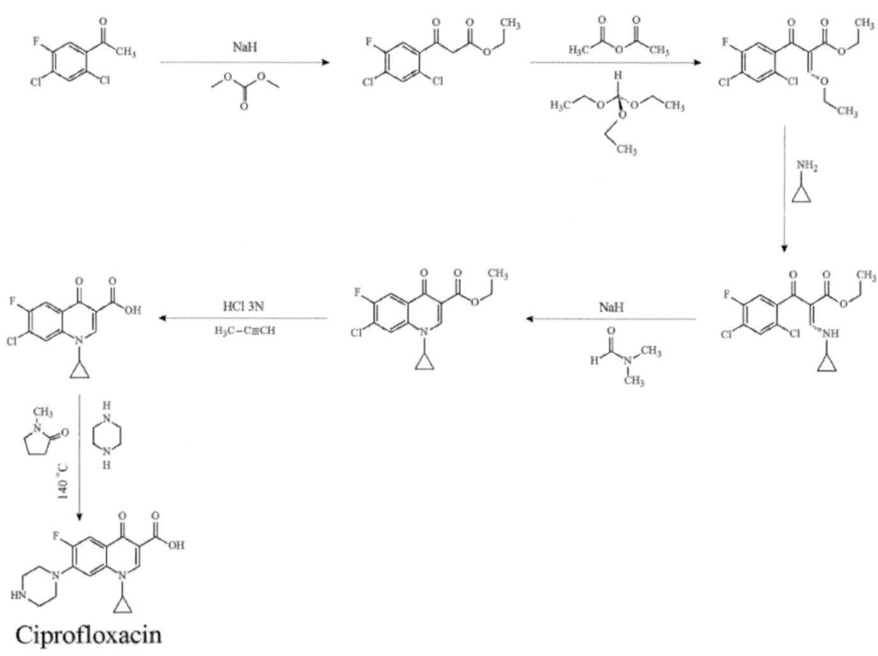

Ciprofloxacin

Figure 2. Synthetic route of ciprofloxacin performed by Bayer AG [45].

Table 3. Action spectrum of ciprofloxacin [37–39, 43]

Gram-Positive	Gram-negative
Gardnerella vaginalis	Escherichia coli
Staphylococcus aureus	Klebsiella pneumoniae
Staphylococcus epidermidis	Klebsiella oxytoca
β-Streptococos hemolítico	Citrobacter freundii
Streptococcus pneumoniae	Enterobacter cloacae
Enterococcus faecalis	Serratia marcescens
Enterococcus faecium	Proteus mirabilis
Bacteroides vulgatus	Proteus mirabilis
Bacteroides asaccharolyticus	Acinetobacter baumannii
Clostridium difficile	Pseudomonas aeruginosa
Mycobacterium xenopi	Campylobacter jejuni
Mycobacterium avium	Helicobacter pylori
Mycobacterium tuberculosis	Haemophilus influenzae
	Moraxella catarrhalis
	Neisseria gonorrhoeae
	Haemophilus ducreyi
	Gardnerella vaginalis
	Bacteroides fragilis
	Ureaplasma urealyticum

Ciprofloxacin inhibits the interaction of two essential topoisomerase enzymes in the replication of bacterial DNA, DNA-gyrase and topoisomerase IV, which have similar structures, but different functions. DNA-gyrase acts in conjunction with the ω protein, a type I topoisomerase, in establishing the super-helical density of the bacterial chromosome. In addition, gyrase alleviates torsional stress, which is found at the beginning of the transcription complex and the replication fork [15, 37, 47–49].

Topoisomerase IV exhibits the function of removing nodes that accumulate in the bacterial chromosome following basic cellular processes, but also separates the template tape from the new DNA strand formed after replication [15, 37, 47–49].

Cirprofloxacin acts on DNA-gyrase in gram-positive bacteria. There are studies indicating that ciprofloxacin binds to the gyrase-DNA complex, thus forming the gyrase-DNA-ciprofloxacin complex by changing the conformation of the enzyme, which in turn generate complexes dependent on Ca^{2+} ions and alter the cleavage rate of ATP, causing a rupture of the double strand due to increased torsional strain as the replication fork walks over the DNA of the bacterium, thereby leading to cellular lysis [47, 49, 50].

In gram-negative bacteria, ciprofloxacin acts on the enzyme topoisomerase IV. The interaction between ciprofloxacin and the DNA molecule is performed by π-π integers, and by Van der Waals forces. This occurs through the formation of a bond between a Mg^{2+} ion with the oxygen bound in C4 and the oxygen belonging to the carboxylic grouping in C3. This connection is mediated by four water molecules, characterizing an octahedral geometry to this complex, presented in Figure 3. Two of these water molecules bind to the amino acid residues Ser87 and Glu88, and the presence of the piperidic group at C7 combine with with Arg418 [51].

This brings a change in the tertiary structure of the enzyme present in the ciprofloxacin-topoisomerase IV-DNA complex, which is linked to the intersection of the template ribbon and the new DNA strand, consequently compromising enzymatic activity and binding of the double strand of DNA, causing a rupture of the tapes, cleaving the tape template as well as the new tape and preventing the formation of a new cell [47, 50, 52].

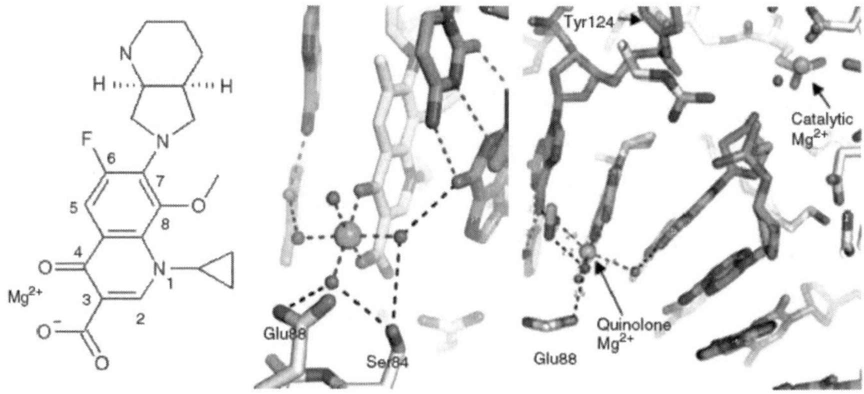

Figure 3. Interaction between ciprofloxacin and the amino acids belonging to topoisomerase IV [51].

Table 4. Main infections that use ciprofloxacin as treatment

Clinical Indications	Infections	References
Urinary Tract	Urinary Tract Infection and Prostatitis	[53–60]
Gastrointestinal Tract	Diarrhea and abdominal infection	[61–66]
Respiratory Tract	Cystic fibrosis, upper respiratory tract infections	[67–72]

Table 5. Maximum acceptable limits (MLR) for ciprofloxacin in various food samples [81]

Animal	MLR	Target Fabric
Porcine, rabit	100 μg kg^{-1}	Muscle
	100 μg kg^{-1}	Fat
	200 μg kg^{-1}	Liver
	300 μg kg^{-1}	Kidneys
Bovine, ovine, Caprine	100 μg kg^{-1}	Muscle
	100 μg kg^{-1}	Fat
	300 μg kg^{-1}	Liver
	200 μg kg^{-1}	Kidneys
	100 μg kg^{-1}	Milk
Poultry	100 μg kg^{-1}	Muscle
	100 μg kg^{-1}	Skin and fat
	200 μg kg^{-1}	Liver
	300 μg kg^{-1}	Kidney
All other food producing species	100 μg kg^{-1}	Muscle
	100 μg kg^{-1}	Fat
	200 μg kg^{-1}	Liver
	200 μg kg^{-1}	Kidney

In view of the wide spectrum of action of ciprofloxacin, it is an ideal treatment for various diseases in humans. Table 4 shows the main diseases in which ciprofloxacin is used for treatment.

Ciprofloxacin is also used in livestock, for example, in beef cattle it is used as treatment for diseases of the gastrointestinal tract and respiratory tract, and in dairy cattle it is used against mastitis [73–75]. In poultry, ciprofloxacin is used to treat diseases of the respiratory tract and skin infections, but most often in the form of enrofloxacin, which is metabolized by the liver and biotransformed in the ciprofloxacin [76–79].

The administration of ciprofloxacin in humans is performed orally, and is rapidly absorbed by the gastrointestinal tract, and exhibits an average absolute bioavailability of 80%. The maximum serum concentration is reached approximately on average from 60 to 120 minutes after oral administration. The serum balance concentration after 12 hours in an individual with normal renal function for the dose 250 mg of ciprofloxacin is 0.2 μg mL^{-1}. Four metabolites were identified in human urine:formilciprofloxacin, sulfociprofloxacin, desenoethyleneprodyloxacin and oxociprofloxacin. However, they presented low concentration and low antibacterial action [80].

Although ciprofloxacin exhibits a broad spectrum of action and has a rapid effect on infections, ciprofloxacin is often prescribed by physicians as an extremely effective way of treating bacterial infections. However, there are studies that indicate some undesired side effects in patients who have been given ciprofloxacin.

In Europe, the European Union member countries have a specific body responsible for monitoring chemical residues in different matrices called the European Environment Agency. This comittee has a common chemical residue monitoring program that has set forth the maximum acceptable limits (MLR) of ciprofloxacin in different food samples, which are outlined in Table 5.

Some studies also demonstrate the correlation between the use of ciprofloxacin for treatment of bacterial infections and the rupture of the Achilles tendon. The symptoms appear, on average, six days after the start of the medication, which are pain, swelling, redness and stiffness in the region. Recovery of the affected area can occur with early diagnosis and discontinuation of ciprofloxacin. In cases of a ruptured tendon, the usual orthopedic treatment must be performed [82–84].

Theoretically, ciprofloxacin should have no effect on human cells, due to the low homology between the enzymes topoisomerase and gyrase. However, there are studies that show that ciprofloxacin has effects on the fibroblast homeostasis present in the tissues of tendons. Another effect observed is that ciprofloxacin undergoes a chelating reaction when it comes in contact with some metals, such as Mg^{2+}; Al^{2+}; Ca^{2+}. This chelation affects the synthesis of collagen and causes cartilage degradation. These observations were found through studies conducted using laboratory animals and *in vitro* cultured fibroblast cells [85–89].

An additional side effect caused by ciprofloxacin is peripheral neuropathy. This disease is characterized by destruction of the peripheral nerve, which carries the nerve impulses of the brain and spinal cord to the limbs of the body. The antibiotic acts on $GABA_A$ receptors by inhibiting it from mediating the transport of one of the main neurotransmitters of the brain, aminobutyric acid. By inhibiting this reaction te following symptoms occur: weakness, pain, burning sensation, change in sensation of touch and heat, difficulty in movement, loss of muscle mass. Symptoms that usually affect arms and legs may be irreversible [90–94].

Liver damage was also observed in subjects that were given Ciprofloxacin. The mechanism of how liver damage occurs is still unknown, but is side effect of hepatocellular necrosis is observed after the use of ciprofloxacin. This adverse effect can damage the liver function and in extreme cases cause cirrhosis or hepatitis [95–102].

In addition to the effects discussed above, ciprofloxacin also exhibits a danger to the environment when compared to other molecules of different classes of antibiotic classes, because it can lead to the emergence of strains that are resistant to bacteria or superbugs. The development of analytical methods for controlling the residues of ciprofloxacin dispersed in the environment is of utmost importance because these methods allow the possibility to monitor the residue levels of this antibiotic, thus guarding against all the harmful effects that it can cause [103–111].

METHODS OF DETECTION FOR CIPROFLOXACIN

There are several techniques employed to determine the amount of ciprofloxacin in different matrices. The most widely used method is high-performance liquid chromatography (HPLC).

Early reports regarding the detection of ciprofloxacin were published in 1985. Initially, researchers developed chromatographic methods to analyze the pharmacokinetics and the influence of food intake on the absorption of the antibiotic in biological fluids, such as urine, serum and bile. For these biological fluids, isocratic chromatography on a reversed-phase analytical column with ultraviolet and/or fluorescence detection was used [112–114]. Gau et al. [115] used the same technique in order to replace the microbiological assays that, according to the authors, did not distinguish the drug from its metabolites.

New biological samples were analyzed in subsequent studies, such as saliva, blister fluid and sputum [116]. In addition, a need arose to develop chromatographic methods that could differentiate ciprofloxacin from antibiotics of the same class and similar structures, such as norfloxacin, pefloxacin and ofloxacin [117–119].

In the following years, no new method for the detection of ciprofloxacin was developed. Several publications [120–134] discussed the use of the HPLC technique for the separation and quantification of this antibiotic, with only a few differences among them.

In 1993, Altria and Chanter [135] reported the detection of quinolone antibiotics, like ciprofloxacin, using capillary electrophoresis (CE). This method was able to withstand pH extremes and presented acceptable levels of precision, linearity, limits of detection and quantification. CE was used for determining both drug content and levels of related impurities present in drug substances. The authors concluded that CE of basic drug compounds at low pH offered a useful alternative and complement to HPLC.

A luminescence detection procedure for the in vivo liquid chromatographic determination of ciprofloxacin was proposed by Rieutord et al. [136] Fluoroquinolone compounds are chelated in the presence of lanthanide ions, then, the ion terbium was used to chelate with ciprofloxacin and monitored using a reverse-phase eluent. With the proposed method, the luminescence detection allowed the quantification of 0.25 pmol L^{-1} ciprofloxacin.

Ciprofloxacin was one of 38 antibiotics evaluated by a multiple bioassay technique with standard solutions. Using this method, the antibiotics were assayed on seven plates prepared with different media and microorganisms. According to the authors, this technique can be used after a screening test to identify groups of antibiotics and, then, the samples can follow more specific techniques for complete identification and quantification [137].

Volmer et al. [138] used liquid chromatography coupled with electrospray ionization tandem mass spectrometry (LC/MS/MS) for simultaneous detection of 15 quinolone antibiotics, including ciprofloxacin. Until this publication, all previous works found employed UV-Vis or fluorescence detectors. However, in the following years, it was possible to find a range of articles which employ the HPLC-coupled mass spectroscopic technique for the determination of ciprofloxacin [139–151].

Since using the HPLC technique to detect ciprofloxacin is broad and recurrent, the authores will highlight when alternative techniques are employed. For example, an article published by Bannefeld et al. [152], reported a method to determine plasma concentrations of ciprofloxacin and its metabolite desethyleneciprofloxacin (M1) by CE with HeCd laser-induced fluorescence.

A terbium-sensitized luminescence method was described for the determination of the sum of residues of enrofloxacin and its major metabolite ciprofloxacin in edible animal tissues. Several parameters affecting both detection and extraction were studied. However, in this case, HPLC was not used. Instead, the samples, after undergoing an appropriate treatment process, were subjected to fluorescence measurements, with emission intensity at 549 nm and an excitation wavelength of 276 nm [153].

A fluorescence method was developed using functionalized nano-CdS nanoparticles to interact with ciprofloxacin, aiming to enhance the fluorescence intensity signals of the fluoroquinolone compound. When the proposed method was applied in human serum samples, the recovery was between 95–105% and the relative standard deviation was low [154].

The fluorescence property of ciprofloxacin was also analyzed by Chen et al. [155]. The antibiotic presented an increase in the fluorescence intensity in the presence of Cu^{2+}-gold nanoclusters, which are stabilized by bovine serum albumin.

Snitkoff et al. [156] developed an immunoassay based on enzyme linked antibodies (EIA) for the detection of ciprofloxacinin serum and dialysate samples. This assay is able to present results with a high degree of specificity and able to process multiple samples at a time. According to the authors, the serum proteins do not interfere with sample quantification and do not require sample treatment. The immunoassay was selective for ciprofloxacin and its level of sensitivity was found to be picogram of the analyte.

El-Ansary et al. [157] were able to differentiate some drugs, among them ciprofloxacin, by employing an indirect method. The ion-association complexes of the analytes with $[Co(NO_2)_6]^{3-}$ were precipitated and the excess unreacted cobalt complex was detected using atomic absorption spectrometry (AAS). The method was applied to drugs in pure solution, pharmaceutical preparations, and urine. The paper mentions that the results were precise, accurate and sensitive. However, there were no results describing the selectivity of the proposed method. A similar work was proposed by Salem et al. [158] to determine ten different fluoroquinolones. However, the precipitant agents were silver nitrate, copper acetate and ferric chloride.

In 2000, Rizk et al. [159] studied electrochemical techniques to determine three quinolone antibacterials: norfloxacin, ciprofloxacin and sparfloxacin. These compounds were complexed with nickel (II) and monitored using direct current, differential pulse and alternating current polarography. The method described was applied to determine the drugs in bulk and tablet formulations. The recovery and sensitivity were favorable compared to those given by a reference method. However, the selectivity of the method was also not mentioned.

Another work that describes the discernment of ciprofloxacin by complexation was reported by Djurdjević et al. [160] The antibiotic was distinguished in serum without previous extraction using iron(III) nitrate as the chromogenic agent. The solution containing the metal complexed with ciprofloxacin was measured by spectrophotometric technique at a wavelength of 430 nm. The method exhibited a limit of detection of 0.2 $\mu mol\ L^{-1}$.

The solid-phase spectrofluorimetry was employed to develop a method for the differentiation of ciprofloxacin. The analyte was fixed on Sephadex SP C-25 gel and was measured directly after packing the gel beads in a silica gel, using a solid-phase attachment. It was used to analyze human urine and serum samples and yielded recovery levels around 100% in all cases [161].

A flow-injection chemiluminescence method was developed for the differentiation of fluoroquinolones, including ciprofloxacin, in pharmaceutical preparations, based on the reaction of sulphite with cerium (IV) sensitized by these compounds. The paper stated that the results coincide with those obtained by official methods [162]. The chemiluminescence method using flow injection also was reported by Aly et al. [163]. The authors were able to discern three fluoroquinolone antibiotics, among them ciprofloxacin. However, in this paper, the compounds were reacted with tris(2,2'-bipyridyl) ruthenium(II) and Ce(IV) and found in dosage forms and biological fluids.

The strains of three microorganisms (*Micrococcus luteus*, *Bacillus cereus* and *Escherichia coli*) were used to detect residues of antibiotics with low limits of detection by Okerman et al. [164]. Each antibiotic group presented distinct inhibition patterns typical for each microorganism. Ciprofloxacin, which belongs to the fluoroquinolones class of antibiotics, gives only inhibition zones on plates with *E. coli*, whose limit of detection is 0.5 ng.

Another method proposed to determine ciprofloxacin in edible meat was developed by Duan and Yuan using an indirect competitive enzyme-linked immunosorbent assay (ELISA) [165]. The authors carried out the conjugation of analyte with bovine serum albumin (BSA) and the human serum albumin (HSA) to produce a specific antibody for ciprofloxacin. The indirect competitive ELISA did not present crossreactivity with antibiotics.

An indirect ELISA was also reported by Li et al. [166]. The goal was to detect and quantify 13 fluoroquinolone antibiotics while simultaneously using specific polyclonal antibody. While, Gomes and Ferreira [167] developed an ELISA assay for ciprofloxacin using antibody fragments, instead of whole antibodies.

Antibodies were also used in a high-performance immunoaffinity chromatography column for the analysis of several fluoroquinolones antibiotics. For this, a column with anti-sarafloxacin antibodies was employed to bind to the fluoroquinolones compounds, and then detected through fluorescence [168].

Some research describes screening methods for detection of ciprofloxacin in different samples. For example, [169] et al. used thin layer chromatography to separate β-lactam and fluoroquinolone antibiotics. While, Myllyniemi et al. [170] developed an indirect conductometric method, which used the conductance variation between the growth stages of the bacterium to relate to the presence of certain antibiotics, among them ciprofloxacin.

Liquid chromatography mass spectrometry was previously described and was widely used for the determination of ciprofloxacin in several matrices. However, in 2003, McCourt et al. [171] employed a capillary zone electrophoresis-electrospray ionisation tandem mass spectrometric (CZE–ESI-MS–MS) method for the evaluation of some fluoroquinolones. According to the authors, it was the first work that used this technique to detect ciprofloxacin.

Pascual-Reguera [172] used a spectrophotometric continuous flow sensor to quantify ciprofloxacin in pharmaceutical preparations. The proposed sensor principle consists of injecting the sample and transporting the analyte by a constant flow to a cationic exchanger gel, in which the analyte is retained, and monitoring is performed with an absorbance signal at 277 nm. After the measurement, the gel is regenerated for the next analysis.

Thin-layer chromatography (TLC) was reported by Choma et al. [173], who described a semiquantitative method to determine ciprofloxacin by combining TLC with microbiological detection, known as thin-layer chromatography–bioautography (TLC–B). This method consists of placing the TLC plates in a bacterial growth medium seeded with an appropriate bacterial strain. Information about the type and amount of antibiotic present are provided by the position of the growth inhibition zones.

The electrochemical techniques were further explored to detect ciprofloxacin without the need to use a metal coupled to the analyte to monitor the electron transfer. Pellegrini et al. [174] developed an electrochemical biosensor for the antibiotics identification of tetracyclines and quinolones, in which ciprofloxacin is found. The sensor monitored carbon dioxide production relative to the inhibition of microbial growth.

Another work reported the qualitative detection of three pharmaceutical compounds: 5-aminosalicylic acid, ciprofloxacin and azithromycin. The analytes were mechanically immobilized on the surface of the paraffin impregnated graphite electrode and detection was performed using square-wave voltammetry [175].

An enzymatic biosensor for ciprofloxacin based on catechol mediation was developed using a rotating disk electrode and continuous flow/stopped-flow/continuous-flow processing. The enzyme used was horseradish peroxidase (HRP), which was immobilized on the surface of a glassy carbon electrode. This enzyme, in the presence of its substrate (hydrogen peroxide), oxidized the catechol. When ciprofloxacin is presented in the solution, the mediator reacted with the piperazine group of the analyte, forming piperazine-quinone derivatives, which decreased the peak current. In this way, the application of the sensor in different pharmaceutical samples containing the target antibiotic was performed [176, 177].

Yi and Li [178] described a voltammetric sensor for ciprofloxacin based on the interaction between the antibiotic and the surfactant cetyltrimethylammonium bromide (CTAB). The authors employed the differential pulse voltammetry technique to monitor the oxidation peak of the analyte using a carbon paste electrode. In the absence of surfactant, the peak presented was poorly defined. However, when the CTAB was presented in thc solution, the oxidation peak was well-defined and sensitive to ciprofloxacin.

Two different researchers employed voltammetric techniques using multi-wall carbon nanotube film modified on glassy carbon electrode

(MWCNT/GCE). Fotouhi and Alahyari [179] reported an electrochemical method to detect only ciprofloxacin. While Ensafi et al. [180] developed a sensor that detected enrofloxacin and ciprofloxacin simultaneously, using a least-squares support vector machine. In another method found, this same electrode was modified with $MgFe_2O_4$ nanoparticles to develop a voltammetric sensor for ciprofloxacin. The composite films facilitate interfacial electron transfer and electrocatalytic activity in the oxidation of ciprofloxacin [181].

Zhang et al. [182] described a similar procedure to determine electrocatalytic oxidation of ciprofloxacin, however, modification of the glassy carbon electrode was achieved using poly(alizarin red)/electrodeposited graphene (PAR/EGR) composite film. The sensor was applied to detect the analyte in presence of ascorbic, uric acid, and dopamine.

A potentiometric ion-selective membrane electrode for ciprofloxacin was proposed using polyvinyl chloride membrane and ciprofloxacin-tetraphenylborate complex to provide the electroactive signal [183].

A label free impedimetric immunosensor was reported for the detection of ciprofloxacin [184]. The impedance technique measures the charge transfer resistance (R_{ct}). In general, there is an increase of the R_{ct} value for every modification on the electrode surface. Thus, it is not necessary to use a labeling compound, e.g., an enzyme, to monitor the electrochemical signal. For the development of this sensor, anti-ciprofloxacin antibodies were immobilized onto a poly(pyrrole-N-hydroxysuccinimide) film, which was electropolymerized on the surface of a gold electrode. After, the antibiotic present in the sample was bound to antibodies and the R_{ct} was monitored. The method was quite sensitive, with detected concentrations in the order of 10 pg mL^{-1} ciprofloxacin.

Tsekenis et al. [185] also described a label free immunosensor for ciprofloxacin using alternating current (ac) impedance. However, in this study, a screen-printed carbon electrode was used as a substrate and an anti-ciprofloxacin antibody was immobilized onto a polyaniline, which was electrodeposited on the electrode surface.

To quantify fluoroquinolone antibiotics in milk samples, an amperometric magneto-immunosensor (AMIS) was developed by Pinacho et al. [186]. The procedure to build the sensor consists of the biomofidication of antibodies for fluoroquinolones compounds on magnetic beads. Then, after the immunoreaction, a magnetic graphite–epoxy composite electrode captures the magnetic beads with the analyte.

The determination of fluoroquinolone compounds can also be performed using a DNA-based electrochemical sensor. The sensor proposed by Abnous et al. [187] acts according to the interaction between the fluoroquinolone antibiotic and an aptamer used as a molecular recognition probe. In the presence of the analyte, the aptamer changes the conformation and does not allow the binding of single stranded DNA. In this manner, the electron transfer of the redox probe has a much greater ability to reach the electrode surface and, consequently, yield a high current signal. On the other hand, in the absence of analyte, the aptamer maintains the original conformation and encourages binding of the single stranded DNA. With this procedure, the electrode surface is heavily blocked, and the electron transfer of the redox probe has difficulty in reaching the electrode surface, therefore generating a low current signal.

As described previously, most of published studies regarding the determination of ciprofloxacin, uses the HPLC technique with different detectors to identify and quantify the antibiotic in different samples. However, in general, the studies are very similar, and therefore not cited in this chapter. However, some studies are highlighted due to their innovation, such as the paper reported by Yan et al. [188], whose work used molecularly imprinted polymer (MIP) as solid-phase extraction (SPE) for a selective sample cleanup. It should be emphasized that MIP can also be used as a pre-treatment step, employed as SPE, in the technique of capillary electrophoresis [189].

MIP is a biomimetic material that recognizes a specific compound or a class of compounds. The MIP is produced through the growth of a structural polymer around a molecule used as a template. In the MIP's synthesis, functional monomers are used to provide chemical interactions between the template and the polymer. After the template removal, a cavity is formed into the polymeric structure, whose shape and size of these cavities are analogous to the molecule used as template. MIPs are inspired by the antigen-antibody complexes, since both have complementary chemical interaction and are able to shape to the compound of interest [190, 191].

In the paper published by Yan et al., ofloxacin was used as template for MIP synthesis and this material presented high selectivity for five fluoroquinolones, including ciprofloxacin. The authors compared the imprinted polymer with a conventional SPE and the MIP had a superior performance [188].

Further work on the synthesis of MIP for ciprofloxacin has been reported, in which enrofloxacin is used as a template for the cleaning and preconcentration of fluoroquinolone antibiotics [192]. Alternatively, ciprofloxacin was also used as a template for more specific and efficient retention to the MIP cavities [193].

An improvement in the use of MIP in pretreatment of samples was the development of magnetic MIPs, which are imprinted polymers with a magnetic core, as proposed by Chen et al. [194]. The advantage of this material is the facilitated separation of the adsorbent material, in which ciprofloxacin is absorbed by the magnetic polymer cavities from the sample by application of a magnetic field, due to the magnetic nanoparticle in the core of polymers.

In addition to being employed as solid phase extraction to cleanup and preconcentration before the HPLC analysis, the MIP can be used as a stationary phase in chromatography [195–197].

Yan and Row [195] described the synthesis and application of a ciprofloxacin-imprinted monolithic column. This method was used to distinguish ciprofloxacin in urine samples. According to the authors, samples could be directly injected into the column due to the porous structure and flow-through channels existing in the network skeleton of the monolithic MIP, which resulted in a rapid, efficient, precise and selective analysis.

MIP can be also used as a recognition system in the development of sensors [198, 199]. This MIP application was described by Oliveira et al.

[198] to detect ciprofloxacin in fish and in pharmaceuticals. To achieve this detection, MIP was attached to the electrode surface in a poly(vinyl chloride) membrane.

Electropolymerization technology is an alternative to synthetizing MIP on the electrode surface. The procedure is very simple and preparation of the sensor is only requires one electroactive monomer in combination with the template in a convenient electrolyte solution. Then immerse the electrode in this solution and carry out successive cyclic voltammogram measurements [191, 200]. Yan et al. [201] developed an electrochemical sensor for ciprofloxacin based on MIP synthetized by electropolymerization. For this process, pyrrole and o-phenylenediamine were used as monomers to form the polymeric film on the pencil graphite electrode.

Another way to use HPLC for the analysis of ciprofloxacin was the use of ionic liquids as additives of the mobile phase. Herrera-Herrera et al. [202] evaluated four different ionic liquid to separate seven fluoroquinolone antibiotics. The ionic liquids helped improve the performance of this method, since an increase in peak resolution was observed.

A multi-analyte screening optical sensor for the most frequently used antibiotics in the veterinary field, among them ciprofloxacin, was developed using specific antibodies as bioreceptors. This sensor uses the evanescent-wave principle, which consists of varying the refractive index proximal to the modified substrate surface. The sensor was able to detect more than 30 different antibiotics and presented satisfactory results when applied in milk samples [203].

Fourier-transform infrared (FTIR) spectroscopy was reported as an accurate and sensitive technique to quantify ciprofloxacin in tablet samples, using the carbonyl group signal at 1707 cm^{-1} [204].

He et al. [205] developed a method to detect three antibiotics (enrofloxacin, ciprofloxacin and chloramphenicol) using Surface-enhanced Raman spectroscopy (SERS) coupled with dendritic silver nanosubstrates. SERS is a technique that involves both electromagnetic enhancement and chemical charge transfer effect. This method was able to identify and characterize these antibiotics quickly and accurately. Guo et al. [206] used the magnetic-MIP technology to enhance the sensitiveity of the SERS technique and developed a method to detect ciprofloxacin.

CONCLUSION

This chapter presented an analysis of the presence of ciprofloxacin in different organisms, citing its discovery, microbiological action and application in the treatment of animal and human infections, as well as the main methods of detection and quantification of the antibiotic ciprofloxacin in several matrices. The techniques used were not detailed, as the objective was to present a survey of the different methodologies that can be used to determine this antibiotic. Electrochemical techniques (voltammetry, amperometry and electrochemical impedance), optical (fluorescence, chemiluminescence and SERS) and separation techniques (HPLC and capillary electrophoresis) have been widely used since 1985. High performance liquid chromatography - mainly with UV detection, fluorescence and MS - should be highlighted because this technique has the highest number of publications in detecting ciprofloxacin.

New compounds, such as biological materials, nanomaterials and molecularly printed polymers, have been associated with these techniques and have been shown to improve the performance of these methods. Therefore, there are still many possibilities available to develop new methodologies for the discernment of ciprofloxacin in a variety of matrices.

REFERENCES

[1] Connor, W. R. 1984. *Thucydides.* Princeton: Princeton University Press. (Connor 1984, 1-280).

[2] Ujvari, tefan C. 2009. *A História Da Humanidade Contada Pelos Vírus: Bactérias, Parasitas E Outros Microorganismos*: São Paulo: CONTEXTO. (Ujvar 2009, 1-202).

[3] Martin, S. *A Short History of Disease: Plagues, Poxes and Civilisation.* London: Oldcastle Books. (Martin 2015, 1-320).

[4] Austin, S. 2003. "A Pest in the Land: New World Epidemics in a Global Perspective Citation." *Journal of the Royal Anthropological Institute - Wiley* 12:219–269. Accessed February 28, 2018. doi: 10.1111/j.1467-9655.2006.00289_1. x.

[5] Darling, R. G., Catlett, C. L., Huebner, K. D., Jarrett, D. G. 2002. "Threats in Bioterrorism I: CDC Category a Agents." *Emergency Medicine Clinics of North America* 20:273–309. Accessed February 28, 2018. doi: 10.1016/S0733-8627(02)00005-6.

[6] Slack, P. 1989. "The Black Death Past and Present: Some Historical Problems." *Transactions of the Royal Society of Tropical Medicine and Hygiene* 83:461–463. Accessed February 28, 2018. doi: 10.1016/ 0035-9203(89)90247-2.

[7] *U. S. C. Bureau*, World Population: Historical Estimates of World Population https://www.census.gov/population/international/data/worldpop/table_history.php.

[8] Farhi, D., Dupin, N. 2010. "Origins of Syphilis and Management in the Immunocompetent Patient: Facts and Controversies." *Clinics in Dermatology* 28:533–538. Accessed February 28, 2018. doi: 10.1016/j.clindermatol. 2010.03. 011.

[9] Armelagos, G. J., Zuckerman, M. K., Harper, K. N. 2012. "The Science Behind Pre-Columbian Evidence of Syphilis in Europe: Research by Documentary." *Evolutionary anthropology* 21:50–57. Accessed February 28, 2018. doi: 10.1002/evan.20340.

[10] Lobdell, J. E., Owsley, D. 1974. "The Origin of Syphilis." *Journal The Journal of Sex Research* 10:76–79. Accessed February 28, 2018. doi: 10.1080/00224497409550828.

[11] Gaul, J. S., Grossschmidt, K., Gusenbauer, C., Kanz, F. 2015. "A Probable Case of Congenital Syphilis from Pre-Columbian

Austria." *Anthropologischer Anzeiger* 72:451–472. Accessed February 28, 2018. doi: 10.1127/anthranz/2015/0504.

[12] Fracastoro, G. *Syphilis, sive morbus Gallicus*, [Syphilis, or the French Disease] Veronae, 1530.

[13] Maatouk, I., Moutran, R. 2014. "History of Syphilis: Between Poetry and Medicine." *Journal of Sexual Medicine* 11:307–310. Accessed February 28, 2018. doi: 10.1111/jsm.12354.

[14] Parascandola, L. J. 2009. "From Mercury to Miracle Drugs: Syphilis Therapy over the Centuries." *American Institute of the History of Pharmacy* 51:14–23. Accessed February 28, 2018. PMID: 20027915.

[15] Tortora, G. J. and Funke, B. R., and Case, C. L. 2007. *Microbiologia, 1 -579*. Porto Alegre: Artmed Editora SA. (Tortora and Funk and Case 2007, 10).

[16] Dobell, C. and Leeuwenhoek, A. Van. 1932. *Antony van Leeuwenhoek and his "Little Animals", Being Some Account of the Father of Protozoology and Bacteriology and His Multifarious Discoveries in These Disciplines, 1-520*. New York: Harcourt, Brace and company. (Dobell and Leeuwenhoek 1932, 1).

[17] Dictionary, O. E. *Etymology of the word bacteria* https://web.archive.org/web/20061118024752/http://www.etymonline.com/index.php?term=bacteria.

[18] Boone, D. R. and Castenholz, R. W. and Garrity, G. M. 2001. *Bergey's Manual of Systematic Bacteriology: The Archaea and the Deeply Branching and Phototrophic Bacteria, 1-722*. New York: Springer-Verlag New York. (Bonne and Castenholz and Garrity 2001, 2).

[19] Parke, E. C. 2014. "Flies from Meat and Wasps from Trees: Reevaluating Francesco Redi's Spontaneous Generation Experiments." *Studies in History and Philosophy of Science Part C: Studies in History and Philosophy of Biological and Biomedical Sciences* 45:34–42. Accessed February 28, 2018. doi: 10.1016/j.shpsc.2013.12.005.

[20] Redi, F. 2016. *Esperienze Intorno Alla Generazione Degli Insetti,* [Experiences around the generation of insects] 1-240. Pisa: Editrice. (Redi 2015, 5).

[21] Schaechter, M. 2009. *Encyclopedia of Microbiology, 45-56.* Cambridge: Academic Press. (Schaechter 2009, 3).

[22] Pasteur, L. 1864. "On Spontaneous Generation." *Sorbonne Scientific Soirée* 1:257–264. Accessed February 28, 2018.

[23] Ross, L. N., Woodward, J. F. Koch's Postulates: An Interventionist Perspective. *Stud. Hist. Philos. Sci. Part C Stud. Hist. Philos. Biol. Biomed. Sci.* 2016, *59*, 35–46. Accessed February 28, 2018. doi: 10.1016/j.shpsc.2016.06.001.

[24] Ross, L. N., Woodward, J. F. 2016. "Koch's postulates: An interventionist perspective." *Studies in History and Philosophy of Science Part C: Studies in History and Philosophy of Biological and Biomedical Sciences 59*:35–46. Accessed February 28, 2018. doi: 10.1016/j.shpsc.2016.06.001.

[25] Singh, V. P., Proctor, S. D., Willing, B. P. 2016. "Koch's Postulates, Microbial Dysbiosis and Inflammatory Bowel Disease." *Clinical Microbiology and Infection* 22:594–599. Accessed February 28, 2018. doi: 10.1016/j.cmi.2016.04.018.

[26] Neville, B. A., Forster, S. C., Lawley, T. D. 2018. "Commensal Koch's Postulates: Establishing Causation in Human Microbiota Research." *Current Opinion in Microbiology* 42:47–52. Accessed February 28, 2018. doi: 10.1016/j.mib.2017.10.001.

[27] Rang, H. P., and Dale, M. M., and Flower, R. J., Henderson, G. 2016. *Rang and Dale's Pharmacology, 1-776* London: Churchill Livingston. (Rang and Dale and Flower 2016, 8).

[28] Aminov, R. I. 2010. "A Brief History of the Antibiotic Era: Lessons Learned and Challenges for the Future." *Frontiers in Microbiology* 1:134. Accessed February 28, 2018. doi: 10.3389/fmicb.2010.00134.

[29] Williams, K. 2009. "The Introduction of "chemotherapy" Using Arsphenamine – the First Magic Bullet." *Journal of the Royal*

Society of Medicine 102:343–348. Accessed February 28, 2018. doi: 10.1258/jrsm.2009.09k036.

[30] Frith, J. 2013. "Arsenic – the " Poison of Kings " and the " Saviour of Syphilis."" *Journal of Military and Veterans' Health* 21:11–18. Accessed February 28, 2018.

[31] Tan, S. Y., Tatsumura, Y. 2015. "Alexander Fleming (1881-1955): Discoverer of Penicillin." *Singapore Medical Journal* 56:366–367. Accessed February 28, 2018. doi: 10.11622/smedj.2015105.

[32] Fleming, A. 1929. "On the Antibacterial Action of Cultures of a Penicillium, with Special Reference to Their Use in the Isolation of B. influenzae." *British Journal of Experimental Patholog* 10:226–236. Accessed February 28, 2018.

[33] Sykes, R. 2001. "Penicillin: From Discovery to Product." *Bulletin World Health Organization* 79:778–779. Accessed February 28, 2018.

[34] Wong, W. R., Oliver, A. G., Linington, R. G. 2012. "Development of Antibiotic Activity Profile Screening for the Classification and Discovery of Natural Product Antibiotics." *Chemistry & Biology* 19:1483–1495. Accessed February 28, 2018. doi: 10.1016/j.chembiol.2012.09.014.

[35] Bisacchi, G. S. 2015. "Origins of the Quinolone Class of Antibacterials: An Expanded "Discovery Story."" *Journal of Medicinal Chemistry* 58: 4874–4882. Accessed February 28, 2018. doi: 10.1021/jm501881c.

[36] Lesher, G. Y., Froelich, E. J., Gruett, M. D., Bailey, J. H., Brundage, R. P. 1962. "1,8-Naphthyridine Derivatives. A New Class of Chemotherapeutic Agents." *Journal of Medicinal Chemistry* 5:1063–1065. Accessed February 28, 2018. doi: 10.1021/jm01240a021.

[37] Aminov, R. 2017. "*History of Antimicrobial Drug Discovery-Major Classes and Health Impact*." 133:4–19. Accessed February 28, 2018. doi: 10.1016/j.bcp.2016.10.001.

[38] Van Bambeke, F., Michot, J. M., Van Eldere, J., Tulkens, P. M. 2005. "Quinolones in 2005: An Update." *Clinical Microbiology and*

Infection 11:256–280. Accessed February 28, 2018. doi: 10.1111/j. 1469-0691.2005.01131.x.

[39] Appelbaum, P. C., Hunter, P. A. 2000. "The Fluoroquinolone Antibacterials: Past, Present and Future Perspectives." *International Journal of Antimicrobial Agents* 16:5–15. Accessed February 28, 2018. doi: 10.1016/S0924-8579(00)00192-8.

[40] Irikura, T. *Piperazinyl Derivatives of Quinoline Carboxylic Acids*. US4146719 A, 1979.

[41] Koga, H., Itoh, A., Murayama, S., Suzue, S., Irikura, T. 1980. "Structure-Activity Relationships of Antibacterial 6,7- and 7,8-Disubstituted 1 -A1 Kyl- 1,4-Dihydro-4-Oxoquinoline-3-Carboxylic Acids." *Journal of Medicinal Chemistry* 9:1358–1363. Accessed February 28, 2018. doi: 10.1021/jm00149a003.

[42] Domagala, J. M., Hanna, L. D., Heifetz, C. L., Hutt, M. P., Mich, T. F., Sanchez, J. P., Solomon, M. 1986. "New Structure-Activity Relationships of the Quinolone Antibacterials Using the Target Enzyme. The Development and Application of a DNA Gyrase Assay." *Journal of Medicinal Chemistry* 29:394–404. Accessed February 28, 2018. doi: 10.1021/jm00153a015.

[43] Shah, P. M. 1991. "Ciprofloxacin." *International Journal of Antimicrobial Agents* 1:75–96. Accessed February 28, 2018. doi: 10.1016/0924-8579(91)90002-U.

[44] Avataneo, R. *Pharmaceutical Composition for Topical Use*. EP0763359 A1, 1997.

[45] Clinton, S. N. A *Continuous Process Towards The Synthesis*, Virginia Commonwealth University, 2015.

[46] *Pubchem - open chemistry database*. Bethesda. National Center for Biotechnology Information, U.. No Title https://pubchem.ncbi.nlm. nih.gov/compound/2764#section=Top.

[47] Levine, C., Hiasa, H., Marians, K. J. 1998. "DNA Gyrase and Topoisomcrase IV: Biochemical Activities, Physiological Roles during Chromosome Replication, and Drug Sensitivities." *Biochimica et Biophysica Acta (BBA) - Gene Structure and*

Expression 1400:29-43. Accessed February 28, 2018. doi: 10.1016/S0167-4781(98)00126-2.

[48] Champoux, J. J. DNA Topoisomerases: Structure, Function, and Mechanism. *Annu. Rev. Biochem.* 2001, *70*, 369–413. Accessed February 28, 2018. doi: 10.1021/bi5000564.

[49] Aldred, K. J., Kerns, R. J., Osheroff, N. 2014. " Mechanism of Quinolone Action and Resistance." *Biochemistry* 53:1565-1574. Accessed February 28, 2018. doi: 10.1021/bi5000564.

[50] Drlica, K. 1999. "Mechanism of Fluoroquinolone Action." *Current Opinion in Microbiology* 2:504–508. Accessed February 28, 2018. doi: 10.1016/S1369-5274(99)00008-9.

[51] Wohlkonig, A., Chan, P. F., Fosberry, A. P., Homes, P., Huang, J., Kranz, M., Leydon, V. R., Miles, T. J., Pearson, N. D., Perera, R. L., et al. 2010. "Structural Basis of Quinolone Inhibition of Type IIA Topoisomerases and Target-Mediated Resistance." *Nature Structural & Molecular Biology* 17:1152-1153. Accessed February 28, 2018. doi: 10.1038/nsmb.1892.

[52] Anderson, V. E., Gootz, T. D., Osheroff, N. 1988. "Topoisomerase IV Catalysis and the Mechanism of Quinolone Action." *The Journal of Biological Chemistry.* 273:17879–17885. Accessed February 28, 2018. doi: 10.1074/jbc.273.28.17879.

[53] Talan, D. A., Naber, K. G., Palou, J., Elkharrat, D. 2004. "Extended-Release Ciprofloxacin (Cipro XR) for Treatment of Urinary Tract Infections." *International Journal of Antimicrobial Agents* 23:54-66. Accessed February 28, 2018. doi: 1 10.1016/j.ijantimicag.2003.12.005.

[54] Stein, G. E., Schooley, S., McMillan, J. 1998. "Urinary Pharmacodynamics of Low-Dose Ciprofloxacin and Ofloxacin." *Diagnostic Microbiology & Infectious Disease* 30:261–265. Accessed February 28, 2018. doi: 10.1016/S0732-8893(98)00002-9.

[55] Naber, K. G. 2001. "Which Fluoroquinolones Are Suitable for the Treatment of Urinary Tract Infections?" *International Journal of Antimicrobial Agents* 17:331-341. Accessed February 28, 2018. doi: 10.1016/S0924-8579(00)00362-9.

[56] Gluhovschi, G., Gadalean, F., Gluhovschi, C., Velciov, S., Petrica, L., Bob, F., Bozdog, G., Kaycsa, A. 2016. “Is Ciprofloxacin Safe in Patients with Solitary Kidney and Upper Urinary Tract Infection?” *Biomedicine & Pharmacotherapy* 84:366-372. Accessed February 28, 2018. doi: 10.1016/j.biopha.2016.09.052.

[57] Osonwa, U. E., Ugochukwu, J. I., Ajaegbu, E. E., Chukwu, K. I., Azevedo, R. B., Esimone, C. O. 2017. “Enhancement of Antibacterial Activity of Ciprofloxacin Hydrochloride by Complexation with Sodium Cholate.” *Bulletin of Faculty of Pharmacy, Cairo University* 55:233-237. Accessed February 28, 2018. doi: 10.1016/j.bfopcu.2017.09.006.

[58] Cal, C., Sayiner, A. A., Ozyurt, C., Cureklibatir, I., Ozacar, T., Badak, Z. 1997. “Ciprofloxacin Treatment in Chronic Prostatitis.” *Clinical Microbiology and Infectious Diseases.* 3:314–316. Accessed February 28, 2018. doi: 10.1111/j.1469-0691.1997.tb00619.x.

[59] Naber, K. G., Busch, W., Focht, J. 2000. “Ciprofloxacin in the Treatment of Chronic Bacterial Prostatitis: A Prospective, Non-Comparative Multicentre Clinical Trial with Long-Term Follow-Up. The German Prostatitis Study Group.” *International Journal of Antimicrobial Agents* 14:143–149. Accessed February 28, 2018. doi: 10.1016/S0924-8579(99)00142-9.

[60] Stratton, C. 1992. “Fluoroquinolone Antibiotics: Properties of the Class and Individual Agents.” *Clinical Therapeutics.* 14:348-75, discussion 347. Accessed February 28, 2018. PMID:1638577.

[61] Kusachi, S., Sumiyama, Y., Takahashi, Y., Kato, K., Mashita, K., Takeyama, H., Oda, S., Kobayashi, S. 2012. “Evaluation of the Efficacy and Safety of Intravenous Ciprofloxacin versus Meropenem in the Treatment of Postoperative Infection.” *Journal of Infection and Chemotherapy* 18:152–159. Accessed February 28, 2018. doi: 10.1007/s10156-011-0307-1.

[62] MADAN, A. 2004. “Use of Ciprofloxacin in the Treatment of Hospitalized Patients with Intra-Abdominal Infections.” *Clinical*

Therapeutics. 26:1564–1577. Accessed February 28, 2018. doi: 1 10.1016/j.clinthera.2004.10.013.

[63] Hsieh, W.-J., Lin, H.-C., Hwang, S.-J., Hou, M.-C., Lee, F.-Y., Chang, F.-Y., Lee, S.-D. 1998. "The Effect of Ciprofloxacin in the Prevention of Bacterial Infection in Patients with Cirrhosis after Upper Gastrointestinal Bleeding." *The American Journal of Gastroenterology*. 93:962–966. Accessed February 28, 2018. doi: 10.1111/j.1572-0241.1998.00288.x.

[64] DuPont, H. L. 1991. "Use of Quinolones in the Treatment of Gastrointestinal Infections." *European Journal of Clinical Microbiology and Infectious Diseases* 10:325–329. Accessed February 28, 2018. PMID: 1864292.

[65] Mikamo, H., Ninomiya, M., Tamaya, T. 2003. "Pharmacokinetics of Single-Dose Intravenous Ciprofloxacin in Blood and Ascites of Patients with Pelvic Peritonitis." *Journal of Infection and Chemotherapy* 9:276–277. Accessed February 28, 2018. doi: 10.1007/s10156-003-0250-X.

[66] Petruccelli, B. P., Murphy, G. S., Sanchez, J. L., Walz, S., DeFraites, R., Gelnett, J., Haberberger, R. L., Echeverria, P., Taylor, D. N. 1992. "Treatment of Traveler's Diarrhea with Ciprofloxacin and Loperamide." *The Journal of Infectious Diseases* 165:557–560. Accessed February 28, 2018. doi: 10.1093/infdis/165.3.557.

[67] Antonela Antoniu, S. 2012. "Inhaled Ciprofloxacin for Chronic Airways Infections Caused by *Pseudomonas Aeruginosa*." *Expert Review of Anti-infective Therapy* 10:1439–1446. Accessed February 28, 2018. doi: 10.1586/eri.12.136.

[68] Torge, A., Wagner, S., Chaves, P. S., Oliveira, E. G., Guterres, S. S., Pohlmann, A. R., Titz, A., Schneider, M., Beck, R. C. R. 2017. "Ciprofloxacin-Loaded Lipid-Core Nanocapsules as Mucus Penetrating Drug Delivery System Intended for the Treatment of Bacterial Infections in Cystic Fibrosis." *International Journal of Pharmaceutics* 527:92–102. Accessed February 28, 2018. doi: 10.1016/j.ijpharm.2017.05.013.

[69] Chono, S., Tanino, T., Seki, T., Morimoto, K. 2007. "Pharmacokinetic and Pharmacodynamic Efficacy of Intra-pulmonary Administration of Ciprofloxacin for the Treatment of Respiratory Infections." *Drug Metabolism and Pharmacokinetics 22*:88–95. Accessed February 28, 2018. doi: 10.2133/dmpk.22.88.

[70] Cios, A., Wyska, E., Szymura-Oleksiak, J., Grodzicki, T. 2014. "Population Pharmacokinetic Analysis of Ciprofloxacin in the Elderly Patients with Lower Respiratory Tract Infections." *Experimental Gerontology* 57:107–113. Accessed February 28, 2018. doi: 10.1016/j.exger.2014.05.013.

[71] Park, S. Y., Kim, T., Kim, M.-C., Sung, H., Kim, M.-N., Kim, S.-H., Lee, S.-O., Choi, S.-H., Woo, J. H., Kim, Y. S., et al. 2017. "Ciprofloxacin Treatment for Cryptogenic Klebsiella Pneumoniae Liver Abscesses." *Journal of Infection* 75:590–593. Accessed February 28, 2018. doi: 1 10.1016/j.jinf.2017.10.004.

[72] Principi, N., Esposito, S. 2015. "Approprieate Use of Fluoriquinolones in Children." *International Journal of Antimicrobial Agents* 45:341–346. Accessed February 28, 2018. doi: 10.1016/j.ijantimicag.2015.01.004.

[73] Jinqing, J., Haitang, Z., Zhixing, A., Zhiyong, X., Xuefeng, Y., Huaguo, H., Ziliang, W. 2012. "Development of an Heterologous Immunoassay for Ciprofloxacin Residue in Milk." *Physics Procedia* 25:1829–1836. Accessed February 28, 2018. doi: 10.1016/j.phpro.2012.03.318.

[74] Jorge, L. L., Rezende, M. L. G. 2012. "Avaliação Da Eficácia Terapêutica da Ciprofloxacina, Administrada Pela via Intramamária, Em Vacas Em Lactação [Evaluation of the Therapeutic Efficacy of Ciprofloxacin, Administered by the Intramammary Route, in Lactating Cows]." *A Hora Veterinária* **2012**, *32* (190), 23–27.

[75] Admas, H. R. 2003. *Farmacologia e terapêutica em veterinária,* [Pharmacology and veterinary therapeutics] 1-1004. Rio de Janeiro: Guanabara Koogan. (Admas 2003, 8).

[76] Fluoroquinolones, I. V. S. on, Ford, R., Co., V. L. S. *Third International Veterinary Symposium on Baytril: Proceedings,*

Princeton, N. J., Ed., Veterinary Learning Systems: Sevile, 1999, pp 11–12.

[77] Morales-Gutiérrez, F. J., Barbosa, J., Barrón, D. 2015. "Metabolic Study of Enrofloxacin and Metabolic Profile Modifications in Broiler Chicken Tissues after Drug Administration." *Food Chemistry.* 172:30–39. Accessed February 28, 2018. doi: 10.1016/j.foodchem.2014.09.025.

[78] Devreese, M., Antonissen, G., De Baere, S., De Backer, P., Croubels, S. 2014. "Effect of Administration Route and Dose Escalation on Plasma and Intestinal Concentrations of Enrofloxacin and Ciprofloxacin in Broiler Chickens." *BMC Veterinary Research* 10:289. Accessed February 28, 2018. doi: 10.1186/s12917-014-0289-1.

[79] Sidhu, P. K., Landoni, M. F., Aliabadi, F. S., Lees, P. 2010. "PK-PD Integration and Modeling of Marbofloxacin in Sheep." *Research in Veterinary Science* 88:134–141. Accessed February 28, 2018. doi: 10.1016/j.rvsc.2009.05.013.

[80] Bergan, T., Thorsteinsson, S. B., Solberg, R., Bjornskau, L., Kolstad, I. M., Johnsen, S. 1987. "Pharmacokinetics of Ciprofloxacin: Intravenous and Increasing Oral Doses." *The American Journal of Medicine* 82:97-102. Accessed February 28, 2018. PMID: 3578334.

[81] Commission Regulation (EU), *On pharmacologically active substances and their classification regarding maximum residue limits in foodstuffs of animal origin* https://ec.europa.eu/health/sites/health/files/files/eudralex/vol-5/reg_2010_37/reg_2010_37_en.pdf (accessed Jan 6, 2018).

[82] Lewis, T., Cook, J. 2014. "Fluoroquinolones and Tendinopathy: A Guide for Athletes and Sports Clinicians and a Systematic Review of the Literature." *Journal of Athletic Training* 49:422–427. Accessed February 28, 2018. doi: 10.4085/1062-6050-49.2.09.

[83] Corrao, G., Zambon, A., Bertù, L., Mauri, A., Paleari, V., Rossi, C., Venegoni, M. 2006. "Evidence of Tendinitis Provoked by Fluoroquinolone Treatment a Case-Control Study." *Drug Safety*

29:889–896. Accessed February 28, 2018. doi: 10.2165/00002018-200629100-00006.

[84] Williams, R. J., Attia, E., Wickiewicz, T. L., Hannafin, J. A. 2000. "The Effect of Ciprofloxacin on Tendon, Paratenon, and Capsular Fibroblast Metabolism." *The American Journal of Sports Medicine* 28:364–369. Accessed February 28, 2018. doi: 10.1177/03635465 000280031401.

[85] Melhus, A. 2005. "Fluoroquinolones and Tendon Disorders." *Expert Opinion on Drug Safety* 4:299–309. Accessed February 28, 2018. doi: 10.1517/14740338.4.2.299.

[86] Tsai, W., Yang, Y. 2011. "Fluoroquinolone-Associated Tendinopathy." *Chang Gung Medical Journal* 34: 461–467. Accessed February 28, 2018. PMID: 22035890.

[87] van der Linden, P. D., van Puijenbroek, E. P., Feenstra, J., Veld, B. A., Sturkenboom, M. C., Herings, R. M., Leufkens, H. G., Stricker, B. H. 2001. "Tendon Disorders Attributed to Fluoroquinolones: A Study on 42 Spontaneous Reports in the Period 1988 to 1998." *Arthritis & Rheumatology* 45:235–239. Accessed February 28, 2018. doi: 10.1002/1529-0131(200106)45:3<235::AID-ART254> 3.0.CO,2-7.

[88] Burkhardt, J. E., Hill, M. A., Carlton, W. W. 1992. "Morphologic and Biochemical Changes in Articular Cartilages of Immature Beagle Dogs Dosed with Difloxacin." *Toxicologic Pathology* 20:246–252. Accessed February 28, 2018. doi: 10.1177/ 019262339202000211.

[89] Tsai, W., Yang, Y. 2011. "Fluoroquinolone-Associated Tendinopathy." *Chang Gung Medical Journal* 34: 461–467. Accessed February 28, 2018. PMID: 22035890.

[90] Aoun, M. 1992. "Peripheral Neuropathy Associated with Fluoroquinolones." *Lancet* 340:127. Accessed February 28, 2018. doi: 10.1016/0140-6736(92)90460-K.

[91] Hedenmalm, K., Spigset, O. 1996. "Peripheral Sensory Disturbances Related to Treatment with Fluoroquinolone." *Journal*

of Antimicrobial Chemotherapy 37:1–7. Accessed February 28, 2018. PMID: 8722551.

[92] Ali, A. K. 2014. "Peripheral Neuropathy and Guillain-Barré Syndrome Risks Associated with Exposure to Systemic Fluoroquinolones: A Pharmacovigilance Analysis." *Annals of Epidemiology* 24:279–285. Accessed February 28, 2018. doi: 10.1016/j.annepidem.2013.12.009.

[93] Grill, M. F., Maganti, R. K. 2011. "Neurotoxic Effects Associated with Antibiotic Use: Management Considerations." *British Journal of Clinical Pharmacology* 72:381–393. Accessed February 28, 2018. doi: 10.1111/j.1365-2125.2011.03991.x.

[94] Ghavanini, A. A. 2017. "Do Fluoroquinolones Cause Neuropathy?" *Jornaul Neurology. e Neurosurgery* 3:2–4. Accessed February 28, 2018. doi: 10.19080/OAJNN.2017.02.555604.

[95] Unger, C., Al-Jashaami, L. S. 2016. "Ciprofloxacin Exposure Leading to Fatal Hepatotoxicity: An Unusual Correlation." *American Journal of Case Reports* 17:676–681. Accessed February 28, 2018. doi: 10.12659/AJCR.899080.

[96] Alshammari, T. M., Larrat, E. P. 2014. "The Risk of Hepatotoxicity with Fluoroquinolones : A National Case-Control Safety Study." *American Journal of Health-System Pharmacy* 71:37–43. Accessed February 28, 2018. doi: 10.2146/ajhp130165.

[97] Adikwu, E., Brambaifa, N. 2012. "Ciprofloxacin Cardiotoxicity and Hepatotoxicity in Humans and Animals." Pharmacology & Pharmacy 3:207–213. Accessed February 28, 2018. doi: 10.4236/pp.2012.32028 P.

[98] Andrade, R. J., Tulkens, P. M. 2011. "Hepatic Safety of Antibiotics Used in Primary Care." *Journal of Antimicrobial Chemotherapy* 66:1431–1446. Accessed February 28, 2018. doi: 10.1093/jac/dkr159.

[99] Villeneuve, J.-P., Davies, C., Côté, J. 1995. "Suspected Cirpofloxacin-Induced Hepatotoxicity." *Annals of Pharmacotherapy* 29:257–259. Accessed February 28, 2018. doi: 10.1177/106002809502900305.

[100] Qutrio Baloch, Z., Raza, M. A., Abbas, S. A., Bukhari, S. Ciprofloxacin-Induced Hepatotoxicity in a Healthy Young Adult. *Cureus* 2017, *9* (2), 8–11. Accessed February 28, 2018. doi: 1 10.1016/j.cld.2012.03.002.

[101] Zimmerman, H. 2012. "Drug-Induced Liver disease." *Clinics in Liver Disease* 4:73–96. Accessed February 28, 2018. doi: 1 10.1016/j.cld.2012.03.002.

[102] Fuchs, S., Simon, Z., Brezis, M. 1994. "Fatal Hepatic Failure Associated with Ciprofloxacin." *The Lancet* 343:738–739. Accessed February 28, 2018. doi: 10.1016/S0140-6736(94)91624-1.

[103] Ore, J., Bricheux, G., Togola, A., Bonnet, J. L., Donnadieu-bernard, F., Nakusi, L., Forestier, C., Traore, O. 2016. "C Ciprofloxacin residue and antibiotic-resistant biofilm bacteria in hospital effluent." *Environmental Pollution* 214:635–645. Accessed February 28, 2018. doi: 10.1016/j.envpol.2016.04.033.

[104] Wang, H., Hu, C., Liu, L., Xing, X. 2017. "Interaction of Ciprofloxacin Chlorination Products with Bacteria in Drinking Water Distribution Systems." *Journal of Hazardous Materials* 339:174–181. Accessed February 28, 2018. doi: 10.1016/ j.jhazmat.2017.06.033.

[105] Davids, M., Gudra, D., Radovica-Spalvina, I., Fridmanis, D., Bartkevics, V., Muter, O. 2017. "The Effects of Ibuprofen on Activated Sludge: Shift in Bacterial Community Structure and Resistance to Ciprofloxacin." *Journal of Hazardous Materials* 340:291–299. Accessed February 28, 2018. doi: 10.1016/j.jhazmat. 2017.06.065.

[106] Wang, H., Shen, Y., Hu, C., Xing, X., Zhao, D. 2018. "Sulfadiazine/ciprofloxacin Promote Opportunistic Pathogens Occurrence in Bulk Water of Drinking Water Distribution Systems." *Environmental Pollution* 234:71–78. Accessed February 28, 2018. doi: 10.1016/j.envpol.2017.11.050.

[107] Van Alphen, N. A., Gonzalez, A., McKenna, M. C., McKenna, T. K., Carlsen, B. T., Moran, S. L. 2014. "Ciprofloxacin-Resistant Aeromonas Infection Following Leech Therapy for Digit

Replantation: Report of 2 Cases." *Journal of Hand Surgery* 39:499–502. Accessed February 28, 2018. doi: 10.1016/j.jhsa.2013.11.041.

[108] Moreira da Silva, R. C. R., de Oliveira Martins Júnior, P., Gonçalves, L. F., de Paulo Martins, V., de Melo, A. B. F., Pitondo-Silva, A., de Campos, T. A. 2017. " Ciprofloxacin resistance in uropathogenic Escherichia coli isolates causing community-acquired urinary infections in Brasília, Brazil.." *Journal of Global Antimicrobial Resistance* 9:61–67. Accessed February 28, 2018. doi: 10.1016/j.jgar.2017.01.009.

[109] Zhang, W., Zhang, Y., Wang, X., Ding, F., Fu, Y., Zhao, J., Song, W., Opiyo, O. J., Zhang, F., Chen, X. 2017 " Siderophores in Clinical Isolates of Klebsiella Pneumoniae Promote Ciprofloxacin Resistance by Inhibiting the Oxidative Stress." *Biochemical and Biophysical Research Communications* 491:855–861. Accessed February 28, 2018. doi: 10.1016/j.bbrc.2017.04.108.

[110] Wang, Y., Zhang, A., Yang, Y., Lei, C., Jiang, W., Liu, B., Shi, H., Kong, L., Cheng, G., Zhang, X., et al. 2017. "Emergence of Salmonella Enterica Serovar Indiana and California Isolates with Concurrent Resistance to Cefotaxime, Amikacin and Ciprofloxacin from Chickens in China." *International Journal of Food Microbiology*, 262:23–30. Accessed February 28, 2018. doi: 10.1016/j.ijfoodmicro.2017.09.012.

[111] El Kary, N., El Rassy, E., Azar, N., Choucair, J. 2016. "Ciprofloxacin and Imipenem Resistance and Cross-Resistance in Pseudomonas Aeruginosa: A Single Institution Experience." *American Journal of Infection Control* 44:1736–1737. Accessed February 28, 2018. doi: 10.1016/j.ajic.2016.04.246.

[112] Weber, A., Chaffin, D., Smith, A., Opheim, K. E. 1985. "Quantitation of Ciprofloxacin in Body Fluids by High-Pressure Liquid Chromatography" *Antimicrobial Agents Chemotherapy* 27:531–534. Accessed February 28, 2018. doi: 10.1128/AAC.27.4.531.

[113] Jehl, F., Gallion, C., Debs, J., Brogard, J. M., Monteil, H., Minck, R. 1985. "High-Performance Liquid Chromatographic Method for

Determination of Ciprofloxacin in Biological Fluids." *Journal of Chromatography B: Biomedical Sciences and Applications* 339:347–357. Accessed February 28, 2018. PMID: 3159745.

[114] Joos, B., Ledergerber, B., Flepp, M., Bettex, J. D., Lüthy, R., Siegenthaler, W. 1985. "Comparison of High-Pressure Liquid Chromatography and Bioassay for Determination of Ciprofloxacin in Serum and Urine." *Antimicrobial Agents Chemotherapy* 27:353–356. Accessed February 28, 2018. PMID: 3158274.

[115] Gau, W., Ploschke, H. J., Schmidt, K., Weber, B. 1985. "Determination of Ciprofloxacin (Bay O 9867) in Biological Fluids by High-Performance Liquid Chromatography." *Journal of Liquid Chromatography* 8:485–497. Accessed February 28, 2018. doi: 10.1080/01483918508067095.

[116] Vallée, F., LeBel, M., Bergeron, M. 1986. "Determination of Ciprofloxacin in Biological Samples by Reversed-Phase High Performance Liquid Chromatography." *Therapeutic Drug Monitoring* 8:340–345. Accessed February 28, 2018. PMID: 2944255.

[117] Morton, S. J., Shull, V. H., Dick, J. D. 1986. "Determination of Norfloxacin and Ciprofloxacin Concentrations in Serum and Urine by High-Pressure Liquid Chromatography." *Antimicrobial Agents and Chemotherapy* 30:325–327. Accessed February 28, 2018. doi: PMID: 3767345.

[118] Schönfeld, W., Knöller, J., Bremm, K. D., Dahlhoff, A., Weber, B., König, W. 1986. "Determination of Ciprofloxacine, Norfloxacine, and Ofloxacine by High Performance Liquid Chromatography." *Zentralblatt für Bakteriologie, Mikrobiologie und Hygiene. Series A: Medical Microbiology, Infectious Diseases, Virology, Parasitology* 261:338–344. Accessed February 28, 2018. doi: 10.1016/S0176-6724(86)80051-7.

[119] Groeneveld, A. J. N., Brouwers, J. R. B. J. 1986. "Quantitative Determination of Ofloxacin, Ciprofloxacin, Norfloxacin and Pefloxacin in Serum by High Pressure Liquid Chromatography."

Pharmaceutisch Weekblad Scientific Edition 8:79–84. Accessed February 28, 2018. doi: 10.1007/BF01975486.

[120] Scholl, H., Schmidt, K., Weber, B. 1987. "Sensitive and Selective Determination of Picogram Amounts of Ciprofloxacin and Its Metabolites in Biological Samples Using High-Performance Liquid Chromatography and Photothermal Post-Column Derivatization." *Journal of Chromatography B: Biomedical Sciences and Applications* 416:321–330. Accessed February 28, 2018. PMID: 3611263.

[121] Nilsson-Ehle, I. 1987. "Assay of Ciprofloxacin and Norfloxacin in Serum and Urine by High-Performance Liquid Chromatography." *Journal of Chromatography B: Biomedical Sciences and Applications* 416:207–211. Accessed February 28, 2018. doi: 10.1016/0378-4347(87)80504-2.

[122] Awni, W. M., Clarkson, J., Guay, D. R. P. 1987. "Determination of Ciprofloxacin and Its 7-Ethylenediamine Metabolite in Human Serum and Urine by High-Performance Liquid Chromatography." *Journal of Chromatography B: Biomedical Sciences and Applications* 419:414–420. Accessed February 28, 2018. doi: 10.1016/0378-4347(87)80309-2.

[123] Myers, C. M., Blumer, J. L. 1897. "High-Performance Liquid Chromatography of Ciprofloxacin and Its Metabolites in Serum, Urine and Sputum." *Journal of Chromatography Biomedical Applications.* 422:153–164. Accessed February 28, 2018. PMID: 3437004.

[124] Tyczkowska, K., Hedeen, K. M., Aucoin, D. P., Aronson, A. L. 1989. "High-Performance Liquid Chromatographic Method for the Simultaneous Determination of Enrofloxacin and Its Primary Metabolite Ciprofloxacin in Canine Serum and Prostatic Tissue." *Journal of Chromatography B: Biomedical Sciences and Applications 493*:337–346. Accessed February 28, 2018. doi: 10.1016/S0378-4347(00)82739-5.

[125] Griggs, D. J., Wise, R. 1989. "A Simple Isocratic High-Pressure Liquid Chromatographic Assay of Quinolones in Serum." *Journal*

of Antimicrobial Chemotherapy 24:437–445. Accessed February 28, 2018. PMID: 2808195.

[126] Naora, K., Katagiri, Y., Ichikawa, N., Hayashibara, M., Iwamoto, K. 1990. "Simultaneous High-Performance Liquid Chromatographic Determination of Ciprofloxacin, Fenbufen and Felbinac in Rat Plasma." *Journal of Chromatography B: Biomedical Sciences and Applications* 530:186–191. Accessed February 28, 2018. doi: 10.1016/S0378-4347(00)82320-8.

[127] El-Yazigi, A., Al-Rawithy, S. 1990. "A Direct Liquid Chromatographic Quantitation of Ciprofloxacin in Microsamples of Plasma with Fluorometric Detection." *Therapeutic Drug Monitoring* 12:378–381. Accessed February 28, 2018. doi: 10.1097/00007691-199007000-00014.

[128] Katagiri, Y., Naora, K., Ichikawa, N., Hayashibara, M., Iwamoto, K. 1990. "High-Performance Liquid Chromatographic Determination of Ciprofloxacin in Rat Brain and Cerebrospinal Fluid." *Chemical and Pharmaceutical Bulletin* 38:2884–2886. Accessed February 28, 2018. PMID: 2076578.

[129] Bauer, J. F., Howard, S., Schmidt, A. 1990. " High-Performance Liquid Chromatographic Determination of Several Quinolone Antibacterials in Medicated Fish Feed." *Journal of Chromatography* 514:348–354. Accessed February 28, 2018.

[130] Teja-Isavadharm, P., Keeratithakul, D., Watt, G., Webster, H. K., Edstein, M. D. 1991. "Measurement of Ciprofloxacin in Human Plasma, Whole Blood, and Erythrocytes by High-Performance Liquid Chromatography." *Therapeutic Drug Monitoring* 13:263–267. Accessed February 28, 2018. doi: 10.1097/00007691-199105000-00014.

[131] Pou-Clave, L., Campos-Barreda, F., Pascual-Mostaza, C. 1991. "Determination of Ciprofloxacin in Human Serum by Liquid Chromatography." *Journal of Chromatography B: Biomedical Sciences and Applications* 563:211–215. Accessed February 28, 2018. doi: 10.1016/0378-4347(91)80298-Q.

[132] Mack, G. 1992. "Improved High-Performance Liquid Chromatographic Determination of Ciprofloxacin and Its Metabolites in Human Specimens." *Journal of Chromatography B: Biomedical Sciences and Applications* 582:263–267. Accessed February 28, 2018. doi: 10.1016/0378-4347(92)80331-J.

[133] Jim, L. K., El-Sayed, N., Al-Khamis, K. I. 1992. "A Simple High-Performance Liquid Chromatographic Assay for Ciprofloxacin in Human Serum." *Journal of Clinical Pharmacy and Therapeutics banner* 17:111–115. Accessed February 28, 2018. doi: 10.1111/j.1365-2710.1992.tb01277.x.

[134] Lovdahl, M., Steury, J., Russlie, H., Canafax, D. M. 1993. "Determination of Ciprofloxacin Levels in Chinchilla Middle Ear Effusion and Plasma by High-Performance Liquid Chromatography with Fluorescence Detection." *Journal of Chromatography A* 617:329–333. Accessed February 28, 2018. doi: 10.1016/0378-4347(93)80508-2.

[135] Altria, K. D., Chanter, Y. L. 1993. Validation of a Capillary Electrophoresis Method for the Determination of a Quinolone Antibiotic and Its Related Impurities." *Journal of Chromatography A* 652:459–463. Accessed February 28, 2018. doi: 10.1016/0021-9673(93)83266-U.

[136] Rieutord, A., Vazquez, L., Soursac, M., Prognon, P., Blais, J., Bourget, P., Mahuzier, G. 1994. "Fluoroquinolones as Sensitizers of Lanthanide Fluorescence: Application to the Liquid Chromatographic Determination of Ciprofloxacin Using Terbium." *Analytica Chimica Acta* 290:215–225. Accessed February 28, 2018. doi: 10.1016/0003-2670(94)80058-8.

[137] Calderön, V., González, J., Díez, P., Berenguer, J. A. 1996. "Evaluation of a Multiple Bioassay Technique for Determination of Antibiotic Residues in Meat with Standard Solutions of Antimicrobials." *Food Additives & Contaminants* 13:13–19. Accessed February 28, 2018. doi: 10.1080/02652039609374377.

[138] Volmer, D. A., Mansoori, B., Locke, S. J. 1997. "Study of 4-Quinolone Antibiotics in Biological Samples by Short-Column

Liquid Chromatography Coupled with Electrospray Ionization Tandem Mass Spectrometry." *Analytical Chemistry 69*:4143–4155. Accessed February 28, 2018. doi: 10.1021/ac970425c.

[139] Delepine, B., Hurtaud-Pessel, D., Sanders, P. 1998. "Simultaneous Determination of Six Quinolones in Pig Muscle by Liquid Chromatography-Atmospheric Pressure Chemical Ionisation Mass Spectrometry." *Analyst* 123:2743–2747. Accessed February 28, 2018. PMID: 10435336.

[140] Morgan, J., Joyce-Menekse, M. E., Rowlands, R. T., Gilbert, I. H., Lloyd, D. 2001. "Rapid and Sensitive Quantitation of Antibiotics in Fermentations by Electrospray Mass Spectrometry." *Rapid Communications in Mass Spectrometry* 15:1229–1238. Accessed February 28, 2018. doi: 10.1002/rcm.368.

[141] van Vyncht, G., Jànosi, A., Bordin, G., Toussaint, B., Maghuin-Rogister, G., De Pauw, E., Rodriguez, A. R. 2002. "Multiresidue Determination of (Fluoro)quinolone Antibiotics in Swine Kidney Using Liquid Chromatography-Tandem Mass Spectrometry." *Journal of Chromatography A* 952:121–129. Accessed February 28, 2018. doi: 10.1016/S0021-9673(02)00092-4.

[142] Schneider, M. J., Donoghue, D. J. 2002. "Multiresidue Analysis of Fluoroquinolone Antibiotics in Chicken Tissue Using Liquid Chromatography-Fluorescence-Multiple Mass Spectrometry." *Journal of Chromatography B* 780:83–92. Accessed February 28, 2018. doi: 10.1016/S1570-0232(02)00437-3.

[143] Ballesteros, O., Toro, I., Sanznebot, V., Navalon, A., Vilchez, J., Barbosa, J. 2003. "Determination of Fluoroquinolones in Human Urine by Liquid Chromatography Coupled to Pneumatically Assisted Electrospray Ionization Mass spectrometry." *Journal of Chromatography B* 798:137–144. Accessed February 28, 2018. doi: 10.1016/j.jchromb.2003.09.019.

[144] Batt, A. L., Aga, D. S. 2005. "Simultaneous Analysis of Multiple Classes of Antibiotics by Ion Trap LC/MS/MS for Assessing Surface Water and Groundwater Contamination." *Analytical*

Chemistry 77:2940–2947. Accessed February 28, 2018. doi: doi.org/ 10.1021/ac048512.

[145] Segura, P. A., García-Ac, A., Lajeunesse, A., Ghosh, D., Gagnon, C., Sauvé, S. 2007. "Determination of Six Anti-Infectives in Wastewater Using Tandem Solid-Phase Extraction and Liquid Chromatography–tandem Mass Spectrometry." *Journal of Environmental Monitoring* 9:307–313. Accessed February 28, 2018. doi: doi.org/ 10.1039/B618801J.

[146] Krebber, R., Hoffend, F. J., Ruttmann, F. 2009. "Simple and Rapid Determination of Enrofloxacin and Ciprofloxacin in Edible Tissues by Turbulent Flow Chromatography/tandem Mass Spectrometry (TFC-MS/MS)." *Analytica Chimica Acta* 637:208–213. Accessed February 28, 2018. doi: doi.org/10.1016/j.aca.2008.11.006.

[147] Babić, S., Mutavdžić Pavlović, D., Ašperger, D., Periša, M., Zrnčić, M., Horvat, A. J. M., Kaštelan-Macan, M. 2010. "Determination of Multi-Class Pharmaceuticals in Wastewater by Liquid Chromatography–tandem Mass Spectrometry (LC–MS–MS)." *Analytical and Bioanalytical Chemistry* 398:1185–1194. Accessed February 28, 2018. doi: 10.1007/s00216-010-4004-1.

[148] López Zavala, M. Á., Reynoso-Cuevas, L. 2015. "Simultaneous Extraction and Determination of Four Different Groups of Pharmaceuticals in Compost Using Optimized Ultrasonic Extraction and Ultrahigh Pressure Liquid Chromatography–mass Spectrometry." *Journal of Chromatography A* 1423:9–18. Accessed February 28, 2018. doi: 10.1016/j.chroma.2015.10.051.

[149] Imamoglu, H., Oktem Olgun, E. 2016. "Analysis of Veterinary Drug and Pesticide Residues Using the Ethyl Acetate Multiclass/Multiresidue Method in Milk by Liquid Chromatography-Tandem Mass Spectrometry." *Journal of Analytical Methods in Chemistry* 2170165:1–17. Accessed February 28, 2018. doi: 10.1155/2016/2170165.

[150] Szerkus, O., Jacyna, J., Gibas, A., Sieczkowski, M., Siluk, D., Matuszewski, M., Kaliszan, R., Markuszewski, M. J. 2017. "Robust HPLC–MS/MS Method for Levofloxacin and Ciprofloxacin

Determination in Human Prostate Tissue." *Journal of Pharmaceutical and Biomedical Analysis* 132:173–183. Accessed February 28, 2018. doi: 10.1016/j.jpba.2016.10.008.

[151] Wang, Z., Li, Y., Chang, Q., Kang, J., Pang, G.-F. 2018. "A Detection and Confirmation Strategy for Screening of Veterinary Drugs in Honey by Liquid Chromatography Coupled Quadrupole Time-of-Flight Mass Spectrometry." *Analytical Methods* 10:59–68. Accessed February 28, 2018. doi: 10.1039/C7AY02440A.

[152] Bannefeld, K. H., Stass, H., Blaschke, G. 1997. "Capillary Electrophoresis with Laser-Induced Fluorescence Detection, an Adequate Alternative to High-Performance Liquid Chromatography, for the Determination of Ciprofloxacin and Its Metabolite Desethyleneciprofloxacin in Human Plasma." *Journal of chromatography. B, Biomedical sciences and applications* 692:453–459. Accessed February 28, 2018. PMID: 9188836.

[153] Hernández-Arteseros, J. a, Compañó, R., Prat, M. D. 1998. "Determination of Ciprofloxacin and Enrofloxacin in Edible Animal Tissues by Terbium-Sensitized Luminescence." *Analyst* 123:2729–2732. Accessed February 28, 2018. PMID: 10435333.

[154] Li, D., Yan, Z.-Y., Cheng, W.-Q. 2008. "Determination of Ciprofloxacin with Functionalized Cadmium Sulfide Nanoparticles as a Fluorescence Probe." *Spectrochimica Acta. Part A, Molecular and Biomolecular Spectroscopy* 71:1204–1211. Accessed February 28, 2018. doi: 10.1016/j.saa.2008.03.024.

[155] Chen, Z., Qian, S., Chen, J., Cai, J., Wu, S., Cai, Z. 2012. "Protein-Templated Gold Nanoclusters Based Sensor for Off–on Detection of Ciprofloxacin with a High Selectivity." *Talanta* 94:240–245. Accessed February 28, 2018. doi: 10.1016/j.talanta.2012.03.033.

[156] Snitkoff, G. G., Grabe, D. W., Holt, R., Bailie, G. R. 1998. "Development of an Immunoassay for Monitoring the Levels of Ciprofloxacin Patient Samples." *Journal of Immunoassay* 19:227–238. Accessed February 28, 2018. doi: 10.1080/01971529808005483.

[157] El-Ansary, A. L., El-Hawary, W. F., Issa, Y. M., Ahmed, A. F. 1999. "Application of Ion-Pairs in Pharmaceutical Analysis. Atomic Absorption Spectrometric Determination of Promazine, Chlorpromazine, Promethazine, Imipramine and Ciprofloxacin Hydrochlorides with Sodium Cobaltinitrite." *Analytical Letters* 32:2255–2269. Accessed February 28, 2018. doi: 10.1080/00032719908542968.

[158] Salem, H., Khater, W., Fada, L. 2007. "Atomic Absorption Spectrometric Determination of Certain Fluoroquinolones in Pharmaceutical Dosage Forms and in Biological Fluids." *American Journal of Pharmacology and Toxicology* 2:65–74. Accessed February 28, 2018. doi: 10.3844/ajptsp.2007.65.74.

[159] Rizk, M. S., Belal, F., Ibrahim, F. A., Ahmed, S. M., Sheribah, Z. A. 2000. "Polarographic Determination of Some 4-Quinolone Antibacterials via Their Ni(II)-Complexes." *Electroanalysis* 12:531–534. Accessed February 28, 2018. doi: 10.1002/(SICI)1521-4109(200005)12:7<531::AID-ELAN531>3.0.CO,2-D.

[160] Djurdjević, P., Todorović, M., Stankov, M. J., Odović, J. 2000. "Spectrophotometry Determination of Ciprofloxacin in Serum Using Iron(III) Ion as Chromogenic Agent." *Analytical Letters* 33:657–665. Accessed February 28, 2018. doi: 110.1080/00032710008543081.

[161] Navalón, A., Ballesteros, O., Blanc, R., Vílchez, J. L. 2000. "Determination of Ciprofloxacin in Human Urine and Serum Samples by Solid-Phase Spectrofluorimetry." *Talanta* 52:845–852. Accessed February 28, 2018. doi: 10.1016/S0039-9140(00)00437-9.

[162] Rao, Y., Tong, Y., Zhang, X., Luo, G., Baeyens, W. R. G. 2000. "Flow-Injection Chemiluminescence Determination of Fluoroquinolones." *Analytical Letters* 33:1117–1129. Accessed February 28, 2018. doi: 10.1080/00032710008543113.

[163] Aly, F. A., Al-Tamimi, S. A., Alwarthan, A. A. 2001. "Chemiluminescence Determination of Some Fluoroquinolone Derivatives in Pharmaceutical Formulations and Biological Fluids

Using [Ru(bipy)32+]-Ce(IV) System." *Talanta 53*:885–893. Accessed February 28, 2018. doi: 10.1016/S0039-9140(00)00590-7.

[164] Okerman, L., Croubels, S., De Baere, S., Hoof, J. Van, De Backer, P., De Brabander, H. 2001. "Inhibition Tests for Detection and Presumptive Identification of Tetracyclines, Beta-Lactam Antibiotics and Quinolones in Poultry Meat." *Food Additives and Contaminants* 18:385–393. Accessed February 28, 2018. doi: 10.1080/02652030010024320.

[165] Duan, J., Yuan, Z. 2001. "Development of an Indirect Competitive ELISA for Ciprofloxacin Residues in Food Animal Edible Tissues." *Journal of Agricultural and Food Chemistry* 49:1087–1089. Accessed February 28, 2018. doi: 10.1021/jf000091j.

[166] Li, Y., Ji, B., Chen, W., Liu, L., Xu, C., Peng, C., Wang, L. 2008. "Production of New Class-Specific Polyclonal Antibody for Determination of Fluoroquinolones Antibiotics by Indirect Competitive ELISA." *Food and Agricultural Immunology* 19:251–264. Accessed February 28, 2018. doi: 10.1080/095401008 02471538.

[167] Brás Gomes, F. B. M., Riedstra, S., Ferreira, J. P. M. 2010. "Development of an Immunoassay for Ciprofloxacin Based on Phage-Displayed Antibody Fragments." *Journal of Immunological Methods 358*:17–22. Accessed February 28, 2018. doi: 10.1016/j. jim.2010.03.021.

[168] Holtzapple, C. K., Buckley, S. A., Stanker, L. H. 2001. "Determination of Fluoroquinolones in Serum Using an on-Line Clean-up Column Coupled to High-Performance Immunoaffinity-Reversed-Phase Liquid Chromatography." *Journal of Chromatography B: Biomedical Sciences and Applications* 754:1–9. Accessed February 28, 2018. doi: 10.1016/S0378-4347(00)00575-2.

[169] Thangadurai, S., Shukla, S. K., Anjaneyulu, Y. 2002. "Separation and Detection of Certain β-Lactam and Fluoroquinolone Antibiotic Drugs by Thin Layer Chromatography." *Analytical Sciences.*

18:97–100. Accessed February 28, 2018. doi: 10.2116/analsci.18.97.

[170] Myllyniemi, A.-L., Sipilä, H., Nuotio, L., Niemi, A., Honkanen-Buzalski, T. 2002. "An Indirect Conductimetric Screening Method for the Detection of Antibiotic Residues in Bovine Kidneys." *Analyst* 127:1247–1251. Accessed February 28, 2018. doi: 10.1039/B204175H.

[171] Mccourt, J., Bordin, G., Rosarodriguez, A. 2003. "Development of a Capillary Zone Electrophoresis–electrospray Ionisation Tandem Mass Spectrometry Method for the Analysis of Fluoroquinolone Antibiotics." *Journal of Chromatography A* 990:259–269. Accessed February 28, 2018. doi: 10.1016/S0021-9673(03)00050-5.

[172] Pascual-Reguera, M. I., Pérez Parras, G., Molina Díaz, A. 2004. "A Single Spectroscopic Flow-through Sensing Device for Determination of Ciprofloxacin." *Journal of Pharmaceutical and Biomedical Analysis.* 35:689–695. Accessed February 28, 2018. doi: 10.1016/j.jpba.2004.03.002.

[173] Choma, I. M., Choma, A., Komaniecka, I., Pilorz, K., Staszczuk, K. 2004. "Semiquantitative Estimation of Enrofloxacin and Ciprofloxacin by Thin-Layer Chromatography–Direct Bio-autography." *Journal of Liquid Chromatography & Related Technologies* 27:2071–2085. Accessed February 28, 2018. doi: 10.1081/JLC-120039419.

[174] Pellegrini, G. E., Carpico, G., Coni, E. 2004. "Electrochemical Sensor for the Detection and Presumptive Identification of Quinolone and Tetracycline Residues in Milk." *Analytica Chimica Acta* 520:13–18. Accessed February 28, 2018. doi: 10.1016/j.aca.2004.04.052.

[175] Komorsky-Lovrić, Š., Nigović, B. 2004. "Identification of 5-Aminosalicylic Acid, Ciprofloxacin and Azithromycin by Abrasive Stripping Voltammetry." *Journal of Pharmaceutical and Biomedical Analysis* 36:81–89. Accessed February 28, 2018. doi: 10.1016/j.jpba.2004.05.008.

[176] Torriero, A., Ruizdiaz, J., Salinas, E., Marchevsky, E., Sanz, M., Raba, J. 2006. "Enzymatic Rotating Biosensor for Ciprofloxacin Determination." *Talanta* 69: 691–699. Accessed February 28, 2018. doi: 10.1016/j.talanta.2005.11.005.

[177] Torriero, A. A. J., Salinas, E., Raba, J., Silber, J. J. 2006. "Sensitive Determination of Ciprofloxacin and Norfloxacin in Biological Fluids Using an Enzymatic Rotating Biosensor." *Biosensors and Bioelectronics* 22:109–115. Accessed February 28, 2018. doi: 10.1016/j.bios.2005.12.004.

[178] Yi, H., Li, C. 2007. "Voltammetric Determination of Ciprofloxacin Based on the Enhancement Effect of Cetyltrimethylammonium Bromide (CTAB) at Carbon Paste Electrode." *Russian Journal of Electrochemistry 43*: 1377–1381. Accessed February 28, 2018. doi: 10.1134/S1023193507120075.

[179] Fotouhi, L., Alahyari, M. Electrochemical Behavior and Analytical 2010. "Application of Ciprofloxacin Using a Multi-Walled Nanotube Composite Film-Glassy Carbon Electrode." *Colloids Surfaces B: Biointerfaces* 81:110–114. Accessed February 28, 2018. doi: 10.1016/j.colsurfb.2010.06.030.

[180] Ensafi, A. A., TAEI, M., Khayamian, T., Hasanpour, F. 2010. "Simultaneous Voltammetric Determination of Enrofloxacin and Ciprofloxacin in Urine and Plasma Using Multiwall Carbon Nanotubes Modified Glassy Carbon Electrode by Least-Squares Support Vector Machines." *Analytical Sciences* 26:803–808. Accessed February 28, 2018. doi: 10.2116/analsci.26.803.

[181] Ensafi, A. A., Allafchian, A. R., Mohammadzadeh, R. 2012. "Characterization of MgFe2O4 Nanoparticles as a Novel Electrochemical Sensor: Application for the Voltammetric Determination of Ciprofloxacin." *Analytical Sciences* 28:705–710. Accessed February 28, 2018. doi: 10.2116/analsci.28.705.

[182] Zhang, X., Wei, Y., Ding, Y. 2014. "Electrocatalytic Oxidation and Voltammetric Determination of Ciprofloxacin Employing Poly(alizarin Red)/graphene Composite Film in the Presence of Ascorbic Acid, Uric Acid and Dopamine." *Analytica Chimica Acta*

835:29–36. Accessed February 28, 2018. doi: 10.1016/j.aca.2014.05.020.

[183] Mahmoud Nejem, R., Mohamed Issa, M., Stefan-van Staden, R.-I., Baroud, H. 2012. "A Novel Ciprofloxacin Selective Membrane Electrode." *Current Pharmaceutical Analysis* 8:334–338. Accessed February 28, 2018. doi: 10.2174/157341212803341591.

[184] Ionescu, R. E., Jaffrezic-Renault, N., Bouffier, L., Gondran, C., Cosnier, S., Pinacho, D. G., Marco, M. P., Sánchez-Baeza, F. J., Healy, T., Martelet, C. 2007. "Impedimetric Immunosensor for the Specific Label Free Detection of Ciprofloxacin Antibiotic." *Biosensors and Bioelectronics* 23: 549–555. Accessed February 28, 2018. doi: 10.1016/j.bios.2007.07.014.

[185] Tsekenis, G., Garifallou, G. Z., Davis, F., Millner, P. A., Pinacho, D. G., Sanchez-Baeza, F., Marco, M. P., Gibson, T. D., Higson, S. P. J. 2008. "Detection of Fluoroquinolone Antibiotics in Milk via a Labeless Immunoassay Based upon an Alternating Current Impedance Protocol." *Analytical. Chemical* 80: 9233–9239. Accessed February 28, 2018. doi: 10.1021/ac8014752.

[186] Pinacho, D., Sánchez-Baeza, F., Pividori, M.-I., Marco, M.-P. 2014. "Electrochemical Detection of Fluoroquinolone Antibiotics in Milk Using a Magneto Immunosensor." *Sensors 14*:15965–15980. Accessed February 28, 2018. doi: 10.3390/s140915965.

[187] Abnous, K., Danesh, N. M., Alibolandi, M., Ramezani, M., Taghdisi, S. M., Emrani, A. S. 2017. "A Novel Electrochemical Aptasensor for Ultrasensitive Detection of Fluoroquinolones Based on Single-Stranded DNA-Binding Protein." *Sensors Actuators B Chemica* 240:100–106. Accessed February 28, 2018. doi: 10.1016/j.snb.2016.08.100.

[188] Yan, H., Qiao, F., Kyung, H. R. 2017. "Molecularly Imprinted-Matrix Solid-Phase Dispersion for Selective Extraction of Five Fluoroquinolones in Eggs and Tissue." *Analytical. Chemical 79*:8242–8248. Accessed February 28, 2018. doi: 10.1021/ac070644q.

[189] Lombardo-Agüí, M., Gámiz-Gracia, L., Blanco, C. C., García-Campna, A. M. 2010. "Laser Induced Fluorescence Coupled to Capillary Electrophoresis for the Determination of Fluoroquinolones in Foods of Animal Origin Using Molecularly Imprinted Polymers." *Journa of Chromatography A* 1217:2237–2242. Accessed February 28, 2018. doi: 10.1016/j.chroma.2010.02.016.

[190] Foguel, M. V., Pedro, N. T. B., Wong, A., Khan, S., Zanoni, M. V. B., Sotomayor, M. D. P. T. 2017. 2017. "Synthesis and Evaluation of a Molecularly Imprinted Polymer for Selective Adsorption and Quantification of Acid Green 16 Textile Dye in Water Samples." *Talanta* 170:244-251. Accessed February 28, 2018. doi: 10.1016/j.talanta.2017.04.013.

[191] Pupin, R. R. R., Monteiro, G. C. C., Foguel, M. V. V., Bolzani, V. S. S., Pividori, M. I. I., Sotomayor, M. P. T. D. P. T. Molecularly Imprinted Polymers (MIP): From the Bulk Syhthesis to Hybrid Material to Classic and New Applications. In *Molecularly Imprinted Polymers (MIPs): Challenges, Uses and Prospects*, Quinn, T., Ed., Nova Science Publishers: Hauppauge, 2017, pp 44–118.

[192] Benito-Peña, E., Urraca, J. L., Sellergren, B., Moreno-Bondi, M. C. 2008. "Solid-Phase Extraction of Fluoroquinolones from Aqueous Samples Using a Water-Compatible Stochiometrically Imprinted Polymer." *Journal of Chromatography A 1208:*62–70. Accessed February 28, 2018. doi: 10.1016/j.chroma.2008.08.109.

[193] Yan, H., Row, K., Yang, G. 2008. "Water-Compatible Molecularly Imprinted Polymers for Selective Extraction of Ciprofloxacin from Human Urine." *Talanta 75*:227–232. Accessed February 28, 2018. doi: 10.1016/j.talanta.2007.11.002.

[194] Chen, L., Zhang, X., Xu, Y., Du, X., Sun, X., Sun, L., Wang, H., Zhao, Q., Yu, A., Zhang, H., et al. 2010. "Determination of Fluoroquinolone Antibiotics in Environmental Water Samples Based on Magnetic Molecularly Imprinted Polymer Extraction Followed by Liquid Chromatography-Tandem Mass Spectrometry."

Analytica Chimica Acta 662: 31–38. Accessed February 28, 2018. doi: 10.1016/j.aca.2010.01.001.

[195] Yan, H., Qiao, F., Row, K. H. 2009. "Molecularly Imprinted Monolithic Column for Selective On-Line Extraction of Enrofloxacin and Ciprofloxacin from Urine." *Chromatographia* 83: 1612-1112. Accessed February 28, 2018. doi: 10.1365/s10337-009-1244-3.

[196] Rodríguez, E., Navarro-Villoslada, F., Benito-Peña, E., Marazuela, M. D., Moreno-Bondi, M. C. 2011. "Multiresidue Determination of Ultratrace Levels of Fluoroquinolone Antimicrobials in Drinking and Aquaculture Water Samples by Automated Online Molecularly Imprinted Solid Phase Extraction and Liquid Chromatography." *Analytical Chemistry* 83: 2046–2055. Accessed February 28, 2018. doi: 10.1021/ac102839n.

[197] Lv, Y.-K., Yang, L., Liu, X.-H., Guo, Z.-Y., Sun, H.-W. 2013. "Preparation and Evaluation of a Novel Molecularly Imprinted Hybrid Composite Monolithic Column for on-Line Solid-Phase Extraction Coupled with HPLC to Detect Trace Fluoroquinolone Residues in Milk." *Analytical Methods* 5: 1848-1855. Accessed February 28, 2018. doi: 10.1039/C3AY26431A.

[198] Oliveira, H. M. V., Moreira, F. T. C., Sales, M. G. F. 2011. "Ciprofloxacin-Imprinted Polymeric Receptors as Ionophores for Potentiometric Transduction." *Electrochimica Acta* 56:2017–2023. Accessed February 28, 2018. doi: 10.1016/j.electacta.2010.11.082.

[199] Kamel, A. H., Mahmoud, W. H., Mostafa, M. S. 2011. "Biomimetic Ciprofloxacin Sensors Made of Molecularly Imprinted Network Receptors for Potential Measurements." *Analytical Methods* 3:957-964. Accessed February 28, 2018. doi: 10.1039/C0AY00706D.

[200] Pedroso, M. M., Foguel, M. V., Silva, D. H. S., Sotomayor, M. D. P. T., Yamanaka H. 2017. "Electrochemical Sensor for Dodecyl Gallate Determination Based on Electropolymerized Molecularly Imprinted Polymer." *Sensors Actuators, B Chemical* 253:180-186. Accessed February 28, 2018. doi: 10.1016/j.snb.2017.06.127.

[201] Yan, C. 2016. "Selective Recognition of Ciprofloxacin Hydrochloride Based on Molecular Imprinted Sensor via Electrochemical Copolymerization of Pyrrole and O-Phenylenediamine." *International Journal of Electrochemical Sscience* 11:6466–6476. Accessed February 28, 2018. doi: 10.20964/2016.08.56.

[202] Herrera-Herrera, A. V., Hernández-Borges, J., Rodríguez-Delgado, M. Á. 2008." Ionic Liquids as Mobile Phase Additives for the High-Performance Liquid Chromatographic Analysis of Fluoroquinolone Antibiotics in Water Samples." *Analytical and Bioanalytical Chemistry* 392: 1439 - 1446. Accessed February 28, 2018. doi: 10.1007/s00216-008-2442-9.

[203] Adrian, J., Pasche, S., Voirin, G., Adrian, J., Pinacho, D. G., Font, H., Sánchez-Baeza, F., Marco, M.-P., Diserens, J.-M., Granier, B. 2009. "Wavelength-Interrogated Optical Biosensor for Multi-Analyte Screening of Sulfonamide, Fluoroquinolone, β-Lactam and Tetracycline Antibiotics in Milk." *TrAC Trends in Analytical Chemistry* 28: 769–777. Accessed February 28, 2018. doi: 10.1016/j.trac.2009.04.011.

[204] Pandey, S., Pandey, P., Tiwari, G., Tiwari, R., Rai, A. 2012. "FTIR Spectroscopy: A Tool for Quantitative Analysis of Ciprofloxacin in Tablets." *Indian Journal of Pharmaceutical Sciences 74*: 86-90. Accessed February 28, 2018. doi: 10.4103/0250-474X.102551.

[205] He, L., Lin, M., Li, H., Kim, N. J. 2010. "Surface-Enhanced Raman Spectroscopy Coupled with Dendritic Silver Nanosubstrate for Detection of Restricted Antibiotics." *Journal. Raman Spectroscopy 41*:739–744. Accessed February 28, 2018. doi: 10.1002/jrs.2505.

[206] Guo, Z., Chen, L., Lv, H., Yu, Z., Zhao, B. 2014. "Magnetic Imprinted Surface Enhanced Raman Scattering (MI-SERS) Based Ultrasensitive Detection of Ciprofloxacin from a Mixed Sample." *Analytical Methods* 6:1627–1632. Accessed February 28, 2018. doi: 10.1039/C3AY40866C.

In: Ciprofloxacin
Editor: Mohamed Said Attia
ISBN: 978-1-53614-534-2

Chapter 7

FLUORESCENCE DETECTION OF CIPROFLOXACIN

Subhankar Singha*
Department of Chemistry, School of Molecular Science (BK21PLUS),
Pohang University of Science and Technology (POSTECH),
Pohang, Republic of Korea

ABSTRACT

Ciprofloxacin, a fluoroquinolone antibiotic with broad antibacterial spectrum, is widely used for the treatment of bacterial infection in human. Overdose of ciprofloxacin on the other hand can cause several adverse effects not only to human but also to microorganism present in the environment. Unabsorbed ciprofloxacin in the body is mostly excreted through urine and finally goes to the environment, resulting in a drug resistance pressure on bacteria. Hence simple and efficient detection method of ciprofloxacin is necessary. Accordingly, several detection systems have been developed mostly based on either the inherent fluorescence property of ciprofloxacin or sensitized lanthanide luminescence. These detection systems are advantageous for indirect as well as direct measurement of ciprofloxacin in biological samples, which

* Corresponding Author Email: subhankar@postech.ac.kr.

is highly demanding for easy monitoring the overdoses or abuses of ciprofloxacin. In this review chapter, the reported fluorescence detection systems for ciprofloxacin are discussed in terms of their efficiency and suitability for practical applications.

Keywords: fluoroquinolone, ciprofloxacin, analytical, fluorescence, high performance liquid chromatography (HPLC), lanthanides, tissue, serum, urine

LIST OF ACRONYMS

DNA	deoxyribonucleic acid
°C	degree Celsius
N	nitrogen
pKa_1	acid dissociation constant at logarithmic scale
pI	isoelectric point
pH	power of hydrogen or potential of hydrogen
HPLC	high performance liquid chromatography
TLC	thin-layer chromatography
USP	United States Pharmacopoeia
M	molar
UV	ultraviolet
Vis	visible
n	nano
g	gram
m	milli, meter
L	litre
μ	micro
PET	positron emission tomography
F	fluorine
ELISA	enzyme-linked immunosorbent assay
CO_2	carbon dioxide
C	carbon
H	hydrogen

CE	capillary electrophoresis
MIC	minimal inhibitory concentration
E. coli	Escherichia coli
ppb	parts per billion
min	minute
BALB/c mice	albino, laboratory-bred strain of the house mouse
KLH	keyhole limpet hemocyanin
LC	liquide chromatography
MS	mass spectroscopy
v	volume
%	percent
SDS	sodium dodecyl sulfate
EU	European Union
Eu^{3+}	europium(III) ion
Tb^{3+}	terbium(III) ion
S	singlet
T	triplet
kcal	kilocalorie
mol	mole
P	phosphorescence
F	fluorescence
DO3A	1,4,7,10-tetraazacyclododecane-1,4,7-triacetic acid
Tb-DO3A	terbium(III)-DO3A complex
p	pico
SDBS	sodium dodecylbenzene sulfonate
CPNPs	coordination polymer nanoparticles
Ad	adenine
CdS	cadmium sulfide
K_a	association constant
SP	sulfopropyl

INTRODUCTION

Among the fluoroquinolone antibiotics, ciprofloxacin (1-cyclopropyl-6-fluoro-1,4-dihydro-4-oxo-7-(1-piperazinyl)-3-quinolone carboxylic acid) is the most widely used drug due to its high activity against a broad spectrum of gram-negative and gram-positive bacteria (Sun et al. 2006). Besides the excellent antibiotic activity of ciprofloxacin, there are several adverse effects as observed in human are including DNA damage (Cozzarelli 1980), severe liver damage (Drlica 1984) and hematuria (Gellert 1981). It is also found that ciprofloxacin has lower ability to be absorbed from the gastro-intestinal tract in bioactive form compared to that of the other fluoroquinolones (Gürbay et al. 2006). Accordingly, the renal clearance of ciprofloxacin exceeds normal glomerular filtration rates; resulting in a higher amount of renal tubular secretion (Zimpfer et al. 2004) as well as an abnormal level of ciprofloxacin in urine during faliure of renal function (Garlando et al. 1985). The patients undergoing treatment with ciprofloxacin also experiences adverse reactions involving the gastro-intestinal tract (nausea, vomiting), skin or central nervous system (Brumfitt et al. 1984).

Besides those, there is increasing concern about bacterial resistance to antibiotics including ciprofloxacin by means of mutations altering the A subunit of DNA gyrase and other processes such as reduced drug permeation (Panadero et al. 1995). It is also reported that after oral administration, most of the antibiotics including ciprofloxacin are partially metabolized and a major amount is released via patient excreta into the municipal sewage system. If they are not eliminated during sewage treatment, the drugs that are released into the effluent enter the aquatic environment and eventually reach drinking water. If the concentrations are high enough, effluent from hospitals, municipal sewage and sewage treatment plants may become a reservoir for the selection of resistant bacteria. Taking all these facts into consideration, the data, as well as the risk assessment presented, it is necessary to routinewise analyze the amount of antibiotic drugs and active metabolites in sewage sludge.

Furthermore, ciprofloxacin is also widely used as veterinary drugs for food-producing animals, results an abnormal level of antibiotic in the edible animal products like meat, egg and milk (Kümmerer and Henninger 2003). By considering drug overdose and abuse induced adverse effects, the detection and monitoring of the residue levels of antibiotics spicifically for ciprofloxacin in complex biological matrices are utmost necessary by means of sophisticated analytical methods.

In this chapter, an overview on the reported conventional analytical techniques for detection of ciprofloxacin is discussed along with their advantages and limitations, following the major emphasis on the recently developed highly advantageous fluorescence detection systems.

PHYSICAL PROPERTIES OF CIPROFLOXACIN

Ciprofloxacin is an organic heterocyclic molecule with white coloured, bitter taste, and powder like texture (melts at 313–315°C). It is better to store at 4°C in the dark to minimize photolytic degradation. In general, ciprofloxacin is highly soluble in acetic acid, and slightly soluble in water, methanol, ethanol, or acetone. The octanol-water partition coefficient for ciprofloxacin is lower than one (Hirai et al. 1986). Ciprofloxacin hydrochloride is the pharmaceutical formulation, structure of which is shown in Figure 1. Due to the presence of two ionizable functional groups, the 6-carboxylic group and the N-4 of the piperazine substituent (Figure 1), the dissociation and isoelectric constants for ciprofloxacin reported as $pKa_1 = 6.09$ (corresponds to the dissociation of a proton from the carboxyl group), $pKa_2 = 8.62$ (corresponds to the dissociation of a proton from the N-4 in the piperazinyl group), and $pI = 7.14$ (isoelectric point, obtained by calculating the average of pKa_1 and pKa_2) (Melo et al. 2005;Varanda et al. 2006). Accordingly, at the most physiologically relevant pH, a significant fraction of ciprofloxacin exists as zwitterionic species. Due to the presence of a conjugated electronic structure with donor and acceptor type moieties, ciprofloxacin shows a strong ultra-violet absorption (around 275 nm along with a weak absorption around 318 nm) as well as fluorescence property in water solution (Laignier Cazedey and Nunes Salgado 2012). Because there are several possible protonation equilibria in the ciprofloxacin solution, both the absorption and fluorescence properties show variations depending upon pH of the media. It is found that the fluorescent intensity is relatively stable and strong in the range of pH from 2 to 7. At highly acidic (below pH 2) or basic (above pH 7) medium, the fluorescence property of ciprofloxacin drops sharply (Yang et al. 2003). In acidic solution of pH 0–2, ciprofloxacin emits at 450 nm, and fluorescence intensity is relatively weak and gradually increases with increasing of pH. In the range of pH 2 to pH 4, it shows a strong fluorescence with a maxima at 450 nm. When pH > 4, maximum emission wavelength gradually blue-shifts to 414 nm and fluorescence intensity slightly decreases as pH increases, and at the same time an evident change in ultra-violet absorption spectrum is observed due to the existance of the zwitterionic ion form in that condition. Above pH > 8, the fluorescence intensity decreases again until disappearance as pH increases, indicating that it exists as non-fluorescent anionic form. Fluorescence quantum yield of ciprofloxacin under neutral condition has been measured to be 0.12 in a buffer solution of pH 7.0 using quinine bisulphate as a reference at the maximum excitation wavelength of 275 nm (Liu et al. 2005).

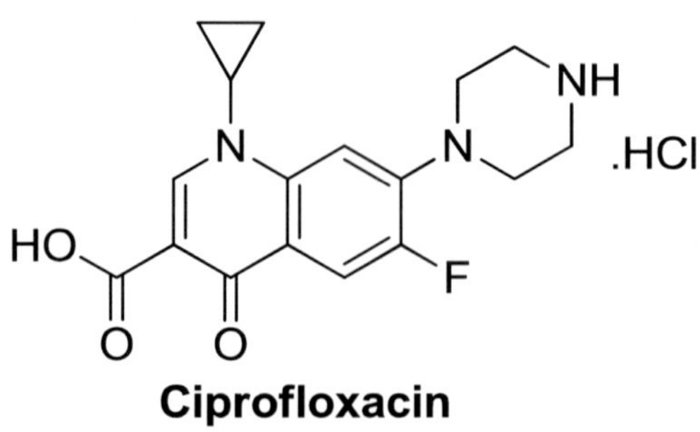

Figure 1. The chemical structure of ciprofloxacin as a hydrochloride salt.

Conventional Analytical Detection of Ciprofloxacin

The strong ultra-violet absorption property of ciprofloxacin has been employed to develop several analytical methods for it's detection mainly using high performance liquid chromatography (HPLC). HPLC is the official method for ciprofloxacin detection in United States Pharmacopoeia, British Pharmacopoeia (United States Pharmacopoeia (USP); 31th ed. United States Pharmacopoeia Convention: Rockville, 2008; British Pharmacopoeia. London: Her Majesty's Stationery Office, 2003). Other than HPLC, diverse conventional analytical or assay methods also have been developed for ciprofloxacin detection in pharmaceutical dosage forms and biological fluids (Sharma et al. 2010). Some of those important analytical procedures are presented here with brief discussion on their promising aspects.

In a simple and sensitive HPLC method, concentration of ciprofloxacin was determined in a canine serum and a prostatic tissue (Tyczkowska et al. 1989). The serum and tissue was sonicated separately in a mixture of 1:1 dilution of acetonitrile and sodium hydroxide (0.1 M) followed by ultrafiltration through a 10,000 molecular mass cut-off filter. Separation of ciprofloxacin from ultrafiltrate was accomplished by ion-paired liquid chromatography using a reversed-phase analytical column, followed by detection with a photometric ultraviolet (UV)-visible detector set at 278.6 nm and confirmed by a photodiode array detector operating from 230 to 360 nm. The limit of detection for ciprofloxacin with this method was 2 ng/mL.

Another HPLC based rapid, accurate, and sensitive method has been developed for the quantitative determination of ciprofloxacin, with high *in vitro* activity against a wide range of Gram-negative and Gram-positive organisms (Samanidou et al. 2003). This method uses a Kromasil 100 C-8 250 mm × 4 mm analytical column and detection was performed with a variable wavelength UV-visible detector at 275 nm, to provide the limit of detection of 0.01 ng per 20 μL injection for ciprofloxacin. It was further applied to detect ciprofloxacin in human blood serum. This method also needs sample pretreatment involving protein precipitation with acetonitrile. Similarly, ciprofloxacin determination using the HPLC technique involving a pump programmed by a system controller, a UV-visible spectrophotometric detector (at 280 nm), and a recorder was also achieved after sample pretreatment with perchloric acid to adjust the pH and mixing phenacetin as the internal standard (Pham et al. 2002). Due to the ease of availability and cheap price, feather meal is currently incorporated into animal feed as a protein source for farming. To ensure delivery of safe foods to consumers, the residual drugs in feathers from treated animals were analysed using HPLC coupled tandem mass spectrometry method. The results show high levels of enrofloxacin and ciprofloxacin through all sampling periods; suggesting that feathers from treated animals should not be fed to food-producing animals (Martin et al. 2007). Several similar HPLC methods are also reported for ciprofloxacin detection either simply by using UV-detection or in combination with various analytical techniques (Szerkus et al. 2017; Kassab et al. 2005; Joos et al. 1985; Scherer et al. 2014; Vella et al. 2015).

Besides HPLC technique, few other conventional methods are also developed. A thin-layer chromatographic (TLC)-densitometric method was shown to identify and quantify ciprofloxacin and its degradation products in pharmaceutical preparations (Krzek et al. 2005). By means of positron emission tomography (PET), the biodistribution and pharmacokinetics of the fluorine-18-labeled (18F)ciprofloxacin in tissue were monitored non-invasively in healthy humans (Brunner et al. 2004). An indirect competitive enzyme-linked immunosorbent assay (ELISA) was developed to detect ciprofloxacin in food animal edible tissues with very high sensityvity (0.32 ng/mL). The method was also specific, accurate, and convenient (Duan and Yuan 2001). As antibiotic residue in meat is a serious public health concern due to its harmful effects on consumer health, in a further report, three analytical methods (ELISA, TLC and HPLC) were used to detect ciprofloxacin residue levels in meat samples. The study showed that the mean ciprofloxacin residue levels were above the recommended limit. Although some of the mean residues levels were below the permissible limits, the co-occurrence of multidrug residues in some of the samples mentioned for concern (Ramatla et al. 2017). The enzymatic degradation of ciprofloxacin by basidiomycetous fungi was studied by monitoring $^{14}CO_2$ production from (14C)ciprofloxacin in liquid cultures to elucidate the structures of the various metabolites by HPLC combined with electrospray ionization mass spectrometry and ^{1}H nuclear magnetic resonance spectroscopy (Heinz-Georg et al. 1999). A molecularly imprinted solid-phase extraction procedure followed by chromatographic analysis was developed for the simultaneous identification of enrofloxacin and its active metabolite, ciprofloxacin, in milk samples. This method is simple and sensitive, and is therefore an alternative tool to the existing HPLC methods for analyzing residual enrofloxacin and ciprofloxacin in biological samples (Yan et al. 2008). Capillary electrophoresis also has been employed for separation, identification, and determination of ciprofloxacin, showing an alternative to liquid chromatography. This capillary electrophoresis (CE) method fulfilled the current European Pharmacopoeia requirements, thus can be applicable to the analysis of different medicinal products containing ciprofloxacin (Michalska et al. 2004). A simple and fast Raman spectroscopy-based procedure was developed to identify the antibiotic susceptibilities and determining the minimal inhibitory concentration (MIC) with a time saving procedure compared to establish the phenotypic methods nowadays used in diagnostics. Micro-Raman spectroscopy was able to detect ciprofloxacin-induced changes in E. coli within a short time of interaction. The method was validated by comparing the data with other well-known procedures (Kirchhoff et al. 2018). A Rayleigh light scattering technique to determine ciprofloxacin lactate in drugs was developed with a detection limit of 6.0 $\mu g\ mL^{-1}$ and a high level of recovery range. The sensitivity of this method compared with HPLC, enables the determination of ciprofloxacin lactate in injections, eye drops and tablets (Xiao et al. 2007). A portable microfluidic system has also been fabricated to detect ciprofloxacin with concentrations down to 1 ppb (McIntosh et al. 2011). In a further development, a rapid (within 3 min), simple, and sensitive gold-based lateral-flow immunochromatography test strip has been used for testing residues of ciprofloxacin in milk samples. A highly sensitive and specific anti-ciprofloxacin antibody was obtained from BALB/c mice with ciprofloxacin-KLH conjugates. As this method provides only preliminary qualitative results, determined positive samples should be further confirmed by some more accurate and quantitative method such as HPLC, LC-MS/MS or an ELISA method (Liu et al. 2014).

For direct quantitation of ciprofloxacin, spectrophotometric methods are important as these can be used in small laboratories without sophisticated and expensive instrumentations. Accordingly, determination of ciprofloxacin by direct measurement of its intrinsic ultraviolet absorption (at 275 nm) is also established recently in ophthalmic solution (Laignier Cazedey and Nunes Salgado 2012). The method is validated through the parameters of linearity, accuracy, precision, limit of detection, limit of quantitation, specificity and robustness.

Though several conventional analytical methods have been developed mainly based on intrinsic ultra-violet absorption property of ciprofloxacin, those suffer from major drawbacks of low sensitivity. Besides, time consuming sample preparation and treatment, expensive instrumentations and reagents, inconvenient reagent pretreatment, and inability to assay real samples are also other limitations. In that respect, fluorescence detection methods are greatly promising for real sample analysis with high sensitivity and selectivity.

Fluorescence Based Detection of Ciprofloxacin

HPLC-Spectrofluorimetry Detection

In recent years, considerable attempts have been made to develop many organic chemosensors to detect antibiotics through the fluorescence responses (Carlucci 1998). In this purpose, fluorescence detection of ciprofloxacin could be an ideal means due to its high sensitivity. Ciprofloxacin, being a quinoline carboxylic acid derivative as well as containing the donor-acceptor type electronic π-conjugated skeleton, shows native fluorescence emission around 440-450 nm upon excitation around 275-280 nm in pure water (Shtykov et al. 2007). Based on the native fluorescence of ciprofloxacin, a large number of analytical methods for ciprofloxacin detection have been developed simply by combination of HPLC with spectrofluorimetry as described below.

In a simple process, ciprofloxacin content in serum was measured by HPLC using an isocratic reversed phase chromatography on a C-18 column (Lavda et al. 2004). A mixture of solvents was used as mobile phase containing acetonitrile–100 mM sodium dihydrogen phosphate buffer (20:80 v/v) adjusted to pH 3.9 with phosphoric acid. Detection was performed by monitoring fluorescence, using an excitation wavelength of 280 nm and a 418 nm long pass emission filter. Similar liquid chromatographic method was also reported for ciprofloxacin detection in biological samples including edible meat food (Nix et al. 1985; Ovando et al. 2004).

An improved HPLC method for analysis of ciprofloxacin and three of its metabolites in plasma, serum and urine samples was also developed (Krol et al. 1995). Instead of the previously used HPLC procedure for the isocratic separation of ciprofloxacin in urine samples using a UV detector, this procedure adopted detection and quantitation based on fluorometric analysis after postcolumn induction of fluorescence, whereas the chromatographic separation technique remain the same. This method was also applicable to the analysis of plasma and serum as well as urine samples. As the metabolites of ciprofloxacin have relatively weak native fluorescence, post-column induction of fluorescence was necessary to enhance the fluorescence signals of the metabolites. The lower quantitation limits of ciprofloxacin and metabolites were in the picogram level per milliliter. This procedure was sufficiently sensitive for the analysis of ciprofloxacin and its metabolites in plasma, serum and urine. The procedure was further used for the analysis of about 5000 samples collected during pharmacokinetic and clinical studies.

Further HPLC-spectrofluorimetry detection was established for ciprofloxacin detection in human serum (Watabea et al. 2010), where the chromatography was performed using a C-8 column with an isocratic mobile phase consisting of triethylamine and acetonitrile. Protein precipitation was conducted using perchloric acid and methanol. The method also showed the within-day and between-day coefficients of variation for three different fluoroquinolones (pazufloxacin, ciprofloxacin, and levofloxacin) were less than 7%, and relative errors ranged from 1.6% to 9.3%. The reliability and validation of this method was established through a good level of recovery experiments in spiked human serum.

A micellar liquid chromatography-fluorescence detection method was developed for the determination of various fluoroquinoles including ciprofloxacin in commercial porcine and bovine meat at an affordable price, which is reasonably interesting in the current context of economic crisis (Terrado-Campos et al. 2017). The quinolones were separated using a mobile phase containing SDS–1-propanol–triethylamine buffered at a pH of 3 using a C-18 column. The method was further validated in terms of selectivity, calibration range, linearity, recovery, precision, decision limit, detection capability, ruggedness and stability. This method can be considered as an interesting alternative for laboratories of public agencies and the agro-food industry to evaluate the compliance of the meat samples with the EU Regulation 37/2010 in terms of antibiotic occurrence, before launching to the market. The simplified sample preparation through extraction by simple shaking and ultrasonication with a minimal participation of the operator was the main feature of this procedure. Moreover, the sample pretreatment is simple, and does not require specific reagents or internal standards treatment before injection, thus reduces significantly the potential sources of variance, and the probability for loss of the analyte to obtain a high sample throughput.

Accurate and precise measurement of plasma drug concentrations is necessary for clinical pharmacokinetic studies of ciprofloxacin. For that purpose, a rapid, selective and sensitive HPLC-fluorimetric method is developed for determination of ciprofloxacin in human plasma (Muchohia et al. 2011). The sample preparation steps include protein precipitation with acetonitrile and quantification purpose needs the internal standard sarafloxacin. A mixture of aqueous orthophosphoric acid-methanol-acetonitrile was used as the mobile phase after adjusting the pH to 3.0 with triethylamine. The signal was monitored by a fluorescence detector (excitation/emission wavelength of 278/450 nm). The limit of detection and quantification were calculated to be 10 ng/mL and 20 ng/mL, respectively. This procedure was also applied for measurement of plasma ciprofloxacin concentrations in a population pharmacokinetics study of ciprofloxacin in malnourished children. Another similar HPLC-fluorimetric method is also developed for ciprofloxacin detection in bovine milk and plasma with the limit of quantitation in milk and plasma are 2 ng/mL and 1 ng/ml, respectively (Idowu and Peggins 2004). This highly sensitive method has been further applied to a study of the pharmacokinetics of enrofloxacin and ciprofloxacin in lactating dairy cows and beef steers.

In spite of several HPLC based analytical methods developed mainly based on intrinsic ultra-violet absorption and/or fluorescence property of ciprofloxacin, majority of those methods suffers from various drawbacks including time consuming sample preparation and treatment, inconvenient reagent pretreatment, and limitation to assay live samples. The widely used HPLC methods for the determination of ciprofloxacin or similar fluoroquinolone derivatives in biological material involve tedious extraction and clean-up steps prior to chromatography. As such, these methods are also not efficient for high throughput analysis for a pharmacokinetic study. The clinical significance of the potency and activities of ciprofloxacin *in vivo* depends on their pharmacology, efficacy, and toxicities; which again depends on their bioavailability or achievable serum levels upon administration in body. Hence, there is a strong need to develop new strategy and well-organized move towards the sensing and delivery of upcoming new antibiotics which can be very easily applied to biological fluids and samples.

Ciprofloxacin Detection Based on Lanthanide Luminescence

Ciprofloxacin shows intrinsic or native fluorescence emission with maximum wavelength around 440-450 nm. Based on the native fluorescence of ciprofloxacin, a large number of HPLC-spectrofluorimetry detection methods are developed as already discussed in the earlier sections. In those existing methods a sample separation process (to remove proteins, amino acids and other biomolecules) is necessary. Accordingly, those methods are difficult to apply for direct biological application due to the high autofluorescence from biological samples at the same shorter wavelength region of ciprofloxacin fluorescence (350-500 nm). To avoid the autofluorescence from biomolecules during bio-analyte detection, emission at longer wavelength (possibly red emission) is preferred. In recent years, use of lanthanides (especially Eu^{3+}, Tb^{3+}) as fluorescence probes offers an excellent possibility for sensitive and selective detection of analytes in biological samples by virtue of lanthanide sensitized luminescence. Several compounds are known to have efficient lanthanide-sensitizing characteristics and can be detected by time-resolved luminescence. The main advantages of this technique include emission at longer wavelength and long luminescence life times, large Stokes shifts, and narrow emission bands, resulting in the elimination of scattering interference and a significant decrease in the background autofluorescence from the biomolecules. Ciprofloxacin, containing the carboxylic and keto-oxygen atoms (Sun et al. 2006), could involve in chelation with lanthanides to act as an antenna via transfer of emission energy of ciprofloxacin to lanthanides (Figure 2), resulting large Stokes shifts and narrow emission bands, which would make them ideal for detection of ciprofloxacin in biological samples without any sample preparation or pretreatment procedures.

Among the lanthanides, europium ion (Eu^{3+}) is well known for its characteristic red luminescence at 615 nm and 591 nm, corresponding to the $^5D_0 \rightarrow {}^7F_2$ and $^5D_0 \rightarrow {}^7F_1$ transitions respectively. Due to the limitation of the direct excitation of Eu^{3+}, a well-established phenomenon of using sensitized excitation of Eu^{3+} could be possible by an excited organic ligand, and the energy transfer occurs from the triplet state of the sensitizer at room temperature (Kaczmarek and Lis 2011). According to the Förster's non-radiation energy transfer theory, the rate of energy transfer depends upon the extent of overlap of the emission spectra of the donor with the excitation spectra of the accepter as well as the distance (Pilehvar et al. 2015). At the same time as the energy transfer occurs from the triplet state of the sensitizer to the lanthanide ion, an organic ligand/dye with high population of the triplet state could serve as an efficient sensitizer. Ciprofloxacin has an intensely populated triplet state due to its relatively low energy gap between the S_1 and T_1 states (11.9 kcal mol^{-1}) and high phosphorescence/fluorescence intensity ratio (*P/F* = 2.92) (Richardson 1982). Accordingly, a co-ordination complex of lanthanide with ciprofloxacin, upon excitation of the ciprofloxacin moiety, would show a sensitized luminescence through Förster's non-radiation energy transfer, where ciprofloxacin acts as energy donor and lanthanide ion acts as energy acceptor (Figure 2). Based on such an antenna effect of ciprofloxacin to induce sensitized lanthanide luminescence, recently several fluorescence detection systems have been developed.

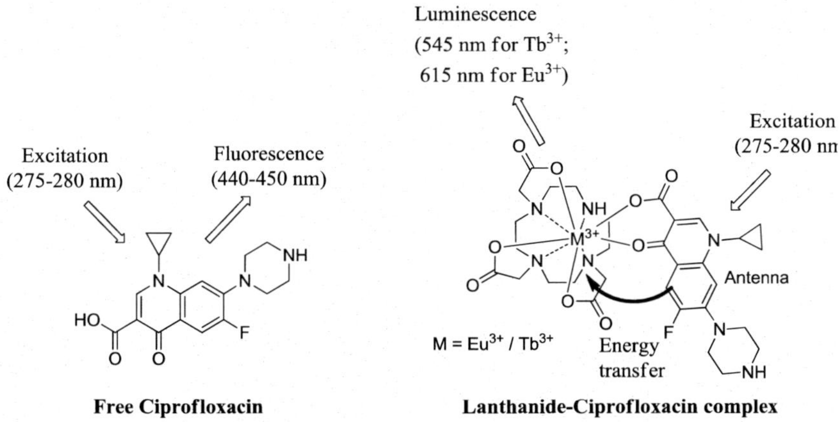

Figure 2. The Förster's non-radiation energy transfer from ciprofloxacin to lanthanide (Eu^{3+}/Tb^{3+}) in a complex to observe antenna sensitized luminescence, resulting emission at long wavelength from that of the free ciprofloxacin.

In a recent report, the screening was performed with Eu^{3+} complexes with various number of free co-ordination sites to find out the best binding sites for ciprofloxacin based upon luminescence intensity of Eu^{3+} at 615 nm after excitation of the ciprofloxacin at 278 nm (Singha and Ahn 2016). Interestingly, a Eu^{3+} complex with two vacant co-ordination sites, can bind to ciprofloxacin to fulfill maximum co-oridantion sites, and finally resulting the antenna effect induced lanthanide emission in the red wavelength region. Although the Eu^{3+} complex shows excellent binding with ciprofloxacin to fulfill the maximum lanthanide coordination sites to result antenna assisted Eu^{3+} emission, but still compared to the native fluorescence of ciprofloxacin the Eu^{3+} emission was too weak, which suggested that the Förster's non-radiation energy transfer from ciprofloxacin to europium is not efficient enough. The less efficient energy transfer could be rationalized from the lower extent of overlap of the emission spectra of the ciprofloxacin with the excitation spectra of the Eu^{3+}, which also suggested the relatively larger energy gap between the triplet state of ciprofloxacin and that of Eu^{3+}. In contrary, a relatively smaller energy gap between the triplet level of ciprofloxacin and the resonance level of terbium (58.2 kcal mol^{-1}) than with europium, could show an efficient energy transfer (Rieutord et al. 1997). Accordingly, terbium (Tb^{3+}) complex of a septadentate ligand, 1,4,7,10-tetraazacyclododecane-1,4,7-triacetic acid (DO3A) was used as receptor to observe ciprofloxacin sensitized lanthanide emission (Singha and Ahn 2016). Upon addition of ciprofloxacin in Tb-DO3A complex, the four intense bands of Tb^{3+} can be recorded with a maximum located at 545 nm ($^5D_4 \rightarrow ^7F_5$ transition). Importantly, the native fluorescence of the ciprofloxacin molecule was drastically decreased in the presence of Tb-DO3A upon excitation of ciprofloxacin, suggesting an efficient Förster's non-radiation energy transfer. The detection method was highly sensitive with limit of detection lowering up to 3 ppb level of ciprofloxacin in buffer solution along with very good selectivity towards ciprofloxacin among the other relevant analytes present in urine. The detection system was also applied for direct detection of ciprofloxacin in urine without any sample pretreatment or separation steps. This simple but efficient detection method is highly promising as it could be useful to measure the amount of excreted ciprofloxacin which was not absorbed in body after taking the drug. So that it would be possible to measure the bioavailability i.e., absorbed amount of ciprofloxacin in body (by excluding the amount of excreted ciprofloxacin from the amount of orally taken drug), which will help to control the dose of the drug, thus drug overdose can be avoided.

The lanthanide luminescence based detection is also used for the in vivo liquid chromatographic determination of ciprofloxacin (Rieutord et al. 1994). Again the initial screening among the three interested lanthanides–samarium, terbium or europium was performed in terms of energy transfer from ciprofloxacin; resulting the most efficient sensitization in case of Tb^{3+}. Interestingly, among the several fluoroquinolones tested, ciprofloxacin was the best sensitizer. Accordingly, the formation of a terbium chelate with ciprofloxacin was demonstrated in a classical reversed-phase eluent (methanol-water (1:1) containing trichloroacetic acid (pH 2.5)) using a postcolumn device upon selective excitation at 320 nm and monitoring the terbium emission at 545 nm. This detection method also showed high sensitivity with the detection of 0.25 pmol of injected ciprofloxacin, thus promising for the determination of this antibiotic drug in biological samples.

The fluorescence characteristics of the terbium-ciprofloxacin complex were also studied thoroughly in terms of the environmental and experimental factors (Wang et al. 2001). It was found that at pH 6.0, the intrinsic fluorescence of Tb^{3+} could be observed at 545 nm upon excitation at 328 nm. Based on this, the determination of trace ciprofloxacin in urine by using simply terbium ion as fluorescent probe has been established with the detection limit of 5.0×10^{-9} mol L^{-1}. Similarly, the effecting parameters were also examined in a terbium-sensitized luminescence method for the determination of the enrofloxacin and its major metabolite ciprofloxacin in edible animal tissues (Hernández-Arteseros et al. 1998). Through an extensive sample pretreatment procedure of extraction in organic solvent followed by dissolving in aqueous nitric acid and defatted with hexane from spiked samples of chicken and trout tissues, the determination of ciprofloxacin was performed in an aqueous micellar medium.

In another approach, ciprofloxacin sensitized terbium(III) luminescence was further used in presence with surfactant such as sodium dodecylbenzene sulfonate (SDBS) to observe a strongly enhanced emission intensity; resulting in a more sensitive detection method of ciprofloxacin with the detection limit of 4.0×10^{-9} mol L^{-1} (Tong et al. 2005). This method was also applied to determine ciprofloxacin in the real pharmaceutical samples. In a similar approach, the effect of surfactants as well as the second ligand on the fluorescence properties of europium(III) complex of ciprofloxacin was also studied; showing the increase of fluorescence intensity by a factor of four in the presence of second ligand such as 1,10-phenanthroline and by a factor of five in presence of sodium dodecylbenzenesulfonate micelles (Shtykov et al. 2007). Due to the enhanced sensitivity, this procedure was also officially tested for determination of antibiotics on the pharmaceutical Ciprolet and blood serum.

Recently, the metal-organic coordination polymers have evolved as a rapidly emerging field due to the very important functional materials with tunable structures and properties. Accordingly, a terbium (Tb^{3+})-based coordination polymer nanoparticles (CPNPs) by employing biomolecule adenine (Ad) as bridging ligand has been developed as a receptor reagent for ciprofloxacin detection in aqueous solution (Hongliang et al. 2013). In presence of ciprofloxacin, a typical emission of Tb^{3+} was observed due to the formation of Ad/terbium-ciprofloxacin complex and the sensitization by ciprofloxacin. A good linearity of terbium emission intensity was observed in the concentration region of 60 nM to 14 μM of ciprofloxacin with the detection limit of 60 nM. The polymer nanoparticle system was enable to detect ciprofloxacin in tablet and urine samples with a satisfactory result. This direct method is advantageous because of the very simple strategy without requiring complicated sample pretreatment processes or special reaction media.

Among the various reported analytical methods, the lanthanide sensitized detection of ciprofloxacin is the most advantageous mainly due to its direct application (without sample pretreatment) and high sensitivity.

Reaction Based Fluorescence Detection of Ciprofloxacin

Compared to the above described lanthanide co-ordination based detection systems, the reaction based systems could provide better selectivity trhough analyte specific reactions. Accordingly, reaction based detection system is advantageous interms of *in vivo* application in complex biomatrix. There are also few reaction based systems reported for ciprofloxacin detection. One of those uses a photonic crystal as sensing material to realize pretreatment-free and label-free detection of ciprofloxacin through Michael addition reaction between the piperazine group of ciprofloxacin and the *ortho*-benzoquinone group present in the photonic crystal (Song et al. 2018). Ciprofloxacin was detected by observing the decreasing emission intensity of the photonic crystal with a limit of detection upto 0.76 μg/L. The method was also applicable to detect ciprofloxacin in fish farming water directly without any sample pretreatment and labeling. The advantageous features of this Michael-addition-mediated detection system are its accuracy, easy preparation, cost-effectiveness, and long-term stability. Such environment friendly and label-free assay method is promising for clinical diagnosis, medicine analysis, food safety, and environmental monitoring.

A reaction based ciprofloxacin detection was also established depending on the chemiluminescence property generated upon reaction with ciprofloxacin. The recent trends in analytical measurement shows chemiluminescence combined with flow injection have various advantages such as sensitivity, speed, easy handling with simple instrumentation. Accordingly, a flow injection chemiluminescence method for determination of ciprofloxacin was reported based on the terbium sensitization in combination with a chemiluminescent method for the determination of fluoroquinolones (Kaczmarek and Lis 2011). The energy transfer to the uncomplexed terbium(III) ions was possible from the excited products of the oxidized ciprofloxacin by the Fenton system, in acidic medium. Under optimum conditions, the detection limits was calculated to be 1×10^{-8} mol L^{-1} for ciprofloxacin. It is a simple, accurate and precise method with a large tolerance to the presence of various interfering substances.

An inorganic nanoparticle based detection system for ciprofloxacin assay is also developed by monitoring the enhanced fluorescence intensity upon interaction of functionalized nano-CdS with ciprofloxacin at pH 7.4. This method provided a new direct quantitative determination for ciprofloxacin in human serum samples without separation of foreign substances. The possible enhancing mechanism is due to the formation of exciplex during reaction between nano-CdS and ciprofloxacin (Dan et al. 2008).

Interaction Based Fluorescence Detection Methods of Ciprofloxacin

There are two reported fluorescence assays of ciprofloxacin, one is based on enzymatic interaction and another is based on solid phase fluorescence interaction.

In an enzymatic host-guest complexation based detection method, fluorescent siderophore pyoverdin, produced from a Pseudomonas monteilii strain, was used for the fluorescent chemosensing of ciprofloxacin in aqueous solution (Pawar et al. 2016). In presence of ciprofloxacin, pyoverdin showed new UV–visible absorption bands at 252 and 321 nm along with a highly selective fluorescence enhancement with a 13 nm blue shift from 458 to 445 nm. The high association constant (K_a) of pyoverdin with ciprofloxacin (1.40×10^5 M^{-1}) enables detection upto micromolar level of ciprofloxacin; thus shows negligible matrix effect and quantitative recovery in the pharmaceutical tablet.

Solid-phase spectrofluorimetry method has also been developed for the determination of trace amounts of ciprofloxacin (Navalón et al. 2000). The intrinsic fluorescence intensity of ciprofloxacin was directly measured after solid-phase attachment on Sephadex SP C-25 gel packed in a 1-mm silica cell. The corresponding emission was followed at 448 nm, upon excitation at 272 nm, which provided a detection limit of 0.1 ng mL^{-1} for ciprofloxacin. The method was highly reliable for ciprofloxacin detection in biological samples such as human urine and serum samples as validated with high recovery levels.

CONCLUSION

Overdose and abuse of antibiotics results excretion of large amount of antibiotics residues in the environment including water as well as edible sources. Such antibiotic contaminations may ultimately cause mutation in the bacteria to generate antibiotic resistant "super bacteria". Ciprofloxacin, as a third-generation synthetic fluoroquinolone antibiotic, is frequently used in medical clinical practice because of its broad-spectrum of antibacterial activity. Besides, overdose of ciprofloxacin not only results in bacterial resistance but also causes DNA damage, severe liver damage, and hematuria in human body. Therefore, it is deemed necessary to develop powerful analytical method to monitor ciprofloxacin through a rapid and simple process. Moreover, determination of ciprofloxacin is also very important for the pharmaceutical quality control.

Accordingly, various methods have been developed to determine the level of ciprofloxacin. Some of those include the conventional analytical methods like high performance liquid chromatography (HPLC) based on the ultraviolet absorption property of ciprofloxacin. To achieve the high sensitivity, fluorescence based detection methods are more advantageous. As ciprofloxacin has intrinsic or native fluorescence, accordingly HPLC methods combined with spectrofluorimetric measurement were also developed. Unfortunately, such widely used HPLC method requires an extensive sample preparation step (to remove proteins and amino acids and other biomolecules). Although few other methods such as flow-injection with chemiluminescence detection, and reaction based sensing systems have been developed, still most of the methods suffer from several limitations such as time consuming procedure or the requirement of expensive and sophisticated instruments as well as limited sensitivity or selectivity for real sample analysis. Moreover, due to the high auto fluorescence from biological samples at the same shorter wavelength region of ciprofloxacin fluorescence, the fluorescence assay is preferred with monitoring the emission in longer wavelength region. In that respect, recently developed lanthanide (Tb^{3+}/ Eu^{3+}) sensitized luminescence based detection systems offer the excellent possibility for sensitive and selective detection of analytes in real biological samples by eliminating the scattering interference and background fluorescence. Based on the initial assessment of better sensitization in case of terbium, several sensitized lanthanides luminescence based systems have been developed. In fact such systems are also used for direct (without any sample pretreatment or separation steps) detection of ciprofloxacin in real samples like urine or plasma with excellent sensitivity as well as high accuracy. These simple but efficient detection methods are highly promising for the possible measurement of the excreted ciprofloxacin in case of overdose, which will help to avoid the drug abuse. In near future, such effective detection methods may find further applications for bioimaging, which may help to understand and monitor *in vivo* drug efficacy as well as pharmacokinetics.

ACKNOWLEDGMENTS

The author gratefully acknowledges the financial support from Basic Science Research Program (2018R1D1A1B07051403) through the National Research Foundation (NRF) of Korea funded by the Ministry of Education.

REFERENCES

Brumfitt, W.; Franklin, I.; Grady, D.; Hamilton-Miller, J. M. T.; Iliffe, A. (1984). Changes in the pharmacokinetics of ciprofloxacin and fecal flora during administration of a 7-day course to human volunteers. *Antimicrob. Agents Chemother.* 26, 757–761.

Brunner, M.; Langer, O.; Dobrozemsky, G.; Muller, U.; Zeitlinger, M.; Mitterhauser, M. et al. (2004) (18F) Ciprofloxacin, a new positron emission tomography tracer for noninvasive assessment of the tissue distribution and pharmacokinetics of ciprofloxacin in humans. *Antimicrob. Agents Chemother.* 48, 3850–3857.

Carlucci, G. (1998) Analysis of fluoroquinolones in biological fluids by high-performance liquid chromatography. *J. Chromatogr. A* 812, 343–367.

Cozzarelli, N. R. (1980). DNA gyrase and the supercoiling of DNA. *Science* 207, 953–960.

Drlica, K. (1984). Biology of bacterial deoxyribonucleic acid topoisomerases. *Microbiol. Rev.* 48, 273–289.

Duan, J.; Yuan, Z. (2001) Development of an indirect competitive ELISA for ciprofloxacin residues in food animal edible tissues. *J. Agric. Food Chem.* 49, 1087–1089.

Garlando, F.; Täuber, M. G.; Joos, B.; Oelz, O.; Lüthy, R. (1985) Ciprofloxacin-induced hematuria. *Infection* 13, 177−178.

Gellert, M. (1981). DNA topoisomerases. *Annu. Rev. Biochem.* 50, 879–910.

Gürbay, A.; Gonthier, B.; Signorini-Allibe, N.; Barret, L.; Favier, A.; Hincal, F. (2006) Ciprofloxacin-induced DNA damage in primary culture of rat astrocytes and protection by Vitamin E. *Neurotoxicology* 27, 6−10.

Heinz-Georg, W.; Stadler, M.; Hans-Volker, T.; Dalhoff, A.; Karl, W. (1999) Degradation of ciprofloxacin by basidiomycetes and identification of metabolites generated by the brown rot fungus Gloeophyllum striatum. *Appl. Environ. Microbiol.* 65, 1556–1563.

Hernández-Arteseros, J. A.; Compañó, R.; Prat, M. D. (1998) Determination of ciprofloxacin and enrofloxacin in edible animal tissues by terbium-sensitized luminescence. *Analyst* 123, 2729–2732.

Hirai, K.; Aoyama, H.; Irikura, T.; Iyobe, S.; Mitsuhashi, S. (1986) Differences in susceptibility to quinolones of outer mermbrane mutants of Salmonella typhimurium and Escherichia coli. *Antimicrob. Agents Chemother.* 29, 535–538.

Idowu, O. R.; Peggins, J. O. (2004) Simple, rapid determination of enrofloxacin and ciprofloxacin in bovine milk and plasma by high-performance liquid chromatography with fluorescence detection. *J. Pharmaceut. Biomed.* 35, 143–153.

Joos, B.; Ledergerber, B.; Flepp, M.; Bettex, J. D.; Luthy, R.; Siegenthaler, W. (1985) Comparision of high-pressure liquid chromatography and bioassay for determination of ciprofloxacin in serum and urine. *Antimicrob. Agents Chemother.* 27, 353–356.

Kaczmarek, M.; Lis, S. (2011) Chemiluminescence determination of fluoroquinolones using Fenton system in the presence of terbium(III) ions. *Analyst* 136, 2592–2597.

Kassab, N. M.; Singh, A. K.; Kedor-Hackmam, E. R. M.; Santoro, M. I. R. M. (2005) Quantitative determination of ciprofloxacin and norfloxacin in pharmaceutical preparations by high performance liquid chromatography. *Braz. J. Pharm. Sci.* 41, 507–513.

Kirchhoff, J.; Glaser, U.; Bohnert, J. A.; Pletz, M. W.; Popp, J.; Neugebauer, U. (2018) Simple ciprofloxacin resistance test and determination of minimal inhibitory concentration within 2 h using raman spectroscopy. *Anal. Chem.* 90, 1811−1818.

Krol, G. J.; Beck, G. W.; Benham, T. (1995) HPLC analysis of ciprofloxacin and ciprofloxacin metabolites in body fluids, *J. Pharmaceut. Biomed.* 14, 181–190.

Krzek, J.; Hubicka, U.; Szczepaniczyk, J. (2005) High-performance thin-layer chromatography with densitometry for the determination of ciprofloxacin and impurities in drugs. *J. AOAC Int.* 88, 1530–1536.

Kümmerer, K.; Henninger, A. (2003) Promoting resistance by the emission of antibiotics from hospitals and households into effluent. *Clin. Microbiol. Infect.* 9, 1203–1214.

Laignier Cazedey, E. C.; Nunes Salgado, H. R. (2012) Spectrophotometric determination of ciprofloxacin hydrochloride in ophthalmic solution. *Adv. Anal. Chem.* 2, 74–79.

Lavda, M.; Clausnitzer, C. E.; Walters, J. D. (2004) Distribution of systemic ciprofloxacin and doxycycline to gingival and gingival crevicular fluid. *J. Periodontol.* 75, 1663–1667.

Li, D.; Yan, Z.-Y.; Cheng, W.-Q. (2008) Determination of ciprofloxacin with functionalized cadmium sulfide nanoparticles as a fluorescence probe. *Spectrochim. Acta A* 71, 1204–1211.

Liu, C. G.; Xu, Y. Z.; Wei, Y. J.; Zhao, J.; Qi, J.; Wang, X. H.; Xu, Z. H.; Wu, J. G. (2005) Spectral properties, protonation and fluorescence quantum yield of ciprofloxacin, *Guang. Pu. Xue. Yu. Guang. Pu. Fen. Xi. (Spectroscopy and Spectral Analysis)* 25, 1446–1450.

Liu, L.; Luo, L.; Suryoprabowo, S.; Peng, J.; Kuang, H.; Xu, C. (2014) Development of an immunochromatographic strip test for rapid detection of ciprofloxacin in milk samples. *Sensors* 14, 16785–16798.

Martin, B. S.; Cornejo, J.; Iraguen, D.; Hidalgo, H.; Anadon, A. (2007) Depletion study of enrofloxacin and its metabolite ciprofloxacin in edible tissues and feathers of white leghorn hens by liquid chromatography coupled with tandem mass spectrometry. *J Food Protect* 70, 1952–1957.

McIntosh, D.; Zhou, Q.; Lara, F. J.; Landers, J.; Campbell, J. C. (2011) Fluorescence detection 400–480nm using microfluidic system integrated GaP photodiodes. *Advances in OptoElectronics* 2011, 491609.

Melo, M. J. P.; Varanda, F. R.; Dohrn, R.; Marrucho, I. M. (2005) Solubility of ciprofloxacin and moxifloxacin in different solvents: the effect of the HCl group. *Enpromer*. 1–5.

Michalska, K. Pajchel, G.; Tyski, S. (2004) Determination of ciprofloxacin and its impurities by capillary zone electrophoresis. *J. Chromatogr. A* 1051, 267–272.

Muchohia, S. N.; Thuoa, N.; Karisa, J.; Muturi, A.; Kokwaro, G. O.; Maitland, K. (2011) Determination of ciprofloxacin in human plasma using high-performance liquid chromatography coupled with fluorescence detection: application to a population pharmacokinetics study in children with severe malnutrition. *J. Chromatogr. B* 879, 146–152.

Navalón, A.; Ballesteros, O.; Blanc, R.; Vílchez, J. L. (2000) Determination of ciprofloxacin in human urine and serum samples by solid-phase spectrofluorimetry. *Talanta* 52, 845–852.

Nix, D. E.; De Vito, J. M.; Schentag, J. J. (1985) Liquid-chromatographic determination of ciprofloxacin in serum and urine. *Clin. Chem.* 31, 684–686.

Ovando, H. G.; Gorla1, N.; Weyers, A.; Ugnia, L.; Magnoli, A. (2004) Simultaneous quantification of ciprofloxacin, enrofloxacin and balofloxacin in broiler chicken muscle. *Arch. Med. Vet.* 1, 93–8.

Panadero, S.; Gómez-Hens, A.; Pérez-Bendito, D. (1995) Stopped flow kinetic determination of nalidixic acid and norfloxacin based on lanthanide-sensitized fluorescence. *Anal. Chim. Acta* 303, 39–45.

Pawar, M. K.; Tayade, K. C.; Sahoo, S. K.; Mahulikar, P. P.; Kuwar, A. S.; Chaudhari, B. L. (2016) Selective ciprofloxacin antibiotic detection by fluorescent siderophore pyoverdin. *Biosens. Bioelectron.* 81, 274–279.

Pham, H. H.; Luo, P.; Genin, F.; Dash, A. K. (2002) Synthesis and characterization of hydroxyapatite-ciprofloxacin delivery systems by precipitation and spray drying technique. *AAPS Pharm Sci Tech* 3, 1–9.

Pilehvar, S.; Gielkens, K.; Trashin, S. A.; Dardenne, F.; Blust, R.; Wael, K. (2015) (Electro)sensing of phenicol antibiotics—a review. *Crit. Rev. Food Sci. Nutr.* 56, 2416–2429.

Ramatla, T.; Ngoma, L.; Adetunji, M.; Mwanza, M. Evaluation of antibiotic residues in raw Meat using different analytical methods. *Antibiotics* 6, 34.

Richardson, F. S. (1982) Terbium(III) and europium(III) ions as luminescent probes and stains for biomolecular systems. *Chem. Rev.* 82, 541−552.

Rieutord, A.; Prognon, P.; Brion, F.; Mahuzier, G. (1997) Liquid chromatographic determination using lanthanides as time-resolved luminescence probes for drugs and xenobiotics: advantages and limitations. *Analyst* 122, 59R–66R.

Rieutord, A.; Vazquez, L.; Soursac, M.; Prognon, P.; Blais, J.; Bourget, P.; Mahuzier, G. (1994) Fluoroquinolones as sensitizers of lanthanide fluorescence: application to the liquid chromatographic determination of ciprofloxacin using terbium. *Anal. Chim. Acta* 290, 215–225.

Samanidou, V. F.; Demetriou, C. E.; Papadoyannis, I. N. (2003) Direct determination of four fluoroquinolones, enoxacin, norfloxacin, ofloxacin, and ciprofloxacin, in pharmaceuticals and blood serum by HPLC. *Anal. Bioanal. Chem.* 375, 623–629.

Scherer, R.; Pereira, J.; Firme, J.; Emos, M.; Lemos, M. (2014) Determination of ciprofloxacin in pharmaceutical formulations using HPLC method with UV detection. *Indian J. Pharm. Sci.* 76, 541–544.

Sharma, P. C.; Jain, A.; Jain, S.; Pahwa, R.; Yar, M. S. (2010) Ciprofloxacin: review on developments in synthetic, analytical, and medicinal aspects. *J. Enzym. Inhib. Med. Ch.* 25, 577–589.

Shtykov, S.; Smirnova, T.; Bylinkin, Y.; Kalashnikova, N.; Zhemerichkin, D. (2007) determination of ciprofloxacin and enrofloxacin by the sensitized fluorescence of europium in the presence of the second ligand and micelles of anionic surfactants. *J. Anal. Chem.* 62, 136−140.

Singha, S.; Ahn, K. H. (2016) Detection of ciprofloxacin in urine through sensitized lanthanide luminescence. *Sensors* 16, 2065.

Song, Y.; Bai, J.; Zhang, R.; He, H.; Li, C.; Wang, J.; Li, S.; Peng, Y.; Ning, B.; Wang, M.; Gao, Z. (2018) Michael-addition-mediated photonic crystals allow pretreatment-free and label-free sensoring of ciprofloxacin in fish farming water. *Anal. Chem.* 90, 1388−1394.

Sun, H. W.; Li, L. Q.; Chen, X. Y. (2006). Flow-injection enhanced chemiluminescence method for determination of ciprofloxacin in pharmaceutical preparations and biological fluids. *Anal. Bioanal. Chem.* 384, 1314−1319.

Szerkus, O.; Jacyna, J.; Gibas, A.; Sieczkowski, M.; Siluk, D.; Matuszewski, M.; Kaliszan, R.; Markuszewski, M. J. (2017) Robust HPLC–MS/MS method for levofloxacin and ciprofloxacin determination in human prostate tissue. *J. Pharmaceut. Biomed.* 132, 173–183.

Tan, H.; Zhang, L.; Ma, C.; Song, Y.; Xu, F.; Chen, S.; Wang, L. (2013) Terbium-based coordination polymer nanoparticles for detection of ciprofloxacin in tablets and biological fluids. *ACS Appl. Mater. Interfaces* 5, 11791−11796.

Terrado-Campos, D.; Tayeb-Cherif, K.; Peris-Vicente, J.; Carda-Broch, S.; Esteve-Romero, J. (2017) Determination of oxolinic acid, danofloxacin, ciprofloxacin, and enrofloxacin in porcine and bovine meat by micellar liquid chromatography with fluorescence detection. *Food Chem.* 221, 1277–1284.

Tong, C. L.; Xiang, G. H.; Liu, W. P. (2005) Study on the determination of ciprofloxacin by the terbium (III) ion fluorescence probe sensitized by the surfactant. *Guang. Pu. Xue. Yu. Guang. Pu. Fen. Xi. (Spectroscopy and Spectral Analysis)* 25, 2061–2064.

Tyczkowska, K.; Hedeen, K. M.; Aucoin, D. P.; Aronson, A. L. (1989) High-performance liquid chromatographic method for the simultaneous determination of enrofloxacin and its primary metabolite ciprofloxacin in canine serum and prostatic tissue. *J. Chromatogr.* 493, 337–346.

Varanda, F.; De Melo, M. J. P.; Caco, A. I.; Dohrn, R.; Makrydaki, F. A.; Voutsas, E. et al. (2006) Solubility of antibiotics in different solvents. 1. Hydrochloride forms of tetracycline, moxifloxacin, and ciprofloxacin. *Ind. Eng. Chem. Res.* 45, 6368–6374.

Vella, J.; Busuttila, F.; Bartolo, N. S.; Sammut, C.; Ferrito, V.; Serracino-Inglott, A.; Azzopardi, L. M.; LaFerla, G. (2015) A simple HPLC–UV method for the determination of ciprofloxacin in human plasma. *J. Chromatogr. B* 989, 80–85.

Wang, L.; Sang, L. H.; Wu, Y. L.; Cheng, X. M.; Su, Z. D.; Yu, A. H. (2001) Determination of ciprofloxacin in urine using terbium ion as fluorescent probe. *Guang. Pu. Xue. Yu. Guang. Pu. Fen. Xi. (Spectroscopy and Spectral Analysis)* 21, 691–693.

Watabea, S.; Yokoyama, Y.; Nakazawa, K.; Shinozaki, K.; Hiraoka, R.; Takeshita, K.; Suzuki, Y. (2010) Simultaneous measurement of pazufloxacin, ciprofloxacin, and levofloxacin in human serum by high-performance liquid chromatography with fluorescence detection. *J. Chromatogr. B* 878, 1555–1561.

Xiao, J. B.; Yang, C. S.; Ren, F. L.; Jiang, X. Y.; Xu, M. (2007) Rapid determination of ciprofloxacin lactate in drugs by the Rayleigh light scattering technique. *Meas. Sci. Technol.* 18, 859–866.

Yan, H.; Tian, M.; Row, K. H. (2008) Determination of enrofloxacin and ciprofloxacin in milk using molecularly imprinted solid-phase extraction. *J. Sep. Sci.* 31, 3015–3020.

Yang, R.; Fu, Y.; Li, L. D.; Liu, J. M. (2003) Medium effects on fluorescence of ciprofloxacin hydrochloride. *Spectrochim. Acta A* 59, 2323–2332.

Zimpfer, A.; Propst, A.; Mikuz, G.; Vogel, W.; Terracciano, L.; Stadlmann, S. (2004) Ciprofloxacin-induced acute liver injury: case report and review of literature. *Virchows Arch.* 444, 87−89.

ABOUT THE EDITOR

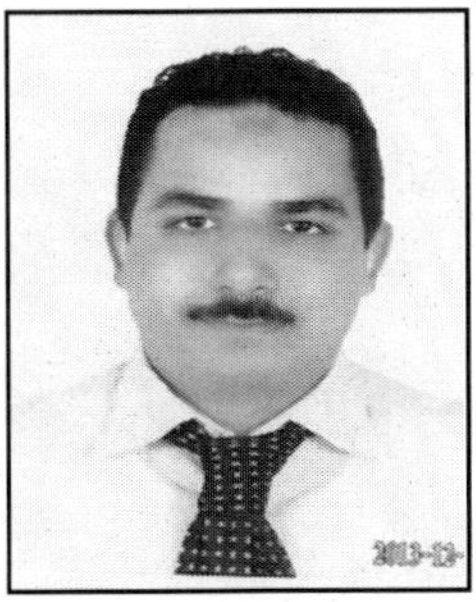

Mohamed Said Attia (M. S. Attia), PhD
Chemistry Department, Faculty of Science, Ain Shams University,
Cairo, Egypt.

Prof. Dr. M. S. Attia received his BS, MS. and PhD degrees from Ain Shams University and he received the professor position in analytical chemistry in 2017. M. S. Attia supervised 70 research students that led to M.S. and Ph.D. degrees being awarded in analytical chemistry (optical sensor for early diagnosis of some diseases), applied spectroscopy, material science and nanosciences, applied photochemistry, and environmental photochemistry including photocatalysis. About 65 research articles have been published in international journals in the last ten years. He also acts as editorial board member of *SpringerPlus* and *Analytical chemistry letters.*

INDEX

#

3-aminopropyltriethoxysilane, 60, 62
3-HQN (3-Hydroxyquinine), 158, 174
4HBA (4-hydroxybenzoic acid), 3, 15, 16

A

A. (Acinetobacter baumannii), 25, 26, 27, 28, 29, 32, 34, 61, 66, 67, 68, 69, 72, 73, 74, 75, 106, 112, 117, 127, 141, 142, 143, 145, 146, 147, 148, 149, 150, 151, 153, 154, 187, 194, 196, 198, 199, 201, 219, 236, 237, 238, 239, 240, 241, 242, 243, 244, 245, 246, 247, 248, 249, 250, 251, 252, 253, 254, 256, 257, 258, 259, 260, 261, 262, 263, 286, 287, 288, 289, 290, 291, 292, 293
AAS (Atomic absorption spectrometry), 204, 226
ABC (ATP-Binding Cassette), 112, 131
absorbance ratio, 164, 166, 167
absorption, 6, 9, 11, 23, 27, 40, 50, 55, 56, 61, 83, 165, 188, 204, 224, 226, 256, 269, 271, 274, 277, 284, 285
ac (Alternating current), 11, 22, 26, 131, 177, 189, 204, 230, 265
accuracy, 86, 87, 89, 90, 95, 98, 104, 109, 162, 163, 164, 274, 283, 286
acetic acid, 168, 269
ACN (Acetonitrile), 82, 83, 84, 85, 88, 109, 156, 169, 170, 171, 172, 173, 174, 175, 271, 272, 275, 276
Ad (adenine), 267, 282
adipose-derived stem cells, 45, 49, 51
adverse effects, 119, 156, 265, 268, 269
age, 79, 92, 94, 99, 121
ALA (alanine), 2, 12, 13, 204
AMIS (Amperometric magneto-immunosensor), 204, 231
amputation, 77, 80, 91, 92, 93, 100
analytical, vi, vii, viii, 65, 73, 82, 83, 107, 153, 156, 159, 160, 162, 163, 168, 182, 183, 184, 185, 189, 193, 194, 195, 196, 203, 204, 223, 224, 253, 254, 255, 256, 257, 259, 260, 262, 263, 266, 269, 271, 272, 274, 275, 277, 282, 283, 285, 290, 291, 295
analytical methods, 156, 159, 204, 223, 269, 271, 272, 274, 275, 277, 282, 285, 290

analytical techniques, 159, 162, 168, 269, 272
antenna, 278, 279, 280
antibacterial agent, 61, 81, 158
antibiotic(s), vii, 4, 25, 26, 27, 29, 32, 38, 41, 42, 52, 59, 60, 61, 62, 63, 64, 66, 68, 69, 77, 80, 81, 92, 106, 107, 109, 112, 113, 115, 119, 126, 128, 130, 131, 133, 135, 138, 139, 141, 142, 148, 151, 155, 158, 178, 180, 182, 189, 194, 198, 201, 203, 212, 214, 215, 216, 223, 224, 225, 226, 227, 228, 229, 230, 231, 232, 233, 234, 237, 238, 241, 246, 247, 252, 253, 257, 258, 260, 261, 263, 265, 268, 272, 274, 276, 277, 281, 282, 285, 288, 290, 292
anxiety and depression, 100
APIs (active pharmaceutical ingredients), 2, 7, 10, 14, 15, 20, 28
ARG (arginine), 2, 12, 13, 21, 204
ASD (amorphous solid dispersions), 2, 12, 13
ASP (aspartic acid), 2, 12, 13, 21
association constant, 267, 284
Asymptomatic PAD, 79
atherosclerotic, 77, 78
ATP (Adenosine triphosphate), 112, 125, 131, 204, 220
ATPS (aqueous two-phase systems), 156, 172, 175
autofluorescence, 278

B

bacteria, 4, 34, 38, 41, 61, 62, 63, 64, 72, 103, 104, 112, 113, 114, 118, 122, 123, 128, 129, 130, 131, 132, 133, 134, 135, 137, 139, 141, 142, 144, 146, 147, 150, 151, 177, 203, 209, 211, 212, 216, 219, 220, 223, 236, 247, 265, 268, 285
bacterial bone infections, 41
bacterial infection, 111, 112, 113, 155, 222, 265
bactericidal activity, 63, 118, 155, 180
bactericidal efficacy, vii, 38
BALB/c mice (albino, laboratory-bred strain of the house mouse), 267, 274
basidiomycetous, 273
BC (Before Christ), 204, 205
BCP (Bromocresol Purple), 156, 165, 167
BCS (Biopharmaceutic Classification Systems), 2, 7, 27
BH (Bromhexine), 157, 165, 166, 188
bile, 168, 224
bioactivity, 44, 47, 48, 49, 53, 64
biocompatibility, v, 37, 38, 40, 43, 44, 48, 49, 73
bioimaging, 286
biological media, 159, 160
biomaterial, 43, 46, 51
biomedical analysis, 160
bivariate analysis, 94
blood, 62, 72, 78, 80, 81, 85, 91, 93, 153, 161, 168, 169, 172, 173, 175, 195, 208, 212, 242, 251, 272, 282, 291
blood serum, 169, 173, 272, 282, 291
Bromocresol Purple, 156, 165
BSA (Bovine serum albumin), 204, 227
BTB (Bromothymol Blue), 157, 165, 167
bulk drug, 156, 163

C

°C (degree Celsius), 266
C (carbon), 6, 8, 9, 17, 18, 22, 23, 25, 26, 28, 31, 32, 41, 64, 67, 68, 70, 71, 73, 74, 75, 79, 82, 84, 86, 87, 91, 93, 95, 96, 98, 99, 104, 105, 106, 108, 109, 110, 123, 143, 144, 145, 146, 148, 149, 150, 151, 152, 153, 154, 160, 180, 185, 188, 192, 195, 198, 199,205, 208, 209, 217, 218, 227, 229, 230, 235, 236, 237, 239, 241,

242, 243, 244, 245, 246, 247, 248, 250, 251, 254, 257, 259, 260, 261, 262, 263, 266, 269, 271, 275, 276, 284, 288, 289, 290, 291, 292
C18 column, 82, 84
C8 column, 169
CA (citric acid), 2, 15, 18
capacitively-coupled contactless conductivity detector, 162
capillary electrophoresis, 159, 162, 204, 224, 231, 234, 267, 273
capsules, 170
carbon electrodes, 160
cardiovascular, 78, 79
cataracts, 100
CdS (cadmium sulfide), 225, 267, 284, 289
CE (capillary electrophoresis), 159, 162, 224, 231, 234, 267, 273
CE (Capillary electrophoresis), 82, 162, 204, 224, 225, 267, 273
cell culture medium (cell lysate), 169, 172
centrifugation, 85, 86, 173, 175
cerebrovascular, 78
cerium (IV) sulphate, 159
chelation, 223, 278
chemicals and consumables, 82
chemiluminescence, 160, 184, 185, 227, 234, 256, 283, 285, 288, 291
chemiluminescence methods, 160
chemometric methods, 161
chemosensors, 274
chitosan dental films, 164
chloroform, 6, 27, 161, 175
chromatographic columns, 163, 169
chromatographic conditions, 84, 88, 170, 171, 172, 173, 174
cigarette smoking, 79, 92
ciprofloxacin activity, 112
ciprolet, 282
CIP-SA (ciprofloxacin with salicylic acid), 3, 22, 23
CL (Chloranilic acid), 157, 165, 167, 189
clindamycin, 81, 150, 214
clinical practice, 158, 176, 285
clinical study, 91, 94
CLS (Classical least squares), 157, 166
CO2 (carbon dioxide), 70, 229, 266
Cocrystals and salts, 14
 2-thiobarbituric acid, 14
 4-hydroxybenzoic acid, 14
 barbituric acid, 14
comorbidity, 100
competitive inhibition, 103
concentration standards, 86, 90
conductivity detector, 159, 162
congestive heart failure, 100, 103
CoNS (Coagulase-Negative Staphylococci), 112, 115, 144, 146, 151
CPNPs (coordination polymer nanoparticles), 267, 282, 291
CTAB (Cetyltrimethylammonium bromide), 204, 229, 259
CWT (Continuous wavelet transform), 157, 166
CYS (cysteine), 3, 12, 13
cytocompatibility, v, 37, 45, 48, 49, 65
CZE–ESI-MS–MS (capillary zone electrophoresis-electrospray ionisation tandem mass spectrometric), 204, 228

D

DAD (Diode Array Detector), 157, 174
D-Ala-D-Ala (D-alanine D-alanine), 204, 214
DANO (Danofloxacin), 157, 172, 195
DCF (Diclofenac), 157, 164, 166, 187
DCM (Dichloromethane), 157, 172
DCM (Dichloromethane), 157
DEA (Diethylamine), 157, 169, 170
debridement, 78, 80, 81, 91, 92, 93, 100
Deg Prod (Degradation product), 157
densitometric, 272

dental films, 164, 166
deproteination, 173, 175
derivative spectrophotometry, 162, 163
detection, vi, 51, 86, 87, 89, 90, 96, 98, 106, 108, 109, 159, 160, 168, 169, 170, 171, 172, 173, 174, 176, 185, 190, 191, 195, 204, 223, 224, 225, 226, 227, 228, 229, 230, 233, 234, 251, 252, 255, 257, 258, 260, 263, 265, 269, 271, 273, 274, 275, 276, 277, 278, 280, 281, 282, 283, 284, 285, 289, 290, 291
determination, 65, 72, 78, 81, 84, 89, 91, 104, 106, 108, 109, 110, 156, 159, 160, 161, 162, 163, 164, 165, 169, 182, 183, 184, 185, 186, 187, 189, 190, 191, 192, 194, 195, 196, 224, 225, 228, 231, 249, 250, 251, 252, 253, 254, 255, 256, 257, 258, 259, 261, 262, 271, 273, 274, 276, 277, 281, 282, 283, 284, 285, 287, 288, 289, 290, 291, 292, 293
Development (HPLC), 7, 13, 21, 37, 40, 56, 59, 77, 79, 80, 81, 82, 84, 86, 88, 89, 91, 94, 95, 97, 102, 103, 106, 107, 109, 116, 154, 156, 159, 162, 163, 166, 168, 169, 170, 172, 178, 179, 184, 185, 186, 187, 188, 189, 190, 191, 192, 193, 194, 195, 196, 199, 205, 210, 212, 213, 215, 216, 223, 224, 225, 230, 231, 232, 233, 234, 238, 239, 243, 254, 255, 257, 258, 262, 266, 271, 272, 274, 275, 276, 277, 278, 285, 287, 288, 289, 291, 292
DEX (dexamethasone), 157, 164, 166, 169, 170, 173, 186, 190, 191
DHPS (Deoxyhypusine synthase), 204, 214
diabetes, 77, 79, 92, 94, 99, 100, 103, 104, 105, 106, 108, 109
DIC (Dicyclomine), 157, 165, 167, 188
Diclofenac, 157, 164, 187
Dicyclomine, 157, 165, 188
DIF (diflunisal), 2, 3, 15, 20, 31
diffuse reflectance infrared fourier transform spectroscopy, 160
dilution, 17, 168, 173, 175, 271
Disodium hydrogen phosphate, 82
dissociation, 26, 43, 205, 214, 269
DNA (Deoxyribonucleic acid), 4, 26, 33, 34, 42, 75, 112, 113, 122, 123, 124, 125, 126, 127, 128, 129, 130, 136, 143, 150, 155, 156, 176, 177, 178, 179, 180, 198, 199, 200, 204, 214, 219, 220, 231, 239, 240, 260, 266, 268, 285, 287
DO3A (1,4,7,10-tetraazacyclododecane-1,4,7-triacetic acid), 267, 280
dosage forms, 159, 163, 227, 271
drug delivery, vii, 38, 40, 41, 48, 52, 53, 59, 61, 64, 105
drug interactions, 103, 156
drugs, 2, 7, 11, 12, 14, 20, 25, 28, 34, 37, 38, 40, 42, 55, 57, 62, 63, 64, 69, 75, 88, 103, 113, 116, 137, 143, 148, 156, 159, 161, 162, 163, 166, 167, 170, 171, 172, 173, 174, 179, 181, 189, 213, 216, 226, 236, 255, 257, 268, 272, 273, 288, 290, 292

E

E. coli (Escherichia coli), 31, 62, 63, 80, 114, 116, 120, 121, 123, 125, 129, 133, 134, 141, 142, 153, 177, 178, 219, 227, 248, 267, 273, 287
ear drops, 164, 166
EDA (Ethylenediamine), 157, 169, 171, 193, 250
EIA (Enzyme-linked antibodies), 204, 226
electrical micro-titration system, 159
electroanalytical methods, 159
electrochemical sensor, 160, 231, 233
electropherogram, 168
electrospray ionization mass spectrometry, 273
ELISA (enzyme-linked immunosorbent assay), 204, 227, 257, 266, 272, 287

ELISA (Enzyme-linked immunosorbent assay), 204
emission, 225, 270, 275, 277, 278, 279, 280, 281, 282, 283, 284, 286, 288
energy transfer, 278, 279, 280, 281, 283
ENRO (enrofloxacin), 106, 157, 172, 173, 185, 195, 221, 225, 230, 232, 233, 244, 250, 254, 255, 258, 259, 262, 272, 273, 277, 281, 287, 288, 289, 290, 291, 292, 293
Enterococcus spp., 80, 115
environmental samples, vii, 159
enzymatic interaction, 284
enzyme metabolism, 103
enzyme-linked immunosorbent assay, 204, 227, 266, 272
EOPO (Thermoseparating copolymers composed of ethylene oxide (EO) and propylene oxide (PO)), 157, 172, 175
EP (efflux pump), 112, 128, 129, 131, 132, 133, 134, 135, 136, 137, 141, 143, 156, 176, 177, 217
esterification reaction, 84
et al. (et alibi (translation and elsewhere)), 8, 9, 10, 11, 12, 13, 14, 16, 17, 18, 19, 20, 21, 22, 23, 30, 32, 38, 39, 40, 41, 42, 44, 45, 46, 47, 48, 49, 50, 51, 52, 53, 54, 55, 56, 57, 59, 60, 61, 62, 63, 70, 78, 79, 80, 81, 83, 84, 85, 86, 87, 88, 90, 102, 103, 105, 106, 107, 108, 109, 114, 115,116, 117, 118, 119, 122, 123, 125, 126, 127, 128, 129, 130, 131, 133, 134, 135, 136, 137, 138, 141, 142, 146, 150, 175, 177, 178, 179, 190, 195, 200, 201, 204, 216, 224, 225, 226, 227, 228, 229, 230, 231, 232, 233, 240, 243, 248, 261, 268, 269, 271, 272, 275, 276, 278, 279, 280, 281, 282, 283, 284, 287, 292
EU (European Union), 222, 244, 267, 276
Eu3+ (europium(III) ion), 267, 278, 279, 286, 290
europium, 267, 278, 280, 281, 282, 290, 291
excitation, 225, 270, 275, 277, 278, 279, 281, 284
extraction, 83, 85, 107, 157, 158, 161, 168, 175, 196, 205, 225, 226, 231, 254, 260, 261, 262, 276, 277, 281
eye drops, 160, 170, 273

F

F (fluorescence), 8, 18, 23, 28, 29, 32, 40, 45, 46, 49, 50, 51, 53, 58, 64, 66, 68, 71, 73, 74, 105, 106, 108, 110, 145, 148, 149, 150, 153, 160, 168, 184, 188, 190, 204, 224, 225, 228, 234, 235, 237, 238, 239, 240, 241, 242, 244, 246, 247, 248, 249, 251, 254, 255, 256, 257, 259, 260, 262, 263, 265, 266, 267, 269, 270, 274, 275, 277, 278, 279, 280, 281, 282, 284, 285, 287, 288, 289, 290, 291, 292, 293
F (fluorine), 8, 18, 23, 28, 29, 32, 40, 41, 45, 46, 49, 50, 51, 53, 58, 64, 66, 68, 71, 73, 74, 105, 106, 110, 113, 145, 148, 149, 150, 153, 184, 188, 190, 216, 235, 237, 238, 239, 240, 241, 242, 244, 246, 247, 248, 249, 251, 254, 255, 256, 257, 259, 260, 262, 263, 266, 267, 272, 279, 287, 289, 290, 291, 292
FA (fumaric acid), 3, 15, 18, 67, 173
Fenton system, 283, 288
FIA (Flow injection analysis), 157, 160, 167
FLD (Fluorescence detector), 157, 168, 170, 172, 173, 174, 176, 190, 225, 277
flow injection analysis, 157, 160
flow rate, 82, 84
fluorescence, vi, 106, 108, 157, 160, 168, 195, 204, 224, 225, 228, 234, 252, 253, 255, 261, 265, 266, 267, 269, 270, 274,

275, 277, 278, 279, 280, 281, 282, 283, 284, 285, 288, 289, 290, 291, 292, 293
fluorescence detection, 106, 108, 168, 224, 266, 269, 274, 279, 288, 289, 292
fluoroquinolone(s), vi, 3, 4, 25, 26, 28, 32, 34, 42, 61, 68, 72, 110, 113, 114, 116, 118, 119, 122, 123, 126, 128, 129, 130, 132, 133, 134, 135, 136, 137, 139, 141, 142, 143, 144, 145, 146, 147, 148, 151, 153, 154, 155, 156, 158, 160, 161, 176, 177, 178, 180, 184, 189, 191, 197, 198, 203, 214, 216, 217, 224, 225, 226, 227, 228, 231, 232, 233, 239, 240, 241, 243, 244, 245, 246, 252, 253, 256, 257, 258, 260, 261, 262, 263, 265, 266, 268, 276, 277, 281, 283, 285, 287, 288, 290, 291
Fontaine system, 79
food, 14, 22, 32, 55, 73, 106, 116, 159, 160, 182, 185, 194, 195, 212, 221, 222, 224, 244, 248, 252, 257, 269, 272, 275, 276, 283, 287, 289, 290, 292
foot ulcers, 80, 105
formic acid, 161, 175
fourier transform infrared spectroscopy, 3, 7, 159, 160
FQ (fluoroquinolone), 3, 4, 20, 22, 23, 25, 26, 28, 32, 34, 42, 61, 68, 72, 113, 114, 116, 118, 119, 122, 123, 126, 128, 129, 130, 132, 133, 134, 135, 136, 137, 139, 141, 142, 143, 144, 145, 148, 151, 154, 156, 158, 177, 197, 198, 224, 225, 227, 228, 231, 232, 233, 239, 240, 241, 244, 245, 253, 256, 257, 258, 260, 261, 262, 263, 265, 266, 268, 277, 285
FTIR (Fourier transform infrared spectroscopy), 3, 7, 8, 9, 12, 17, 19, 21, 22, 23, 159, 160, 183, 204, 233, 263
functionalization, 54, 56, 58, 59, 61, 62, 67, 71

G

g (gram), 4, 38, 41, 55, 61, 62, 101, 102, 111, 112, 113, 114, 115, 116, 117, 119, 123, 128, 129, 130, 131, 134, 135, 136, 137, 138, 141, 142, 144, 145, 147, 148, 149, 150, 151, 175, 176, 178, 203, 216, 218, 219, 220, 230, 266, 268, 271
gender, 79, 92, 94
GLU (gluctamic acid), 205
GLU (glutamic acid), 3, 12, 13, 21
GLY (glycine), 3, 12, 13
gout, 100
gradient elution, 169
gram-negative, 4, 38, 41, 61, 62, 111, 112, 113, 114, 115, 116, 117, 119, 123, 128, 129, 130, 131, 134, 135, 137, 138, 141, 142, 178, 203, 216, 218, 219, 220, 268, 271
gram-positive, 4, 38, 61, 62, 111, 113, 114, 123, 128, 130, 131, 134, 135, 137, 203, 216, 218, 219, 268, 271
graphene, 160, 183, 205, 230, 259
GRAS (generally regarded as safe), 3, 14

H

H (hydrogen), 6, 8, 10, 14, 16, 17, 18, 20, 23, 27, 28, 30, 32, 42, 48, 57, 61, 62, 65, 66, 70, 71, 72, 74, 75, 82, 83, 106, 108, 109, 110, 112, 117, 145, 148, 149, 150, 153, 174, 178, 184, 191, 192, 200, 201, 229, 237, 238, 239, 241, 242, 243, 245, 247, 248, 249, 250, 251, 252, 253, 254, 255, 256, 257, 258, 259, 260, 261, 262, 263, 266, 287, 288, 289, 290, 291, 292, 293
H. (Haemophilus), 27, 28, 32, 42, 48, 62, 65, 66, 70, 71, 72, 74, 75, 106, 109, 110, 112, 117, 118, 120, 145, 147, 148, 149, 150, 153, 201, 219, 237, 238, 239, 241,

242, 243, 245, 247, 248, 249, 250, 251, 252, 253, 254, 255, 256, 257, 258, 259, 260, 261, 262, 263, 287, 288, 289, 290, 291, 292, 293
H2ba (barbituric acid), 3, 15, 17, 30
H2tba (2-thiobarbituric), 3, 15, 17
HA (hippuric acid), 3, 15, 19, 45, 46, 47, 49, 50, 51, 52, 53, 54, 59, 60, 61, 62, 63, 67, 194
Helicobacter pylori, 34, 179, 219
heterocyclic, 269
high performance liquid chromatography (HPLC), 77, 78, 81, 82, 84, 86, 88, 89, 94, 95, 97, 102, 103, 106, 107, 109, 156, 162, 163, 168, 169, 170, 172, 190, 191, 192, 193, 194, 195, 196, 205, 223, 224, 225, 231, 232, 233, 234, 254, 262, 266, 271, 272, 274, 275, 276, 277, 278, 285, 288, 291, 292
High performance liquid chromatography (HPLC), 234
high performance thin layer chromatography, 161
high throughput screening, 78, 81
high-performance liquid chromatography, 106, 108, 159, 162, 205, 223, 287, 288, 289, 292
HILIC columns, 169
homocysteine, 79
homogenate, 88
homogenisation, 88
HPLC (High-performance liquid chromatography), 77, 81, 82, 84, 86, 88, 89, 94, 95, 97, 102, 103, 106, 107, 109, 156, 162, 163, 168, 169, 170, 172, 190, 191, 192, 193, 194, 195, 196, 205, 223, 224, 225, 231, 232, 233, 234, 254, 262, 266, 271, 272, 274, 275, 276, 277, 278, 285, 288, 291, 292
HPLC methods, 78, 81, 156, 169, 170, 172, 272, 273, 277, 285
HPMCAS (hydroxypropyl methylcellulose acetate succinate), 3, 13
HRP (Horseradish peroxidase), 205, 229
HSA (Human serum albumin), 205, 227
HSM (Hot Stage Microscopy), 3, 7, 20
human melanoma cell line A375, 179
human plasma, 86, 107, 108, 109, 161, 169, 172, 173, 174, 276, 289, 292
hydrochloric acid, 84, 217
hydroxyapatite, v, vii, 37, 38, 40, 41, 43, 44, 45, 48, 49, 51, 53, 54, 59, 61, 62, 63, 64, 65, 66, 67, 68, 70, 71, 72, 73, 290
hypercholesterolemia, 100
hyperlipidemia, 100
hypertension, 79, 100, 103, 107
hypothyroidism, 100

I

ILS (Inverse least square), 157, 166
IM (Inner membrane), 112, 138, 139, 140
in vitro, 27, 34, 53, 60, 105, 118, 136, 223, 271
in vivo, 42, 224, 277, 281, 283, 286
INDP (indoprofen), 2, 3, 15, 20, 31
infections, vii, 26, 37, 38, 41, 59, 61, 66, 72, 77, 80, 92, 99, 106, 109, 112, 113, 114, 115, 116, 117, 118, 119, 120, 121, 145, 147, 149, 150, 151, 154, 155, 203, 205, 216, 221, 222, 234, 240, 241, 242, 243, 248
informed consent, 91
infusions, 165, 167
inhibitors of urease, 179
injections, 273
intermittent claudication, 79
internal standard, 82, 83, 85, 157, 161, 169, 175, 272, 276
International Conference on Harmonisation, 107
ion-pair formation methods, 165

IS (Internal standard), 134, 157, 169, 172, 173, 174, 176
isoabsorptive point, 164, 167
isocratic elution, 169
isocratic reversed phase chromatography, 275
isoelectric, 266, 269
IUPAC (International Union of Pure and Applied Chemistry), 205, 218

K

K. (Klebsiella), 29, 30, 31, 32, 34, 71, 73, 74, 107, 109, 112, 116, 120, 121, 133, 141, 144, 145, 146, 147, 148, 150, 152, 153, 196, 219, 235, 237, 239, 240, 241, 243, 244, 245, 246, 247, 248, 249, 250, 251, 252, 255, 257, 258, 260, 261, 262, 287, 288, 289, 290, 291, 292, 293
Ka (association constant), 267, 284
kcal (kilocalorie), 267, 279, 280
kidney, 106, 162, 221, 241, 253
KLH (keyhole limpet hemocyanin), 267, 274
Kruskal Wallis, 94

L

LA (lactic acid), 3, 12, 15, 18
lanthanide(s), 34, 161, 224, 252, 265, 266, 277, 278, 279, 280, 281, 282, 283, 286, 290, 291
lateral-flow immunochromatography, 273
LC (liquide chromatography), 107, 110, 174, 182, 196, 197, 205, 225, 228, 253, 254, 267, 274
LC/MS/MS (Liquid chromatography coupled with electrospray ionization tandem mass spectrometry), 205, 225, 253
LEVO (Levofloxacin), 108, 143, 146, 149, 157, 170, 172, 173, 178, 195, 214, 254, 276, 291, 292
life times, 278
limit of detection (LOD), 86, 87, 89, 90, 96, 98, 160, 176, 226, 227, 271, 274, 277, 280, 283
limit of quantification, 86, 87, 89, 91, 96, 98, 176
LIN (Linezolid), 109, 146, 157, 173, 196
linear equation, 95, 97
linear range, 160, 163, 165
linearity, 86, 89, 90, 95, 97, 224, 274, 276, 282
lipoprotein a, 79
liquid chromatography, 77, 78, 81, 106, 108, 109, 110, 156, 159, 161, 162, 205, 223, 225, 228, 271, 273, 288, 289
liquid–liquid microextraction, 175
LLE (Liquid–liquid extraction), 157, 172, 173, 174, 175
LOME (Lomefloxacin), 157, 178
LPS (Lipopolysaccharide), 112, 138, 141, 214
luminescence (methods), 159, 160, 185, 224, 225, 255, 265, 277, 278, 279, 281, 286, 287, 291

M

M (molar), v, viii, 15, 18, 21, 26, 28, 29, 30, 31, 32, 33, 34, 48, 55, 64, 65, 66, 68, 69, 70, 71, 72, 73, 74, 75, 77, 105, 107, 108, 109, 111, 112, 118, 143, 145, 146, 147, 148, 149, 150, 151, 152, 153, 154, 159, 172, 173, 174, 182, 183, 185, 188, 190, 191, 192, 193, 194, 197, 198, 200, 201, 218, 228, 235, 236, 237, 238, 239, 240, 242, 243, 244, 245, 246, 247, 248, 249, 250, 251, 252, 253, 254, 255, 256, 257, 258, 259, 260, 261, 262, 263, 266, 271,

284, 286, 287, 288, 289, 290, 291, 292, 293, 295
M. (Mycobacteria), v, viii, 26, 28, 29, 30, 31, 32, 33, 34, 48, 55, 64, 65, 66, 68, 69, 70, 71, 72, 73, 74, 75, 77, 107, 109, 111, 112, 118, 143, 145, 146, 147, 148, 149, 150, 151, 152, 153, 154, 182, 185, 191, 192, 193, 194, 197, 198, 200, 201, 218, 235, 236, 237, 238, 239, 240, 242, 243, 244, 245, 246, 247, 248, 249, 250, 251, 252, 253, 254, 255, 256, 257, 258, 259, 260, 261, 262, 263, 286, 287, 288, 289, 290, 291, 292, 293, 295
MA (maleic acid), 3, 15, 18, 19, 22, 106
MAR (Major Facilitator Superfamily Resistance), 112
mass spectrometry, 106, 109, 204, 205, 225, 228, 253, 272, 289
MATE (Multidrug and Toxic Compound Extrusion), 112, 131
matrices, 45, 54, 56, 60, 61, 64, 159, 165, 168, 175, 176, 204, 222, 223, 228, 234, 269
MDR (Multi-Drug Resistant), 112, 116, 131, 133, 135, 137, 150, 178
meat, 169, 172, 195, 209, 227, 236, 252, 257, 269, 272, 275, 276, 290, 292
MEB (Mebeverine hydrochloride), 157, 164, 166
Mebeverin hydrochloride, 164
MeOH (Methanol), 82, 157, 170, 171, 172, 173, 174, 175
MEPS (Microextraction by packed sorbent), 157, 173, 175
MET (Metronidazole), 157, 164, 166, 170, 187, 191
metabolites, 105, 222, 224, 250, 252, 268, 273, 275, 287, 288
methanol, 82, 157
metronidazole, 121, 157, 164, 187, 191
MIC (minimal inhibitory concentration), 13, 134, 136, 177, 267, 273, 288
micellar liquid chromatography, 159, 161, 276, 292
Michael addition, 283
microfluidic system, 273, 289
milk, 162, 169, 172, 173, 194, 195, 221, 231, 233, 243, 254, 258, 260, 262, 263, 269, 273, 277, 288, 289, 293
min (minute), 10, 82, 84, 99, 110, 122, 123, 209, 267, 273
minimal inhibitory concentration, 13, 267, 273, 288
Minimum inhibitory concentration, 41, 103, 104
MIP (Molecularly imprinted polymer), 205, 231, 232, 233, 234, 261
MIPF-SPME (Molecularly imprinted fiber – solid phase microextraction technique), 157, 173, 175
MLR (Maximum acceptable limits), 205, 221, 222
mobile phase, 82, 83, 84, 86, 161, 168, 233, 275, 276
mol (mole), 218, 267, 279, 280, 281, 282, 283
molybdophosphoric acid, 159
monitoring in the environment, 204
MOXI (Moxifloxacin), 127, 147, 157, 174, 178, 184, 200
MRSA (Methicillin-Resistant S. aureus), 112, 115
MS (mass spectroscopy), 168, 169, 174, 176, 182, 192, 196, 197, 204, 205, 225, 228, 234, 254, 267, 274, 291, 295
MSSA (Methicillin-Sensitive S. aureus), 112, 115
MWCNT/GCE (Multi-wall carbon nanotubes film modified on the glassy carbon electrode), 205, 230

N

n (nano), v, 2, 18, 20, 22, 26, 27, 31, 39, 40, 43, 45, 46, 59, 61, 63, 65, 66, 67, 68, 77, 78, 81, 82, 84, 86, 87, 88, 89, 90, 91, 93, 94, 95, 96, 97, 98, 99, 100, 101, 102, 104, 105, 106, 107, 108, 109, 110, 112, 115, 117, 119, 121, 123, 129, 132, 134, 135, 136,141, 143, 145, 147, 149, 150, 151, 153, 154, 159, 160, 161, 162, 163, 168, 169, 177, 178, 179, 180, 181, 182, 183, 184, 185, 186, 187, 188, 189, 190, 191, 192, 193, 194, 195, 196, 197, 198, 201, 204, 213, 214, 215, 216, 221, 222, 223, 224, 225, 226, 227, 228, 229, 230, 231, 232, 265, 266, 275, 283, 284, 288
N (nitrogen), 8, 17, 20, 23, 28, 29, 30, 33, 43, 54, 65, 66, 73, 100, 108, 129, 144, 145, 146, 148, 150, 151, 152, 153, 163, 166, 186, 187, 190, 191, 192, 201, 213, 218, 230, 235, 237, 239, 240, 242, 243, 244, 246, 247, 248, 249, 251, 252, 253, 260, 261, 263, 266, 269, 287, 288, 289, 290, 291, 292
nanocomposites, 38, 41, 48, 51, 54, 63, 64, 67
nanoparticles, v, vii, 37, 38, 39, 41, 48, 52, 54, 55, 59, 62, 63, 64, 65, 66, 67, 68, 71, 73, 160, 178, 183, 225, 230, 255, 259, 289
nanotechnology, vii, 39, 55, 56, 63, 67, 73
native fluorescence, 160, 275, 277, 280, 285
NDA (Nalidixic acid), 157, 173, 214
negatively charged carboxyl group, 168
neuropathy, 80, 92, 94, 99, 107, 223, 245, 246
NGNB (Non-fermenting Gram-negative bacilli), 112
NOR (norfloxacin), 2, 3, 15, 19, 20, 22, 26, 28, 31, 32, 41, 68, 129, 156, 158, 170, 173, 176, 178, 181, 214, 216, 217, 224, 226, 249, 250, 259, 288, 290, 291
nuclear magnetic resonance spectroscopy, 273
number of medications, 78, 94, 99, 101, 102, 103, 104

O

offloading, 80
OFL (Ofloxacin), 26, 28, 68, 82, 83, 146, 147, 149, 156, 158, 170, 173, 174, 178, 184, 197, 240, 249
OMP (Outer Membrane Proteins), 112, 128, 131, 137
ophtalmic solution(s), 163, 165, 167
ORF (Open Reading Frame), 113, 136
ORN (Ornidazole), 158, 161, 165, 167, 169, 171, 173, 184, 187, 191, 192, 196
orthophosphoric acid, 82, 83, 168, 276
osteomyelitis, 37, 41, 60, 61, 68, 113
overlapping spectra, 162, 164
OXO (Oxolinic acid), 158, 172

P

P (phosphorescence), 10, 28, 29, 31, 33, 35, 42, 50, 66, 70, 71, 72, 73, 74, 75, 112, 113, 116, 117, 118, 133, 134, 144, 145, 146, 148, 149, 153, 154, 183, 185, 186, 190, 192, 197, 199, 200, 215, 235, 237, 238, 239, 240, 242, 244, 245, 246, 248, 250, 251, 252, 253, 254, 256,257, 260, 261, 262, 263, 267, 279, 288, 289, 290, 291, 292
p (pico), 8, 11, 50, 51, 52, 94, 267, 271
P. (Pseudomonas), 28, 29, 31, 33, 35, 41, 42, 61, 62, 63, 66, 70, 71, 72, 73, 74, 75, 80, 112, 113, 116, 117, 120, 121, 129, 133, 134, 138, 141, 142, 144, 145, 146, 148, 149, 152, 153, 154, 197, 200, 215,

216, 219, 235, 237, 238, 239, 240, 242, 244, 245, 246, 248, 250, 251, 252, 253, 254, 256, 257, 260, 261, 262, 263, 284, 289, 290, 291, 292
PAR/EGR (Poly(alizarin red)/electrodeposited graphene), 205, 230
partition coefficient, 269
patient profile form, 91, 93
pazufloxacin, 276, 292
PCR (Principal Component Regression), 158, 166
PDA (Photodiode array), 158, 168, 170, 171, 172, 173, 196, 271
peripheral arterial disease (PAD), 77, 78, 79, 80, 81, 82, 91, 92, 93, 94, 99, 100, 101, 102, 103, 104, 106, 107, 108, 109
PET (positron emission tomography), 59, 266, 272, 287
PG (Peptidoglycan), 112, 138, 139, 140, 214
pH (power of hydrogen or potential of hydrogen), 5, 6, 19, 26, 27, 42, 43, 54, 66, 83, 84, 85, 88, 109, 160, 161, 168, 170, 171, 172, 173, 174, 224, 266, 269, 272, 275, 276, 281, 284
pharmaceutical, 2, 7, 12, 13, 14, 15, 18, 21, 22, 23, 25, 28, 29, 30, 32, 37, 65, 107, 156, 160, 162, 163, 168, 170, 175, 176, 182, 183, 184, 185, 186, 187, 188, 189, 190, 191, 192, 193, 195, 196, 197, 213, 215, 217, 226, 227, 228, 229, 239, 251, 255, 256, 258, 260, 263, 269, 271, 272, 282, 284, 285, 288, 291
pharmaceutical analysis, 107, 156, 162
pharmaceutical formulations, 156, 160, 163, 164, 168, 175, 176, 291
pharmacokinetics, 27, 105, 106, 107, 108, 111, 224, 242, 243, 244, 272, 277, 286, 287, 289
phosphate buffer, 82, 83, 84, 85, 160, 161, 168, 170, 171, 172, 173, 275
phosphorescence, 267, 279
photodiode, 158, 168, 196, 271
photodiode array detector, 168, 271
photometric, 271
photonic crystal, 283, 291
Physicochemical properties, 4
  ionization, 4
  pH solubility profile, 4
pI (isoelectric point), 266, 269
pig plasma samples, 162
pKa (Acid dissociation constant), 14, 15, 43, 65, 205, 218, 266
pKa1 (acid dissociation constant at logarithmic scale), 218, 266, 269
plasma, 19, 62, 72, 78, 79, 81, 82, 84, 85, 86, 87, 88, 91, 93, 95, 96, 98, 99, 101, 102, 104, 106, 107, 108, 109, 138, 139, 160, 161, 162, 169, 172, 173, 174, 175, 176, 184, 185, 194, 195, 196, 197, 225, 244, 251, 252, 255, 259, 275, 276, 286, 288
plasma concentration, 19, 81, 87, 101, 102, 225
plasma viscosity, 79
PLS (Partial least squares), 158, 166
polimorphic salt
  maleic acid, 21
  saccharinate, 21
  salicilic acid, 23
polymer nanoparticles, 267
positron emission tomography, 266, 272, 287
potassium bromide, 160
potentiometric titration, 159
PP (Protein precipitation), 84, 88, 158, 172, 173, 174, 175, 195, 276
ppb (parts per billion), 267, 273, 280
precision, 86, 87, 89, 90, 95, 97, 104, 162, 163, 175, 203, 224, 274, 276
predictors, 94, 101
prostatic hyperplasia, 100

protein precipitation, 84, 88, 158, 168, 175, 272, 276
protonation, 43, 139, 270, 289
Pseudomonas aeruginosa, 41, 61, 62, 63, 80, 113, 116, 117, 120, 121, 129, 133, 134, 138, 141, 142, 219
PXRD (powder X ray diffraction), 3, 7, 9, 10, 12, 17, 18, 19, 20, 22
PYR (pyrimethamine), 158, 174

Q

QN (quinine), 158, 171, 173, 192, 196, 270
QRD (Quinolone Resistance Determining Region), 112
quality control, 159, 162, 163, 285
quantitative, 51, 166, 168, 183, 195, 249, 263, 271, 274, 284, 288
quantum yield, 270, 289
quinolones, 34, 66, 112, 113, 129, 143, 148, 150, 151, 155, 162, 177, 178, 180, 181, 182, 201, 216, 229, 238, 242, 250, 253, 256, 257, 276, 287

R

rabbit plasma, 169, 172
radical scavenging potency, 180
radio analytical methods, 159
Raman spectroscopy, 205, 273
rarefaction, 103, 106, 108
Rayleigh light scattering, 273, 292
Rct (charge transfer resistance), 205, 230
recovery, 28, 87, 90, 165, 222, 225, 226, 227, 273, 276, 284, 285
regression coefficient, 101
regression model, vii, 78, 81, 82, 94, 101, 102, 103
Rel sub (Related substances), 158
relative standard deviation, 87, 89, 90, 225
release profile, 53
renal impairment, 100
resistance, v, vii, 48, 61, 64, 66, 72, 103, 111, 112, 113, 114, 115, 116, 117, 122, 123, 128, 129, 130, 131, 132, 133, 134, 135, 136, 137, 141, 142, 143, 144, 145, 146, 147, 148, 149, 150, 151, 153, 154, 155, 176, 177, 197, 198, 205, 230, 240, 247, 248, 265, 268, 285, 288
resistance mechanism, 112, 128, 134, 142, 143, 156, 176, 177
resistant bacteria, 63, 64, 112, 129, 130, 268
resonance level, 280
retention time, 83, 84, 85, 95, 99
reversed phase, 82, 168
RNA (Ribonucleic acid), 127, 204, 205, 214
RND (Resistance Nodulation Division), 113, 131, 132, 133, 134
RP-HPLC, 169, 190, 191, 192, 193
Rutherford system, 79

S

S (singlet), viii, 27, 28, 29, 30, 32, 33, 48, 51, 55, 64, 66, 67, 68, 71, 72, 73, 80, 93, 102, 106, 108, 112, 113, 114, 115, 116, 126, 131, 133, 134, 135, 136, 143, 144, 145, 146, 147, 148, 149, 150, 152, 153, 154, 172, 173, 174, 176, 182, 183, 185, 186, 188, 190, 191, 192, 193, 196, 197, 198, 199, 201, 225, 228, 235, 237, 238, 239, 240, 241, 242, 243, 244, 246, 247, 249, 251, 252, 253, 254, 255, 256, 257, 260, 261, 262, 263, 267, 287, 288, 289, 290, 291, 292, 293, 295
S. (Streptococcus), viii, 27, 28, 29, 30, 32, 33, 48, 51, 55, 64, 66, 67, 68, 71, 72, 73, 112, 113, 114, 115, 116, 118, 120, 121, 123, 128, 133, 134, 135, 136, 143, 144, 145, 146, 147, 148, 149, 150, 151, 152, 153, 154, 182, 186, 190, 191, 192, 198, 199, 201, 219, 235, 237,238, 239, 240,

241, 242, 243, 244, 246, 247, 249, 251, 252, 253, 254, 255, 256, 257, 260, 261, 262, 263, 287, 288, 289, 290, 291, 292, 293, 295
SA (salicilic acid), 3, 15, 23, 192, 236
SAC (saccharin), 2, 3, 15, 22, 23
saliva, 168, 175, 224
Salt
aminoacids, 21
citric acid, 18
diflunisal, 20
fumaric acid, 18
hippuric acid, 19
hydrochloride 1.34-hydrate, 17
indoprofen, 20
lactate, 17
maleic acid, 18
norfloxacin, 19
samarium, 281
sample preparation, 84, 88, 107, 110, 160, 162, 168, 172, 173, 174, 175, 274, 276, 277, 278, 285
Santa Barbara Amouphous-16, 45
SCXRD (single crystal X ray diffraction), 3, 7, 8, 10, 11, 17, 18, 19, 20, 22, 23
SDBS (sodium dodecylbenzene sulfonate), 267, 282
SDM (Sulfadimidine), 82, 83, 158, 172
SDS (sodium dodecyl sulfate), 158, 172, 267, 276
selectivity, 104, 203, 226, 232, 255, 274, 276, 280, 283, 285
sensitivity, 104, 137, 156, 160, 161, 162, 177, 203, 226, 273, 274, 281, 282, 283, 285
sensitizer, 278, 281
separation techniques, 159, 175, 234
SER (serine), 3, 12, 13, 129, 205
SERS (Surface-enhanced Raman spectroscopy), 205, 233, 234, 263
serum, 106, 109, 118, 160, 161, 168, 169, 173, 175, 176, 181, 184, 195, 204, 205, 222, 224, 225, 226, 227, 249, 250, 251, 252, 256, 257, 266, 271, 275, 277, 284, 285, 288, 289, 290, 292
SGF (Savitsky–Golay filters), 158, 166
Silica, v, 37, 43, 52, 61, 65, 66, 67, 68, 71, 72, 73, 74, 75
silica/hydroxyapatite nanoparticles, vii, 38
simultaneous equations, 165, 167
SMR (Small Multidrug Resistance), 113, 131
sodium dodecyl benzene sulfonate, 160
sodium dodecyl sulphate, 158, 161
sodium dodecylbenzene sulfonate (SDBS), 267, 282
sodium-1-octane sulfonate, 169
Solid forms of CIP
amorphization, 7
hydrates and anhydrate, 7
ionized and noionized, 7
solvates, 7
solid phase extraction, 85, 158, 232
solid phase fluorescence, 284
solid state, 1, 2, 3, 5, 7, 8, 9, 10, 11, 20, 24, 25, 32
SOS (Sodium octane sulfonate), 158, 169, 170
SPAR (Sparfloxacin), 146, 147, 149, 158, 174
SPE (Solid phase extraction), 158, 173, 205, 231, 232
SPE (Solid-phase extraction), 205, 231, 273, 293
specificity, 56, 86, 89, 90, 95, 97, 163, 199, 226, 274
spectral methods, 156, 159, 162
spectral waveform analyses, 79
spectrofluorimetric methods, 159, 160
spectrophotometric, 163, 165, 166, 182, 185, 186, 187, 188, 189, 192, 226, 228, 272, 274, 288
SPSS, 93
sputum, 117, 169, 173, 195, 224, 250

ssNMR
solid state nuclear magnetic resonance, 3
stability, 10, 11, 12, 21, 22, 25, 29, 31, 32, 39, 45, 56, 65, 86, 87, 89, 91, 96, 98, 105, 138, 140, 191, 192, 193, 276, 283
stacking–sweeping technique, 162
Staphylococcus aureus, 31, 41, 61, 62, 63, 80, 112, 115, 121, 123, 133, 134, 135, 136, 215, 219
Staphylococcus epidermidis, 41, 120, 121, 219
stationary phase, 169, 170, 171, 172, 173, 174, 232
stock solution, 84, 86, 90, 169
stokes shifts, 278
substances, 12, 14, 22, 131, 158, 159, 161, 162, 168, 193, 213, 224, 244, 284
Sulfadimidine, 82, 83, 158
super bacteria, 285
supramolecular engineering, 2
surface modification, 55, 56
surfactant, 160, 229, 281, 292

T

T (triplet), 30, 34, 46, 67, 68, 70, 71, 74, 105, 106, 109, 131, 135, 143, 145, 146, 148, 150, 154, 184, 186, 189, 192, 194, 237, 239, 240, 241, 242, 243, 244, 245, 246, 247, 248, 253, 258, 259, 260, 261, 262, 267, 278, 280, 286, 287, 288, 290, 291
tablets, 4, 159, 160, 162, 163, 165, 166, 167, 170, 171, 183, 185, 186, 187, 263, 273, 291
Tazobactam, 153
Tb3+ (terbium(III) ion), 267, 278, 279, 280, 281, 282, 283, 286, 288
Tb-DO3A (terbium(III)-DO3A complex), 267, 280
TEA (Triethylamine), 158, 168, 170, 171, 172, 173
terbium, 224, 225, 252, 255, 267, 280, 281, 282, 283, 286, 287, 288, 290, 291, 292
test strip, 273
TeTA (Triethanolamine), 158, 170, 172
Tetrabutylammonium bromide solution, 161
TFA (Trifluoroacetic acd), 158, 173, 174, 175
TG-DSC
thermogravimetry and differential scanning calorimetry, 3
therapeutic effect of drugs, 159
therapeutic target, 179
thin-layer chromatographic, 272
thin-layer chromatography, 159, 161, 205, 228, 266, 288
time-consuming step, 175
time-resolved luminescence, 278, 290
TIN (Tinidazole), 158, 161, 165, 167, 171, 173, 187, 188, 192, 193
tissue concentration, 93, 94, 101, 103
tissue(s), 37, 38, 40, 41, 43, 44, 45, 46, 48, 49, 50, 51, 52, 62, 64, 65, 67, 69, 70, 73, 75, 78, 80, 81, 88, 89, 90, 91, 93, 94, 97, 98, 101, 102, 103, 104, 105, 106, 107, 109, 110, 118, 121, 162, 168, 169, 173, 175, 196, 222, 225, 244, 250, 253, 254, 255, 257, 260, 266, 271, 272, 281, 287, 289, 291, 292
titrimetry, 159
TLC (thin-layer chromatography), 159, 161, 194, 205, 228, 266, 272, 288
TLC–B (Thin-layer chromatography–bioautography), 205, 228
Tosufloxacin, 147, 161
triethylamine, 158, 161, 168, 276, 277
TRIM (Trimethoprim), 158, 173, 195
triplet state, 278, 280
tRNA (Transfer RNA), 205, 214
tumor suppressor pathways, 179

U

UF (Umbeliferone), 158, 172
ultrafiltration, 271
ultra-violet, 269, 271, 274, 277
ultraviolet range, 159
urine, 160, 168, 169, 173, 175, 176, 222, 224, 226, 227, 232, 249, 250, 253, 256, 259, 261, 262, 265, 266, 268, 275, 280, 281, 282, 285, 286, 288, 289, 290, 291, 292
USP (United States Pharmacopoeia), 266, 271
UV (ultraviolet), 159, 162, 163, 165, 168, 204, 224, 266, 271, 274, 285
UV (Ultraviolet), 53, 82, 83, 109, 158, 163, 166, 168, 170, 171, 172, 173, 176, 185, 186, 187, 188, 190, 191, 192, 194, 205, 225, 234, 266, 271, 275, 284, 291, 292
UV-Vis (Ultraviolet–visible.), 185, 205, 225

V

v (volume), 11, 40, 54, 82, 83, 84, 85, 93, 122, 161, 170, 171, 172, 173, 174, 175, 267, 275
validation (HPLC), 22, 77, 81, 82, 84, 86, 88, 89, 91, 94, 95, 97, 102, 103, 106, 107, 109, 156, 162, 163, 168, 169, 170, 172, 177, 184, 186, 187, 188, 190, 191, 192, 193, 194, 195, 196, 197, 205, 223, 224, 225, 231, 232, 233, 234, 252, 254, 262, 266, 271, 272, 274, 275, 276, 277, 278, 285, 288, 291, 292
VAP (Ventilator-Associated Pneumonia), 113, 117
Varian® ProStar HPLC, 82
Vis (visible), 159, 162, 163, 165, 166, 167, 185, 188, 204, 205, 225, 266, 271, 284
voltammetric techniques, 160
VT-PXRD
    variable temperature powder X ray diffraction, 3

W

water bath, 86
water systems, 159
wound debridement, 80
wound management, 80

Z

zwitterionic, 5, 6, 8, 9, 10, 11, 12, 14, 31, 42, 43, 54, 269

Food-Drug Interactions: Pharmacokinetics, Prevention and Potential Side Effects

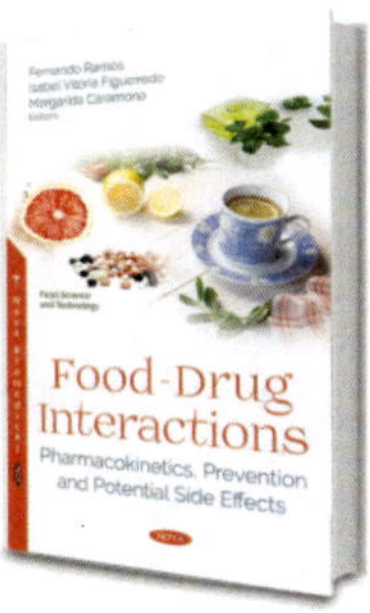

Editors: Fernando Ramos, Ph.D., Margarida Caramona, Ph.D. and Isabel Vitória Figueiredo, Ph.D. (Faculty of Pharmacy, University of Coimbra, Coimbra, Portugal)

Series: Food Science and Technology

Book Description: The objective of this book was to carry out a review on the main drug-food interactions and their impact on health. In this book, the most prevalent chronic pathologies in the population are referenced.

Hardcover ISBN: 978-1-53613-552-7
Retail Price: $195

Pharmaceutical Formulation and Medicinal Chemistry: Mechanisms, Developments and Treatments

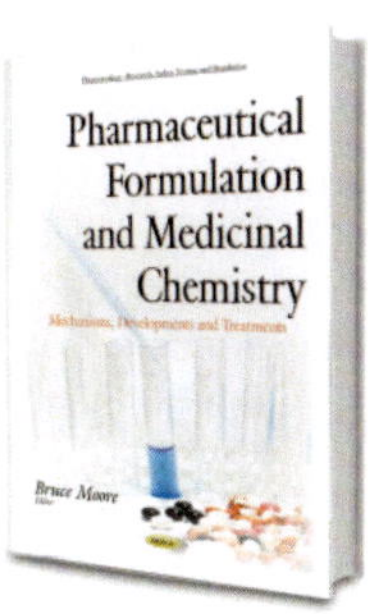

Editors: Bruce Moore

Series: Pharmacology - Research, Safety Testing and Regulation

Book Description: This book reviews research on pharmaceutical formulation and medicinal chemistry. It begins with a summary of old and new discoveries on therapeutic applications of the A3 adenosine receptor in inflammation and cancer, and highlights the most important agonists and antagonists developed for the A3 adenosine receptor, explicitly those in clinical trials for the treatment of inflammation and/or cancer.

Hardcover ISBN: 978-1-63484-082-8
Retail Price: $230